D0875860

ATHLETIC INJURIES
TO THE HEAD, NECK, AND FACE

ATHLETIC INJURIES
TO THE HEAD, NECK, AND FACE

edited by

JOSEPH S. TORG, M.D.

*Professor of Orthopedic Surgery
and
Director, Sports Medicine Center
University of Pennsylvania
School of Medicine
Philadelphia, Pennsylvania*

Lea & Febiger · *1982* · *Philadelphia*

Lea & Febiger
600 Washington Square
Philadelphia, PA 19106
U.S.A.

Library of Congress Cataloging in Publication Data
Main entry under title:

Athletic injuries to the head, neck, and face.

Bibliography: p.
Includes index.
1. Head—Wounds and injuries.   2. Neck—Wounds
and injuries.   3. Face—Wounds and injuries.
4. Sports—Accidents and injuries.   I. Torg,
Joseph S. [DNLM: 1. Athletic injuries.   2. Head
injuries.   3. Facial injuries.   4. Neck—Injuries.
WE 705 T682a]
RD521.A83   617′.51044   81-11784
ISBN 0-8121-0810-8   AACR2

PRINTED IN THE UNITED STATES OF AMERICA

Print No.: 3 2 1

Dedicated to several of those who have helped prepare me to "play the game":

STANLEY PEFFLE, Central High School of Philadelphia

JOHN F. GUMMERE, William Penn Charter School

ARCHIBALD MacINTOSH, Haverford College

JOHN LACHMAN, M.D., Temple University

Preface

The scenario has occurred all too frequently. The youngster, usually a defensive back making a tackle in a high school football game, is involved in a collision with an opponent. A crack is heard and he falls to the ground. The ambulance appears, the fans are silent, and the rescue squad places the motionless body on a stretcher and transports him to the hospital. His neck is broken, the spinal cord injured, and he remains quadriplegic. The usual recriminations follow. It is suggested that the school board eliminate football from the athletic program. A community benefit is held to raise funds for the critically disabled youngster. The money raised, however, is miniscule when compared to the expenses that will be incurred in the immediate treatment, subsequent rehabilitation, and lifelong maintenance of the quadriplegic. Shortly after the injury, the youngster's photograph appears in the local paper. He has a smile on his face and a football, autographed by members of the local professional team, cradled in his paralyzed arm. And it is not long after the injury that the youngster's coach is quoted in the press as describing the tragedy as a "freak injury." And with this explanation of "freak injury," it is business as usual for American football.

It is the purpose and intention of the editor and 22 other contributing authors of this volume that athletic injuries of the neck, head, and face be explained, not on the basis of "freak injury," but rather in accordance with the principle of cause and effect. It is our further intention that existing concepts and principles pertaining to mechanisms of injury, methods of prevention, as well as principles of treatment be reevaluated in terms of scientific evidence. Many concepts that may or may not have been appropriate at a particular point in time are rightfully challenged. This does not mean that we question the diligence, sincerity, or expertise of those who came before us. Rather, many concepts and "facts" pertaining to the particular injuries under discussion require reevaluation in light of the changing circumstances and environment in which they occur.

Using football as an example, we see that when compared to the game played 40 years ago, the participants are larger, stronger, faster, and more skillful in performing their tasks. Rules and techniques have changed. The protective equipment and playing surface have been drastically modified. Medical knowledge, techniques, and expertise have also increased significantly. It is within the area of these changes that we shall attempt to deal with the subject matter, not only as far as injuries that occur in tackle football are concerned, but in all those activities where injuries to the head, neck, and face appear to occur and create a problem because of either their severity or persistence.

The underlying theme and connecting thread of this effort is to, hopefully, effect prevention of injuries by the formulation, propagation, and implementation of principles based on sound, scientific methodology. We recognize that a major problem inherent in the modus operandi of many who are involved in sports medicine has been the reliance on observations that are, at best, anecdotal and lack precision, effort, and accuracy. When millions of our citizens participate in activities that place them at risk of injury, the manner in which these activities are conducted requires thorough and objective scrutiny. And when prevention fails, medical and surgical principles and practices should be no less critically scrutinized.

JOSEPH S. TORG, M.D.

Philadelphia, Pennsylvania

Acknowledgments

Preparation of a text involving contributions from 22 other authors proved to be, to say the least, a significant task. The bulk of the responsibility for communicating with the respective authors, final editing and manuscript preparation, fell on the shoulders of my loyal assistant, Jeanette Bowden. Without her perseverance and patience, this work would never have reached completion. Also, editorial assistance by Marianne Das was invaluable.

Photographic credits are due Otto Lehmann, William Verzyl, and Henry Bacich from the photography staff at the Department of Medical Communications of Temple University School of Medicine.

Don Frey, Head Athletic Trainer at the University of Pennsylvania, and assistant athletic trainers Mitch Biunno, Tom Simmons, Cynthia Mantz, and Phil Frndak were instrumental in assisting with on-field illustrations. Others who participated in this regard are Barbara Maltby, Boris Radisic, and Jim Thornton.

Immeasurable assistance was afforded by John Kotwick in reviewing material pertaining to biomechanics of spine and head injuries.

Joe Vegso, Rich Berggren, and Tina Bonci provided insight, advice, and inspiration.

Significant monetary and moral support was afforded by the Maxwell Football Club and its Executive Council. A special note of thanks is due to Francis "Reds" Bagnell, President, and past president, Lou Elvison.

Carl Brighton, M.D., Chairman of the Department of Orthopedic Surgery at the University of Pennsylvania School of Medicine, Andy Geiger, former Director of Intercollegiate Athletics, and Charles Harris, the current Director of Intercollegiate Athletics at the University, were also supportive of this effort.

Without the interest and contributions of literally thousands of individuals who have participated in supplying information regarding football head and neck injuries to the National Athletic Head and Neck Injury Registry, this effort would have been impossible. To them, a special thanks.

The courage and character demonstrated by Ron Barlow and Boris Radisic, who "paid the price" served as the prime impetus for the initiation and completion of this effort.

Contributors

Alexander J. Brucker, M.D.
Associate Professor of Ophthalmology
University of Pennsylvania
School of Medicine
Philadelphia, Pennsylvania

Leonard A. Bruno, M.D.
Assistant Professor of Neurosurgery
University of Pennsylvania
School of Medicine
Philadelphia, Pennsylvania

Michael H. Bryant, M.D.
Fellow in Sports Medicine
Department of Orthopaedic Surgery
University of Pennsylvania
School of Medicine
Philadelphia, Pennsylvania

Albert H. Burstein, Ph.D.
Professor of Surgery (Orthopaedics)
Cornell University Medical College
Senior Scientist, Department of
*   Biomechanics*
Hospital for Special Surgery
New York, New York

William G. Clancy, Jr., M.D.
Associate Professor of Orthopaedic
*   Surgery*
Head, Section of Sports Medicine
University of Wisconsin
School of Medicine
Madison, Wisconsin

Kenneth S. Clarke, Ph.D.
Professor of Health and Safety
*   Education*
Dean, College of Applied Life Studies
University of Illinois
Champaign, Illinois

Thomas A. Gennarelli, M.D.
Assistant Professor of Neurosurgery
University of Pennsylvania
School of Medicine
Philadelphia, Pennsylvania

Martin S. Greenberg, D.D.S.
Associate Professor of Oral Medicine
University of Pennsylvania
School of Dental Medicine
Chairman, Department of Dental
*   Medicine*
Hospital of the University of
*   Pennsylvania*
Philadelphia, Pennsylvania

Steven D. Handler, M.D.
Assistant Professor of
*   Otorhinolaryngology and Human*
*   Communication*
University of Pennsylvania
School of Medicine
Philadelphia, Pennsylvania

Voigt Hodgson, Ph.D.
Professor of Neurosurgery
Director, Gurdjian-Lissner
 Biomechanics Laboratory
Department of Neurosurgery
Wayne State University
Detroit, Michigan

Robert J. Johnson, M.D.
Professor of Anatomy and Surgery
University of Pennsylvania
School of Medicine
Philadelphia, Pennsylvania

David M. Kozart, M.D.
Associate Professor of Ophthalmology
University of Pennsylvania
School of Medicine
Philadelphia, Pennsylvania

Eric I. Mitchell, M.D.
Fellow in Sports Medicine
Department of Orthopaedic Surgery
University of Pennsylvania
School of Medicine
Philadelphia, Pennsylvania

Charles W. Nichols, M.D.
Associate Professor of Ophthalmology
 and Pharmacology
University of Pennsylvania
School of Medicine
Philadelphia, Pennsylvania

James C. Otis, Ph.D.
Associate Scientist, Research
 Department
Department of Biomechanics
Hospital for Special Surgery,
New York, New York

Helene Pavlov, M.D.
Assistant Professor of Radiology
Cornell University Medical College
Associate Attending Radiologist
Hospital for Special Surgery
New York, New York

Irving M. Raber, M.D.
Assistant Professor of Ophthalmology
University of Pennsylvania
School of Medicine
Philadelphia, Pennsylvania

Richard H. Rothman, M.D., Ph.D.
Professor of Orthopaedic Surgery
University of Pennsylvania
School of Medicine
Chief, Orthopaedics
Pennsylvania Hospital
Philadelphia, Pennsylvania

Carson D. Schneck, M.D., Ph.D.
Professor of Anatomy
Temple University
School of Medicine
Philadelphia, Pennsylvania

Philip Springer, D.M.D.
Clinical Associate in Oral Medicine
Department of Dental Medicine
Hospital of University of Pennsylvania
Philadelphia, Pennsylvania

Joseph S. Torg, M.D.
Professor of Orthopaedic Surgery
Director, Sports Medicine Center
University of Pennsylvania
School of Medicine
Philadelphia, Pennsylvania

Joseph J. Vegso, M.S., A.T., C.
Head Athletic Trainer
Sports Medicine Center
University of Pennsylvania
Philadelphia, Pennsylvania

Sam W. Wiesel, M.D.
Assistant Professor of Orthopaedic
 Surgery
George Washington University
School of Medicine
Washington, D.C.

Contents

IV. FACIAL, ORAL, AND EYE INJURIES

Section I

Prevention

Chapter 1

Problems and Prevention

Joseph S. Torg

A tremendous increase in active participation in recreational and competitive physical activities has occurred over the past several decades. With more leisure time, affluence, and media attention to sports, Americans by the millions are flocking to the playing fields, courts, and trails. Recent estimates place the number of individuals who run and jog on a regular basis to be in the order of 25 million.[6] Another 110 million Americans swim, 65 million bicycle, 26 million play softball, and 25 million iceskate. In addition, 1,300,000 youngsters participate in interscholastic football programs each season.

Associated with large numbers participating in many forms of physical activity, many of which involve body contact, has been a variety of injuries and health problems. It has been estimated that about 17 million Americans seek medical care each year because of such athletic- and recreation-related problems.[5] Because of that need, an area of medical interest referred to as sports medicine has developed. Sports medicine is multidisciplinary in nature. The basic goal is to provide total health care for the athlete through a team effort directed toward injury prevention, treatment, and rehabilitation.

The majority of sports-related injuries involve the musculoskeletal system, and therefore the orthopedic surgeon has assumed a visible and prominent role. However, sports medicine is an area requiring multidisciplinary input and cooperation. It necessarily involves the participation of individuals with medical as well as nonmedical backgrounds. Specifically, sports medicine requires the expertise, knowledge, and cooperation of the physical educator, athletic trainer, exercise physiologist, kinesiologist, biomechanical engineer, and epidemiologist, as well as the pediatrician, family practitioner, radiologist, neurosurgeon, and many other specialists.

Prevention and management of athletic injuries of the head, neck, and face exemplify the interdisciplinary approach to a group of problems confronting the recreational and competitive athlete.

Fortunately, serious athletic injuries to the head, neck, face, and eyes do not occur often. However, in many activities, their occurrence is persistent and demands the attention of those involved with the administration and care of athletes. In some activities, the consequences of these injuries require that they be given a high priority with particular regard to preventing as well as improving methods of medical care. Fatal head injuries resulting from boxing and football; cervical spine injuries with associated neurologic involvement occurring in water sports, use of the trampoline and football; and disabling face and eye injuries in racquet sports and ice hockey are examples of this group.

Head injuries resulting from athletic participation are not a new problem. Gonzales[3] reported that 104 fatal injuries occurred in competitive sports in New York City during the 32-year period from 1918 to 1950. Head injuries accounted for 27 of the 43 deaths that resulted from baseball. Of the 21 deaths that resulted from boxing, the majority were due to closed head injuries.

BOXING

Unterharnscheidt,[15] in his monograph on injuries occurring in boxing, noted that "this sport deserves special attention because, by its intentional destructiveness, it stands apart from all other athletic activities in which injuries are normally of an accidental nature." The validity of this observation has been emphasized by five boxing deaths that occurred in a seven-month period from November 1979 to June 1980. On November 28, 1979, Willie Classen died from head injuries sustained in a professional bout in Madison Square Garden. On January 1, 1980, Tony Thomas, a 20-year-old professional, died in Spartanburg, Virginia from head injuries sustained in a bout on December 22, 1979. On January 9, 1980, Charles Newell, a 26-year-old professional fighter, died in Hartford, Connecticut from injuries sustained in a fight on January 1, 1980. On January 18, 1980, Harlan Hoosier, a 13-year-old amateur, died from injuries sustained January 12 in Lenore, West Virginia. On July 8, 1980, Cleveland Denny died as a result of a "massive brain injury" sustained in a fight on June 20 in Montreal, Canada.

Unterharnscheidt has also described the acute and chronic clinical manifestations of boxing injuries, a description that is simple, lucid, and worthy of consideration:

"Clinically, boxing injuries can be grouped into acute and chronic. The first group includes, for example, cases in which the blow has sufficiently accelerated the head so as to produce cerebral concussion . . . or sudden falls like those in which the boxer is hit much above his center of gravity and is literally knocked off his feet, hitting his occiput in a rapid deceleration trauma.

"The chronic brain lesions of boxers produce a condition known as punchdrunkenness, or chronic progressive traumatic encephalopathy of the boxer. This progressive clinical syndrome becomes noticeable only after a number of years. Frequently, this point coincides with the end of a boxer's active career, or may occur a little later. Clinically the boxer exhibits a combination of extrapyramidal disturbances and cerebellar signs such as disturbed gait and coordination, tremor of the hands and body, and slurred speech."[15]

Although specific head injury fatality rates have not been determined for boxing, in view of the comparatively few participants, and the number of deaths reported in the press, it would appear that they are unacceptably high. Recent published reports indicate that supervision of boxing activities by the state boxing commissions leaves much to be desired.[4] It is necessary to establish and implement criteria as to when a fighter may return after having been rendered unconscious. Also, it is necessary to establish and enforce ringside standards by experienced medical personnel to protect the boxer who has been injured and impaired. As will be emphasized in other chapters, more current diagnostic and treatment methods for the critically head-injured fighter appear to be in order.

FOOTBALL

An annual survey of fatalities that resulted from tackle football has been conducted since 1931. Blyth and Arnold indicated that head and face injuries account for 66% of all football fatalities, while those involving the spine account for 19%.[1]

Consideration of severe head injuries occurring in football should include the total number of direct fatalities, intracranial injuries with associated hemorrhage, and intracranial injuries with hemorrhage resulting in death. Available data permit a nonstatistical comparison of these three entities for two five-year periods: 1959-63 and 1971-75.

For the five years 1959-63, when 820,000 youths were exposed each year, the annual football fatality survey recorded 86 deaths as a direct result of football. During the period from 1971 to 1975, when 1,275,000 players were exposed annually, 77 deaths occurred. When compared on an exposure basis, these figures represent a reduction in the total number of documented direct fatalities. Schneider recorded 139 lesions in which intracranial hemorrhage was a component during the 1959-63 period.[10] The National Football Head and Neck In-

jury Registry has recorded 72 similar lesions during the 1971-75 period.[14] These figures indicate a decrease in injuries in which intracranial hemorrhage was a component.

Schneider reported 65 intracranial injuries that resulted in death during the 1959-63 period.[10] Between 1971 and 1975, 58 similar fatal lesions were registered. When compared on an exposure basis, an apparent decrease in reported deaths had occurred during the more recent five-year period.

Although improvements in the quality of available medical care have played a role, the increased protective capabilities of the helmet-facemask protective system appear to be the major cause of the observed decrease in these three categories. It would appear that a further reduction could be obtained by continuing the enforcement of helmet standards, en-

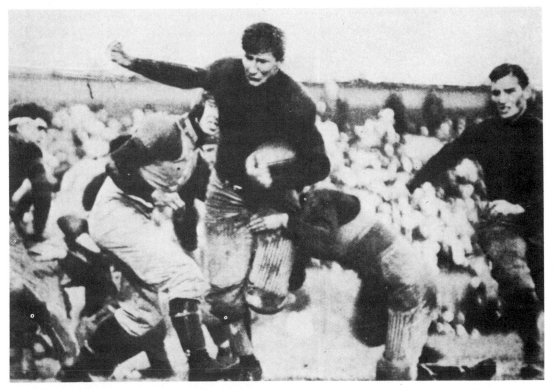

Fig. 1-1. Action photograph of a 1905 Swarthmore-Penn football game. Noteworthy is the absence of protective headgear. The 1905 college season was characterized by 18 deaths and 159 serious injuries, and resulted in President Theodore Roosevelt's order to "adjust rules to eliminate the injury risk."

forcing rules to preclude the use of the head as a primary point of contact in blocking and tackling, and implementing more advanced diagnostic and treatment techniques.

The design of protective head coverings for football has evolved over the past 70 years. In 1905, protection was afforded by a full head of hair (Fig. 1-1). The first "helmet" appeared soon after, and was essentially a pair of heavy-duty leather earmuffs. By 1918, the cranial component was developed and consisted of an outer leather cover and an inner felt lining. In 1932, a more modern helmet appeared that included a primitive suspension webbing. Modest improvements in the design and quality of the suspension system occurred in the early 1940s. The plastic shell, which displayed a significant improvement in design and construction, appeared in 1950.

Early face protectors were improvised to protect a nose that had already been fractured (Fig. 1-2). It was not until the early 1950s that the single-bar and subsequently the double-bar mask were adopted to prevent injuries.

Today, the helmet-facemask protective system consists of a birdcage attached to the polycarbonate shell with a variety of pneumatic, hydraulic, and web suspension systems (Fig. 1-3).

Today's helmet-facemask system provides an extraordinary degree of protection to the head and face. As a result, in recent years coaching methods and playing techniques have developed in which the head and helmet are utilized as a weapon—as a battering ram in blocking and tackling, and for "butting" when running with the ball.

Analysis of severe neck injuries that occur in football requires consideration of two parameters: cervical spine fracture or dislocation, and cervical spine fracture or dislocation with quadriplegia. Available data permit a comparison of these entities for the two five-year periods, 1959-63 and 1971-75.

Between 1959 and 1963, Schneider documented 56 injuries to the cervical spine involving fractures and dislocations.[10] For the five-year period 1971-75, the National Football Head and Neck Injury Registry documented 259 similar

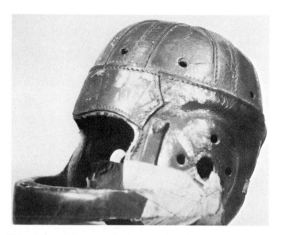

Fig. 1-2. A leather football helmet, vintage 1934. The improvised "single-bar facemask" was constructed by the Temple University trainer-equipment man to protect the fractured nose of a player. Although the single-bar facemask did not become common until 1950, the first such device originated at Temple University 15 years earlier.

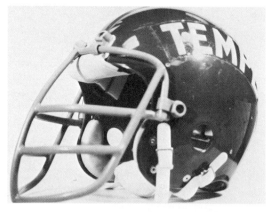

Fig. 1-3. The evolution of the helmet-facemask protective system resulted in a device that effectively protects the head and face from direct-blow injuries. The modern helmet afforded such a high degree of protection that it permitted the head to be used as a battering ram, placing the cervical spine at significant risk of injury.

lesions.[14] These figures demonstrate an increase in documented cervical spine fracture-dislocations during the more recent period.

Schneider documented 30 cases of permanent quadriplegia during the 1959-63 period, while the Registry documented 99 such lesions that occurred between 1971 and 1975. When compared on an exposure basis, these figures represent an increase in documented injuries that resulted in quadriplegia during the more recent five-year period.

Thus, between these two five-year periods, there have been decreases in the total number of fatalities, the total number of closed head injuries associated with intracranial hemorrhage, and the total number of head injuries resulting in death. However, significant increases have occurred in both the number of documented fractures or dislocations involving the cervical spine, and cervical spine fractures or dislocations associated with quadriplegia. This is attributed to the protective capabilities of the modern helmet-face-mask system that adequately protects the head and face, but has encouraged the use of the head as a primary point of contact in blocking, tackling, and head butting. Thus, the head and face are protected by equipment that has permitted the use of techniques that place the cervical spine at risk for considerable injury.

During the 1975 football season, 12 severe neck injuries occurred in Pennsylvania and New Jersey.[13] These injuries included one death, eight cases of quadriplegia, and three cervical spine fractures without neurologic involvement. Determination of the mechanism of injury responsible for the cervical spine fractures or dislocations resulting in quadriplegia is revealing. Six of the eight youngsters were rendered quadriplegic while playing defensive back and making a tackle. In each instance, the head and helmet were used as a battering ram in head tackling. More specifically, striking opponents with the top or crown of the helmet in high-impact situations was implicated as the responsible mechanism.

At the conclusion of the 1975 season, both the National Collegiate Athletic Association (NCAA) and the National Federation of State High School Associations (NFSHSA) adopted rules changes modifying the use of the head in playing techniques. The NCAA football rules committee implemented the following rules additions and modifications for the 1976 season:

1. No player shall intentionally strike a runner with the crown or top of the helmet.
2. No player shall deliberately use his helmet to butt or ram an opponent.
3. Spearing is the deliberate use of the helmet in an attempt to punish an opponent.

Previously, spearing had been limited to situations after "momentum had been stopped."

The National Alliance Football Rules Committee (high school) revised the rules governing butt blocking and face tackling to prohibit "techniques involving a blow with the facemask, frontal area, and top of the helmet driven directly into an opponent as the primary point of contact either in close line play or open field."

The implementation of these rules changes has been associated with a consistent reduction both in cervical spine fracture-dislocations, as well as injuries associated with permanent quadriplegia since the 1977 season (Tables 1-1 and 1-2). Analysis of cervical spine and spinal cord injuries that occur in tackle football has demonstrated that these injuries are primarily technique-related. As a causative factor, the football helmet is considered secondary. That is, it contributes to these injuries only because its protective capabilities permit the head to be used as a battering ram, thus exposing the cervical spine to potential injury. Implementation and enforcement of the aforementioned

TABLE 1-1. Cervical Spine Fracture Dislocations*

	1975	1976	1977	1978	1979	1980
High school	68 (5.70)	95 (7.92)	65 (5.50)	35 (2.91)	32 (2.66)	25 (2.08)
College	23 (30.10)	20 (26.67)	16 (20.30)	7 (9.33)	6 (8.00)	9 (12.00)
Other	1	0	3	3	2	2
Total	92	115	84	45	40	36

* Figures in parentheses represent rate/100,000 participants/season.

rules change is expedient. It is not sufficient for coaches to refrain from teaching techniques utilizing the top or the crown of the helmet as a primary point of contact. Coaches must teach the players *not* to use such techniques.

Analysis of these injuries did not implicate "face in the numbers" blocking and tackling techniques on the line of scrimmage as causing catastrophic cervical spine injuries.

Collision injuries caused by spring-loaded dummies have presented an unusual situation from the standpoint of injury mechanism and prevention.[12] The involved devices were manufactured by an independent commercial firm and marketed throughout the United States without having been subjected to any form of safety control. Both tackling (Fig. 1-4) and blocking (Fig. 1-5) dummies are spring-loaded devices that travel on a suspended railing. Although the dummy itself is made of sponge rubber, the inner core consists of a 3-in. diameter steel pipe. The impact force can be adjusted by changing the springs to strike the subject with either 100, 200, or 300 pounds of force. The object

is for the player to "attack" the dummy after it has been released and neutralize its force by striking it with his head and face, or arms and chest.

As a result of a collision with one of these devices, a 17-year-old high school player sustained comminuted fractures of C3, C4, and C5. Fortunately, the youngster did not have neurologic involvement and recovered with conservative management. Another 17-year-old high school player was not so fortunate. After having been struck on the head with a spring-loaded blocking dummy, he immediately lost consciousness. Two days after the injury, he died. Autopsy revealed hemorrhages in the brain stem and pons, as well as evidence of subarachnoid bleeding.

In response to the apparent danger presented by these devices, the NCAA Committee on Competitive Safeguards and Medical Aspects of Sports issued a position statement "advising against the use of self-propelled mechanized blocking and tackling apparatus because of the apparent undue risk of head or neck injury." These devices are no longer used, and it is hoped that this particular problem has been

TABLE 1-2. Permanent Quadriplegias*

	1975	1976	1977	1978	1979	1980
High school	23 (1.90)	28 (2.23)	14 (1.16)	13 (1.08)	7 (0.58)	10 (0.83)
College	4 (5.30)	7 (9.30)	3 (4.00)	0 (0.00)	3 (4.00)	2 (2.66)
Other	0	0	2	2	0	1
Total	27	35	19	15	10	13

* Figures in parentheses represent rate/100,000 participants/season.

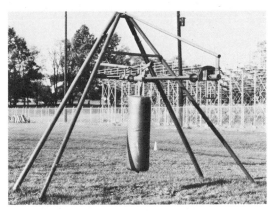

Fig. 1-4. A spring-loaded tackling dummy that was developed and marketed without safety evaluation. Depending on how it is spring-loaded, it can strike with 100, 200, or 300 pounds of force. This device has caused severe neck injuries, including one case of quadriplegia.

solved. However, an issue raised by these injuries is why such an apparently dangerous device was not adequately evaluated from the safety standpoint prior to distribution and use.

WATER SPORTS

The frequency of cervical cord injuries in football has been well publicized. However, a report by Shields et al.,[11] indicates that the majority of injuries to the cervical cord occur during water-related activities. Between June 1, 1964 and December 31, 1973, 1600 patients were admitted to the Spinal Injury Service at Rancho Los Amigos Hospital. Of these, 152, or 9.5% of the patients had been injured in recreational activities. During that period, 118, or 73% of the 152 patients were injured in water-related sports. Diving accidents were the leading cause of injury, and occurred because the patient misjudged the depth and safety of the water at the time of incidence. Most of these patients were injured by diving into shallow water or striking a submerged object. The average depth of the water in which neck injuries occurred was 5 feet. Football accounted for only 16 of the 152 sports-related injuries, or 10% of all sports-related cervical cord injuries, and 1.0% of cervical cord injuries from all causes.

The majority of sports-related spinal cord injuries can be prevented. To accomplish this goal it is necessary to educate swimmers to the dangers inherent in diving. It is equally important that

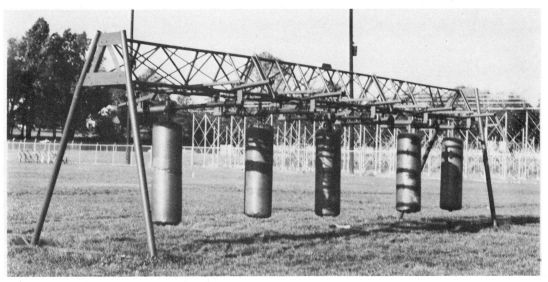

Fig. 1-5. Spring-loaded blocking dummies function on the same principle as the spring-loaded tackling device. The players are expected to meet the moving dummy and neutralize its impact by blocking it with their face, forearm, chest, and shoulders. This particular device was responsible for a brain stem injury resulting in death.

everyone know how these dangers can be avoided. The following guidelines should be observed for safe diving:

1. Do not dive into water that is shallower than twice your height. A 6-foot individual requires 12 feet of depth for safe diving.
2. Do not dive into unfamiliar water. Know the depth and be sure the water is free of submerged objects.
3. Do not assume water is deep enough. Familiar rivers, lakes, bays, and swimming holes change levels. Remember, at low tide there is 6 to 8 feet less depth than at high tide.
4. Do not dive near dredging or construction work. Water levels may change, and dangerous objects may lie beneath the surface.
5. Do not dive until the area is clear of other swimmers.
6. Do not drink and dive. Alcohol distorts judgment.
7. Do not permit or indulge in horseplay while swimming and diving.
8. Do not dive into the ocean surf or lakefront beaches.

Diving is best confined to a properly maintained and supervised pool where the depth has been measured and marked.

TRAMPOLINE

Recently, attention has been called to cervical cord injuries resulting from the use of the trampoline. Rapp et al. reported 34 such cases including 3 deaths that occurred nationally in an exposure group of unspecified size.[9] Of the 34 injuries, 29 occurred in a six-year period. The C5-C6 level was most frequently involved. In 1977, the American Academy of Pediatrics Committee on Accident and Poison Prevention recommended that "trampolines be banned from use as part of physical education programs in grammar school, high school and college, and also be abolished as a competitive sport."[2]

ICE HOCKEY

Injuries to the head and face are prevalent in ice hockey. Those to the intraocular structures present a major problem.

Pashby,[7,8] soliciting information from the Canadian Ophthalmological Society, attempted to document eye injuries in Canada during the 1972-73 and 1974-75 seasons. For the first period, 287 injuries were reported, the majority of which were caused by sticks. Notable is the fact that 13.7% of these injuries resulted in blindness in the injured eye. During the 1974-75 season, a total of 253 injuries were reported and again the majority were due to sticks. Of these, 16% resulted in blindness in the injured eye. Pashby observed that "the number of blinding injuries was a shocking revelation which demanded action." Because of his efforts, great strides have been made in the development of standardized face protectors for forwards and defensemen.

The early development of protective equipment in ice hockey, as well as in most other sports, has been the product of the efforts of various players, coaches, trainers, and craftsmen, with little if any engineering or mechanical input. Jacques Plante, a former great goaltender from Montreal, was responsible for helping to develop the protective facemask. During the early years of his career, Plante suffered four separate fractures of his nose, fractures of both cheek bones, and two separate fractures of his mandible. In addition, he sustained a number of facial lacerations that required more than 250 stitches. In 1956, while playing goalie for Montreal, he experimented with a wire facemask. Because of the distorted optical relationship caused by the wire, and the feeling of "dizziness" that he experienced when wearing the mask, he discarded it. Philip Burchmore, a Canadian who worked with fiberglass, suggested to Plante, in 1957, the feasibility of constructing a fiberglass facemask. Two years later, after he had stopped several more pucks with his face, Plante pursued Burchmore's suggestion. In the spring of 1959, a fiberglass mask was constructed from a plaster mold taken of Plante's face.

Because of strenuous objections from the Montreal coach, the mask was not worn. The coach believed it would obstruct Plante's vision, and equally important, he told Plante that the scars he was accumulating would be "trophies" to be cherished in his later years. Plante acquiesced to the coach's objections. On November 1, 1959, in a game in Madison Square Garden between Montreal and New York, the Rangers' winger Andy Bathgate shot a puck at Plante from a sharp angle. It struck Plante above his upper lip, ripping part of his nose from his face. At that time the teams carried only one goalie and Montreal was vying for an advantaged position in the Stanley Cup Playoff. Plante was taken to the locker room and the laceration was hastily sutured. He agreed to return to the game only if he could wear his fiberglass mask; this time the coach relented. Montreal won the game 4 to 1. While wearing the mask, Plante led Montreal on an 11-game winning streak, and the Canadians swept Chicago and Toronto to win the Stanley Cup in eight games. In addition, for the fifth time in his career, Plante won the Vezina trophy as the National Hockey League's outstanding goalie. However, it was not until 1964, when Detroit Redwings' goalie, Terry Sawchuck, started wearing the fiberglass mask that it became generally accepted.

Plante's performance as a goaltender is documented in the record book. For future generations of hockey players, however, Plante's lasting contribution to the game will be that of a pioneer in protective equipment. Without the benefit of biomechanical, biomaterial, medical, or scientific testing expertise, he helped develop a protective mask that eventually every goalkeeper from the amateur through the professional levels wore.

Unfortunately, the fiberglass goalie mask did not prove to be invulnerable. Bernie Parent, the premiere goalie for the Philadelphia Flyers, sustained a career-ending intraocular injury during the 1978-79 season when the tip of a hockey stick penetrated the visual aperture in his mask, striking him in his eye. Apparently a similar injury had happened to Buffalo's Gerry DesJardin. What is surprising is not that these injuries occurred to Parent and DesJardin, but rather that they have not occurred more frequently. Inspection of the molded fiberglass protective goalie mask reveals that the contour of the device is such that the periocular area has a funnel-like configuration that tends to deflect the end of sticks and pucks directly into contact with the eye, which lies flush against the aperture (Fig. 1-6).

The work of Pashby and his co-workers

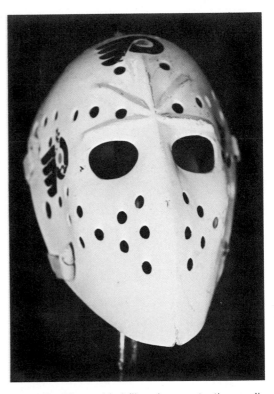

Fig. 1-6. The molded fiberglass protective goalie mask appears invulnerable. However, severe eye injuries resulted from stick ends penetrating the visual aperture.

in Canada, and Vinger in the United States have contributed to the further development and establishment of standards for size, position, visual resolution, prismatic deviation, haze, luminous transmittance, peripheral vision, and penetration for protective masks for goalies, as well as for line players (Fig. 1-7).

RACQUET SPORTS

Increased popularity of racquet sports has also been associated with an awareness of increased ocular hazards to the participants. Vinger and Tolpin reported a prospective study of ocular injuries seen in a suburban practice of 5 ophthalmologists[16]; 59 ocular injuries were seen in a 15-month period and an additional 29 were also documented. Of these 88 injuries, 68 occurred to tennis players. Also to be noted is the danger of ocular injuries on the squash or racquetball court. Protective plastic

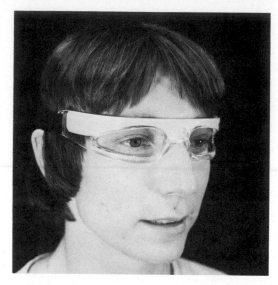

Fig. 1-8. Plastic "goggles" are available and recommended for racquet sports. They allow adequate vision yet prevent the eye from being struck with balls and racquets.

"rims" are currently available for racquetball players, and their use is recommended (Fig. 1-8).

"AN OUNCE OF PREVENTION"

For those responsible for dealing with athletic injuries, whether they occur to the head, neck, face, or other areas of the body, the adage, "an ounce of prevention is worth a pound of cure," is well-taken. The logical sequence in this regard is to first identify the problem by applying sound epidemiologic principles. Once the problem has been identified, either with regard to the severity of the sequelae or frequency of occurrence of the injury, appropriate modifications of conditioning methods, protective equipment, playing technique, and rules modifications should be implemented on the basis of sound scientific methodology. Available expertise in engineering, materials, and medicine precludes an anecdotal approach to these problems. Existing regulatory and administrative bodies for the many amateur, interscholastic, intercollegiate, and professional athletic activities should estab-

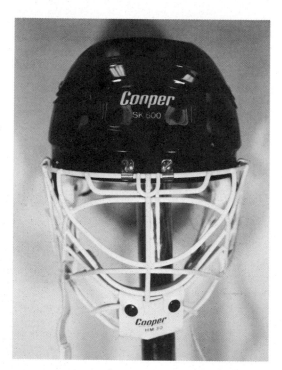

Fig. 1-7. The wire protective goalie mask provides better vision and ventilation, and is firmly attached to the helmet. Presumably, its configuration makes the eye less vulnerable to direct-blow injury.

lish, support financially, and be guided by injury-prevention research commissions. These commissions should consist of experts from both industry and the academic communities working independently to deal with the matter of injury prevention.

The National Operating Committee on Standards for Athletic Equipment (NOCSAE) is the existing prototype for such research commissions. Established in 1970 in response to a concern over the safety of protective equipment used in competitive sports, NOCSAE is a nonprofit corporation. The charter members were the NCAA the NFSHSA, the National Junior College Athletic Association, the Sporting Goods Manufacturers Association, the American College Health Association, and the National Athletic Trainers Association. Subsequently, the National Sporting Goods Dealers Association, the National Athletic Equipment Reconditioners Association, and the National Association for Intercollegiate Athletics were added to the membership. Consisting of representatives from each of these organizations, the group authorized and sponsored in-depth experimentation of protective equipment conducted by the Gurdjian-Lissner Biomechanics Laboratory at Wayne State University in Detroit, Michigan. The objectives of this organization have been to promote, conduct, and foster research; to study, analyze, and collect data and statistics relating to athletic equipment, with the view of encouraging the establishment of safety standards. They also disseminate information and promote, conduct, and further activities designed to increase knowledge and understanding of safety,

comfort, utility, and the legal aspects of athletic equipment. NOCSAE provides a forum with which individuals and organizations may consult and cooperate in considering problems related to athletics. All activities of the organization are for charitable, educational, and scientific purposes.

REFERENCES

1. Blyth, C.S., and Arnold, D.C.: The forty-seventh annual survey of football fatalities: 1931–1978. Athletic Training, 4:234, 1979.
2. Committee on Accident and Poison Prevention of the American Academy of Pediatrics. Am. Acad. Pediatr. News and Comment, 28:5, 1977.
3. Gonzales, T.A.: Fatal injury in competitive sports. J.A.M.A., 146:1506, 1951.
4. Kirshenbaum, J.: Time for reform. Sports Illustrated, 52:12, Feb. 18, 1980.
5. Nicholas, J.A.: Hippocrates, the father of sports medicine. Institute of Sports Medicine and Athletic Training, Lenox Hill Hospital, 1975.
6. Nicholas, J.A.: What sports medicine is about. Community Med., 42:4, 1978.
7. Pashby, T.J.: Eye injuries in Canadian amateur hockey. Am. J. Sports Med., 7:254, 1979.
8. Pashby, T.J., Pashby, R.C., and Chisholm, L.D.: Eye injuries in Canadian hockey. Can. Med. Assoc. J., 113:663, 1975.
9. Rapp, G.F., and Nicely, P.G.: Trampoline injuries. Am. J. Sports Med., 6:269, 1978.
10. Schneider, R.C.: Head and Neck Injuries in Football. Baltimore, Williams & Wilkins, 1973.
11. Shields, C.L., Jr., Fox, J.M., and Stauffer, E.S.: Cervical cord injuries in sports. Phys. and Sportsmed., 6:71, 1978.
12. Torg, J.S., et al.: Collision with springloaded football tackling and blocking dummies. J.A.M.A., 236:1270, 1976.
13. Torg, J.S., et al.: Severe and catastrophic neck injuries resulting from tackle football. J. Am. Coll. Health Assoc., 25:224, 1977.
14. Torg, J.S., et al.: The National Football Head and Neck Injury Registry. Report and conclusions 1978. J.A.M.A., 241:1477, 1979.
15. Unterharnscheidt, F.J.: Injuries due to boxing and other sports. Handbook of Clin. Neurol., 23:527, 1975.
16. Vinger, P.F., and Tolpin, D.W.: Racquet sports: an ocular hazard. J.A.M.A., 239:2575, 1978.

Chapter 2

An Epidemiologic View

Kenneth S. Clarke

The purpose of this chapter is to characterize, with available epidemiologic data, the current picture of athletic injuries to the head, neck, and face. Attention is given to the degree of severity of these injuries in descending order: fatalities, nonfatal catastrophic injuries (e.g., quadriplegia), and potentially catastrophic neurotrauma (e.g., concussion).

EPIDEMIOLOGY

Epidemiology is concerned with studying the distribution of disease or injury within a population and its environment. Its methods are to follow frequencies and patterns of distribution in the search for causative agents (determinants). The goal is to remove or negate the influence of an alleged determinant, and then to observe whether the distribution of that disease or injury has been altered accordingly.

While addressing itself to cause and effect, the epidemiologic model must deal with associations. One must appreciate that a documented association between a hypothesized determinant (e.g., defectively designed helmet) and a particular type of injury (e.g., cerebral neurotrauma) does not constitute proof of cause and effect. A stable lessening of the problem after removing the alleged agent would be strong confirmation of that hypothesis, but

a more powerful argument obtained with epidemiologic data is that of "disconfirmation." If, for example, a particular helmet is alleged to be the cause of serious cerebral neurotrauma because of its defective design, a strong association between the use of that helmet and such injuries *must* be found, or the cause-effect relationship is disconfirmed.

To evaluate injury patterns (frequencies and associations), comparison must be made. Whether the comparison is year to year, sport to sport, squad to squad, helmet to helmet, or male to female, one must have both a reasonable rationale and sufficient data to permit a fair comparison. The epidemiologic model requires a merging of population data, exposure data, injury data, and injury scenario data for that purpose. We first need to characterize the population at risk, and then to reasonably establish the opportunity for them to contract the disease (i.e., the opportunity for them to receive an injury). The experiences recorded as injuries can then be put in perspective with the use of "rates."

For example, 50 athletes attending 5 practices constitute 250 athlete-exposures (i.e., the opportunity for 250 injuries). If 2 were injured, the rate would be 2 cases per 250 athlete-exposures or 80/10,000 athlete-exposures. If variation in length of season between squads is not substantial, a rate of 2 cases per 50 athletes, or 4/100 athletes would also be a legitimate expression. More precise measures of exposure may be warranted for particular detailed investigations.

Other types of rates may be used to help understand a problem. The number of athletes per case (e.g., one football fatality for every 175,000 athletes) gives a probability figure that can be used for describing and comparing an individual's risk in sport. The number of squads per case gives a probability figure helpful to a sponsoring institution's understanding of its relative risk of experiencing a case.

Injury scenario data (related circumstances) are necessary to examine associations of the many potentially preventive or injurious factors, individually and in combination, with the injuries experienced.

The bottom line in epidemiology is knowing the incidence of the problem (frequency of new cases within a population). Without a baseline, the effectiveness of preventive measures cannot be evaluated. But without identifying patterns within the aggregate of injuries as well, there is no beacon for foreseeing the relative merits of suggested preventive measures.

FATALITIES

Football is the only school-college sport for which sufficient mortality incidence data are available (since 1931).[2] That data first received epidemiologic treatment in the mid-1960s.[3] In that study, the football fatality data had been reported by the Metropolitan Life Insurance Company.[11] Table 2-1 presents relative risk obtained when the epidemiologic consideration of population-at-risk to raw totals is added.

The purpose of that study, however, was to demonstrate the epidemiologic tenet of exposure, as well as population, for evaluating the actuarial question of foot-

TABLE 2-1. Average Annual Fatality Rates in Selected Competitive Sports, 1960-64[3]

Sport	Fatalities	Fatality Rate/ 100,000 Participants
Football	26	3.9
Power boating	1	16.7
Auto racing	30	120.0
Horse racing	2	133.3
Motorcycling	5	178.6

ball deaths. The resulting statistical rationale yielded a 1:1 ratio when the fatality rate from football among football players aged 15 to 24 was compared to the fatality rate among all males in that age group from all accidental causes. In other words, when an athlete stepped on the football field in 1964, one of the worst years in modern football in terms of fatalities, he was no higher an insurance risk for traumatic death than his nonparticipating peers. This exercise also yielded a ratio, again controlled for population and exposure, of one football-related fatality for every nine auto-related fatalities among males in that age group, automobile driving being the only alternative activity for which sufficient data were available to permit such a comparison.

The same rationale was applied ten years later using 1974 data.[7] Not only did the actuarial picture for football remain favorable, but the football-auto fatality ratio now was 1:27. During the intervening decade, deaths in football had decreased, while participation (population and exposure) had risen.

Putting these data in another perspective, in high school and college football, one fatality occurred during Fall 1974 for every six million athlete-exposures. In 1964, it had been one fatality for every 1.5 million athlete-exposures; since 1977, it has been one fatality for every ten million athlete-exposures.

Head and Neck Fatalities

From the 1950s through the present, approximately nine of every ten football deaths from traumatic injury have involved the head or neck. However, by distinguishing between head and neck injuries, different frequency patterns are seen (Fig. 2-1). The development of the modern helmet and facemask in the 1950s and 1960s was associated with changes in blocking and tackling techniques (i.e., the helmeted head was brought into contact more purposefully). It is apparent that these changes were accompanied by a substantial increase in deaths from head injuries, while deaths from cervical cord injury remained infrequent, yet persistent over the years. The trend in head-related fatalities was not only reversed by the early 1970s, but after 1976, dropped down to the "infrequent yet persistent" level of neck injuries. Several determinants were undoubtedly responsible.

In the late 1960s NOCSAE initially formed to develop standards against which all football helmet models were to be tested successfully before being marketed. By 1974, these standards were being utilized by all manufacturers, even though the wearing of helmets, which had passed NOCSAE standards, was not to be mandatory until 1978 at the college, and 1980 at the high-school level.

Also, by the late 1960s, an educational campaign against spearing had been intensified by the American Medical Association (AMA), NFSHSA, NCAA, and others.[1] Then, in January 1976, high-school rules, college rules, and coaching ethics were formally adopted to prohibit tackling-blocking techniques in which the helmeted head received the brunt of the initial impact. The primary reason for these rules was the vulnerability of the athlete's cervical spine when he struck his opponent with the top or the crown of the helmet (e.g., NCAA Rule 9-1-2-n and NFSHSA Rule 9-3-1). However, the phrasings and intent were also intended to preclude the deliberate use (and the teaching) of facemask and brow contact (e.g., NCAA Rule 9-1-2-1 and NFSHSA Rule 9-3-2-k). The contention was that by leading with

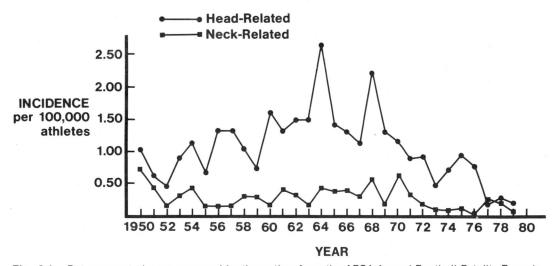

HEAD AND NECK FATALITIES
HIGH SCHOOL AND COLLEGE FOOTBALL
1950-79 SEASONS

Fig. 2-1. Data presented were prepared by the author from the AFCA Annual Football Fatality Reports.

the head, the player cannot always be sure of achieving the desired football position of "head up, neck bulled" at the moment of contact, and improper execution could put his head or neck in a vulnerable position. When the player was not leading with his head, improper execution was not considered as potentially devastating, and the rule was thereby adopted. In 1978, an organized approach to the coach's education of the athlete, concerning the latter's shared responsibility in this regard, was initiated by the NCAA.[14]

To sum up, one can make several observations with respect to fatalities.

(1) The advent of conscious attention to helmet standards in the late 1960s and early 1970s was associated with a distinct decrease in deaths related to head injuries.

(2) The advent of rule changes in 1976 that prohibited leading with the head for contact was associated with another distinct drop in deaths related to head injuries.

(3) The emergence of the facemask in the 1950s and its subsequent continuous use was not accompanied by a sustained increase in the relative frequency of deaths related to neck injuries.

NONFATAL CATASTROPHIC INJURIES

Equivalent trend-line data were not available for nonfatal catastrophic injuries

until recently. In 1976, I surveyed retrospectively (1973-75) spinal cord injuries among the varsity programs of all high schools and colleges in the nation, and found gymnastics had the highest average annual injury rate of all the sports (Table 2-2).[5] Of the others, only football and wrestling showed an annual persistence of such injuries. Of these three sports, only gymnastics and football displayed describable patterns.

Gymnastics

The patterns of injury among all gymnastic events revealed that permanent spinal cord injuries were primarily associated with the trampoline (as a training device), but not to the exclusion of other gymnastic apparatuses (Table 2-3). The vast majority of these injuries occurred when the athlete came down incorrectly on the trampoline. This finding, coupled with a subsequent finding that the stricken trampolinist had invariably been attempting a somersault, resulted in national consensus guidelines in 1978 on the controlled use of the trampoline and minitramp.[15, 18]

Another offshoot of this survey was the advent, in July 1978, of a National Registry of Gymnastic Catastrophic Injuries patterned after the AFCA Football Fatality Report.[9] In its first two years (through June 1980), eleven gymnastic injuries, which resulted in cervical neurotrauma, occurred

TABLE 2-2. Average Annual Incidence of Spinal Cord Injury in School-College–Sponsored Sports, 1973-75[5]

Sport	Athletes/ Case	Programs/ Case
Gymnastics, Men	7,000	281
Gymnastics, Women	24,000	1,113
Football	28,000	403
Wrestling	62,000	1,781
Baseball	177,000	6,254
Basketball, Men	793,000	23,024

TABLE 2-3. Adjusted Proportion of Permanent Spinal Cord Injuries by Type of Event in School-College– Sponsored Gymnastics, 1973-75[5]

Event	Men %	Women %
Trampoline	33	71
Minitramp	11	—
Horizontal bar	22	—
Rings	11	—
Free exercise	22	14
Unevens	—	14

TABLE 2-4. National Incidence of Gymnastic Catastrophic Injuries, July 1978 Through June 1980[9]

Event	Sex	Person	Circumstances	Injury
1. Trampoline	M	Skilled Teenager	Practice, Gymnastics Club	Quadriplegia
2. Trampoline	M	Young Boy	Backyard Recreation	Death
3. Trampoline	M	Skilled Young Adult	Backyard Game of "Horse"	Quadriplegia
4. Trampoline	M	Advanced Beginner Teen	Military Base Recreation	Quadriplegia
5. Trampoline	M	College Asst Instructor	P.E. Class Demonstration	Quadriplegia
6. Minitramp	M	College Cheerleader	Warmup for Football Game	Quadriplegia
7. Minitramp	M	High School Gymnast	Practice for Pep Rally	Quadriplegia
8. Tumbling	F	High School Cheerleader	Cheerleader Practice	Death
9. Trampoline	M	College Gymnast	Practicing Hi-Bar Dismount	Quadriplegia
10. Unevens	F	High School Gymnast	Practicing Routine	Quadriplegia
11. Minitramp	M	College Cheerleader	Unscheduled Practice	Quadriplegia

across the nation: nine developed permanent quadriplegia, and two died. As shown in Table 2-4, most injuries were to skilled performers while practicing; only two injuries occurred under conditions of organized sport, and only one within the context of physical education (to an instructor). This completes only the first two years of a continuing effort, but it appears that catastrophic injuries in gymnastics have lessened substantially since the mid-1970s.

Football

In Fall 1975, while I was preparing the retrospective survey of spinal cord injuries in school sports and physical education, Torg was establishing a National Football Head and Neck Injury Registry patterned after the clinical case-finding method used by Schneider in 1963.[12, 17] Initially, Torg

solicited retrospective documentation of catastrophic cases experienced during the 1971 through 1975 seasons, in order to have a five-year period comparable to that of Schneider (1959-63). In cooperation with the American Football Coaches Association system, he continued to maintain the Registry as a continuous surveillance system, but extended the survey to injuries other than fatalities. Tables 2-5 and 2-6 compare Torg's findings for catastrophic injury patterns in football during 1971-75 with my findings for 1973-75. The high degree of comparability lends credence to the principal injury scenario of a defensive back coming up to make an open-field tackle.

Tables 2-7 and 2-8 display the different

TABLE 2-5. Proportion of Quadriplegic Cases in School-College Football Associated with Tackling

	Torg[17] % (1971-75)	Clarke[5] % (1973-75)
High school	72	83
College	78	83

TABLE 2-6. Proportion of Quadriplegic Cases in School-College Football Associated with Selected Positions

	Torg[17] % (1971-75)	Clarke[5] % (1973-75)
Defensive back		
High school	52	50
College	73	67
Linebacker		
High school	10	29
College	0	0

TABLE 2-7. Comparison of Permanent Cerebral Injuries Nationally in High School-College Football

	Schneider[12] (1959-63)	Torg[17] (1971-75)
Total cases reported	112	72
High school-college cases	87 (est)	65
Average annual incidence/100,000 athletes	2.6 (est)	1.0
Fatal cases	41%	81%

patterns of serious neurotrauma in high school-college football during the 1959-63 and the 1971-75 eras. Essentially, both the frequency of, and mortality from, serious cerebral injuries decreased. Serious cervical cord injuries, on the other hand, had increased (unless disguised by Schneider's 90% response rate). Their predominantly nonfatal nature had precluded detection of this trend via the annual fatality report.

As seen in Table 2-9, however, Torg's Registry reveals a distinct drop in quadriplegia after 1976.[16] The incidence in 1977 and 1978 was half that of 1975 and 1976. Since the rule changes in 1976 required profound adjustments of the athlete, coach, and official to new expectations and different techniques, the one-year lag in its impact was not unexpected.

TABLE 2-8. Comparison of Permanent Cervical Spinal Cord Injuries Nationally in High School-College Football

	Schneider[12] (1959-63)	Torg[17] (1971-75)
Total cases reported	38	99
High school-college cases	30 (est)	95
Average annual incidence/100,000 athletes	0.9 (est)	1.5
Fatal cases	42%	8%

TABLE 2-9. Number of Nonfatal Permanent Neurotrauma Nationally in School-College Football, 1975-78 [16]

	1975	1976	1977	1978	1979	1980
Cerebral						
High school	6	3	3	5	5	2
College	2	1	1	1	0	0
Cervical cord						
High school	23	25	10	11	7	8
College	4	7	2	0	3	2

Calculated as rates,* the current incidence of permanent cervical cord injury, nonfatal and fatal combined, was one per 100,000 athletes in 1977 and 1978, the same as that during the period of the Schneider study (Table 2-8).

Thus, the various efforts in the late 1960s toward the development of mandatory helmet standards, and in the teaching and practice of blocking-tackling techniques, eventually resulted in a decline in the frequency of both fatal and nonfatal catastrophic neurotrauma. This does not mean that all helmets in use at that time were substandard; it means that all helmet models being sold had not yet been subjected to performance tests that would provide confidence that they were not substandard. Similarly, this does not mean that coaches were necessarily teaching an improper technique; it means that improper execution of certain techniques constituted a highly serious hazard.

The Torg vs Schneider data initially suggested that a tradeoff was occurring: the quest for helmet standards was associated with both lowered cerebral injury frequencies and increased cervical cord injuries. To some this meant that the modern helmet was literally causing these injuries (back of helmet forcibly impinging on the spine), instead of, or in addition to,

---

* Calculated by me from the injury data provided by Schneider and Torg, and from the population data found within AFCA Annual Football Fatality Report.

prompting the well-protected athlete to "stick his head-neck in places where he never used to." However, the distinct drop in the frequency of cervical cord injuries since 1976 disconfirms the implication of the helmets as causative agents. The premise for the 1976 rule changes was that helmets can neither cause nor prevent the serious neck injury; it is principally a matter of the blocking-tackling technique. The available epidemiologic data are consistent with that contention.

As was the case for fatalities alone, the trends in relative frequency of all cervical neurotrauma, which by 1978 had returned to that of 1960, do not support an indictment of the facemask as a causative agent.

POTENTIALLY CATASTROPHIC INJURIES

We cannot ignore severe injuries because they are infrequent, nor can we focus only on these injuries. The National Athletic Injury/Illness Reporting System (NAIRS) has been following all athletic injuries in various sports since 1975, including the potentially serious head injuries called concussions.[4]

Concussions

In the NAIRS system, a reportable concussion is any disorientation caused by trauma, which required cessation of play to examine the athlete, no matter how

TABLE 2-11. Average Annual Rate (Cases/100 Athletes) of Concussions in Collegiate Football Accompanied by Proportion of Significant Concussions Associated with Tackling*

Concussions	1975	1976	1977	1978
Reportable	5.8	6.4	6.0	7.0
Significant	0.6	0.7	0.6	0.6
(While tackling)	58%	40%	30%	23%

* From the National Athletic Injury/Illness Reporting System, The Pennsylvania State University, 1979.

momentary the symptoms, and no matter what the subsequent disposition of the athlete with respect to participation. The rate of reportable concussions among the collegiate athletes followed by NAIRS is found in Table 2-10. One concussion in football resulted in death; none of the others produced perceptible permanent brain damage. By both population and exposure, football clearly is the sport most frequently associated with these injuries. Adjusted for exposure, however, the data reveal a difference between Spring football and Fall football. They also show strikingly uniform rates among the other sports.

NAIRS is also able to retrieve injury data by degrees of severity. Customarily, pref-

TABLE 2-10. Average Annual Incidence of Reportable Concussions in Selected College Sports, 1975-77*

	Average Number of Teams	Cases/10,000 Athlete-Exposures	Cases/100 Athletes
Football, Spring	26	11.1	2.2
Football, Fall	49	7.3	6.1
Lacrosse	5	4.1	1.9
Ice hockey	8	3.5	3.7
Softball (Women)	10	3.5	1.7
Wrestling	20	3.0	2.5
Basketball (Women)	21	2.7	2.2
Soccer	13	2.7	1.6

* From the National Athletic Injury/Illness Reporting System, The Pennsylvania State University, 1979. NAIRS data bearing no reference to other published work were prepared by me with the assistance of the NAIRS staff for inclusion in this chapter.

TABLE 2-12.   Average Annual Rate (Cases/1000 Athlete-Exposures) of Significant Concussions by Type and Brand of Helmet in School-College Football, 1975-77[10]

	All Helmets	Helmet												
		#1	#2	#3	#4	#5	#6	#7	#8	#9	#10	#11	#12	#13
Rate	0.1	0.1	0.1	0.1	0.1	0.1	0.1	0.1	0.0	0.1	0.0	0.0	0.1	0.0
Cases	92	7	19	6	24	2	5	19	0	3	3	0	3	0
% Use	100	6.5	22.7	9.9	15.2	2.7	5.8	10.7	3.2	2.7	5.9	0.1	2.1	0.5

erence for analysis is given the *significant injury* (i.e., those keeping the athlete out of participation for at least one week). Table 2-11 reveals that the year-to-year rates of both reportable and significant concussions in football were stable.[10] Since the 1976 rule changes, however, the proportion of significant concussions resulting from tackling has dropped steadily.

Football Helmets. While cerebral concussion is an infrequent occurrence in football, the next concern is whether particular helmets may be contributing to more than their share of these injuries. If a particular helmet is sufficiently defective in design to account for a disproportionate number of these injuries, the rate of concussions would be lowered if that helmet were removed from use.

NAIRS data were examined for this possibility, with Table 2-12 displaying the findings for significant concussions per 1000 athlete-exposures per type and brand of helmet for the seasons of 1975 through 1977.[10] Clearly, these injuries were dis-

tributed randomly through the population proportionate to the frequency of use of each helmet.

NAIRS data also were examined for the association of particular helmets with major cervical spine fractures.[10] These data are presented in view of the contention of some that the back edge of certain helmets can produce a "karate chop" injury to the spine, producing quadriplegia. The data are presented in Table 2-13 in terms of manufacturer only (instead of type and brand), because shell configuration did not vary within brand. Rates were expressed per 100,000 athlete-exposures because of the rarity of these occurrences. The criterion of *major* injury was used (i.e., greater than three weeks' absence from participation).

Only six major vertebral injuries occurred during the three seasons (over one million athlete-exposures) with only one resulting in neurological deficit (which was described as quadriplegia from a "hyperflexion injury").

TABLE 2-13.   Average Annual Rate (Cases/100,000 Athlete-Exposures) of Major Cervical Spine Fractures by Brand of Helmet in School-College Football, 1975-1977[10]

	All Helmets	Helmet						
		#1	#2	#3	#4	#5	#6	#7
Rate	0.5	0.0	0.5	0.0	1.4	2.4	0.0	0.0
Cases	6	0	4	0	1	1	0	0
% Used	100	8.6	60.7	6.6	5.9	3.5	2.9	10.2

The vast number of helmet contacts in a season (giving ample opportunity for a defective design to operate), the infrequency of this type of injury, and the proportionate distribution of these injuries over the helmets being worn, epidemiologically disconfirmed the allegation that the helmet causes cervical injury.

Playing Surface. NAIRS data also made it possible to examine the influence of playing surface on the incidence of selected injuries in college football.[6] The results clearly reveal no undue association of any playing surface with significant concussions, when analyzed on an equivalent exposure basis (Table 2-14). Further, none of the six cervical fractures in Table 2-13 had occurred during participation on an artificial surface, while 35% of the athlete-exposures had been on an artificial surface.

Brachial Plexus ("Burner") Injuries

With the rule changes in 1976 requiring a return to shoulder-blocking and tackling techniques, concern is frequently expressed about an increase in brachial plexus injuries from these changes. The potential for this had been acknowledged by those encouraging the 1976 changes, but the tradeoff between "burners" and quadriplegia presented no argument.

Interestingly, NAIRS data reveal no shift

TABLE 2-15. Rate (Cases/100 Athletes) of Brachial Plexus Injuries in Collegiate Football Accompanied by Proportion of Such Injuries Associated with the Act of Tackling*

	1975	1976	1977	1978
Reportable cases	2.2	2.2	2.2	2.4
(While tackling)	45%	47%	43%	38%
Significant cases	0.5	0.5	0.5	0.7
(While tackling)	31%	40%	47%	27%

* From the National Athletic Injury/Illness Reporting System, The Pennsylvania State University, 1979.

in frequency of reportable or significant brachial plexus injuries after 1976 (Table 2-15). The slight rise in 1978 is currently not significant (i.e., well within the range of normal variation). However, this will be reexamined at the end of the 1980 season to learn whether a trend is in the making.

Table 2-15 also permits examination of this concern by the proportion of such injuries resulting from tackling (the principal activity associated with this injury). A steady increase in this association is seen among significant brachial plexus injuries from 1975 to 1977 (31 to 47%). However, in 1978 this trend was clearly reversed. It is plausible to assume that the new coaching techniques for tackling have evolved into improved methods, or that better neck-conditioning practices have been im-

TABLE 2-14. Annual Rate (Cases/1000 Athlete Exposures) of Significant Concussions by Type of Playing Surface in College Football, 1975-77[6]

	1975	1976	1977
Natural Grass			
Athlete-Exposures	171,386	157,665	318,040
Concussion Rate	0.1	0.1	0.1
Astroturf			
Athlete-Exposures	95,803	87,382	155,027
Concussion Rate	0.0*	0.1	0.1
Tartanturf			
Athlete-Exposures	35,300	28,652	43,161
Concussion Rate	0.0*	0.1	0.1

* Not zero but less than 0.05.

plemented. Again, the patterns associated with this injury continue to be followed by NAIRS.

Facial Injuries

In Table 2-16, the frequency of various facial injuries can be compared in different sports. While ice hockey leads all other sports in frequency of facial injuries, most of this dominance is related to injuries that have few neural implications. Injuries to the eye and orbit are infrequent, yet pose a persistent threat to an athlete participating in any sport. This is one injury category in which Fall football is in last place among the injury-producing sports.

Noncatastrophic injuries with a potential for neurologic impairment can be evaluated only from 1975 to the present. Within this time span, the frequency of these injuries has remained stable at what can be considered a tolerable level. Further, patterns within these frequencies do not implicate a particular type or brand of helmet or playing surface. Much additional analysis of other potential factors is warranted if further practicable preventive measures are to be identified for implementation and evaluation.

TABLE 2-16. Average Annual Rate (Cases/100 Athletes) of Facial Injuries in Selected Collegiate Sports by Category of Injury, 1975-78*

	Eye-Orbit	Maxillo-Facial	Mouth-Teeth	Total
Ice Hockey	3.8	14.3	9.3	27.4
Wrestling	2.8	2.9	2.0	7.7
Basketball	1.3	2.1	2.7	6.1
Field Hockey (W)	1.1	1.7	2.4	5.2
Basketball (W)	1.4	1.0	2.1	4.5
Football, Spring	1.1	2.1	1.1	4.3
Soccer	0.3	1.1	1.1	2.5
Football, Fall	0.3	1.2	0.5	2.0

* From the National Athletic Injury/Illness Reporting System, The Pennsylvania State University, 1979.

CONCLUSIONS

Catastrophic neurotrauma in organized sports is infrequent, yet consistently associated with gymnastics, football, and wrestling. Such injuries occur periodically in other active sports, such as baseball and basketball, but not with the persistence that would enable epidemiologic analysis.

From the catastrophic data at hand, fatal and nonfatal, the recent definitive measures adopted by those sharing responsibility for school and college sports have been followed by a substantial lessening of the problems that had been identified:

1. The recent clarification of guidelines for the controlled use of the trampoline and minitramp in school and college programs has been followed (to date) with a drop in catastrophic injuries from these activities.

2. The decision to promulgate uniform testing standards for football helmets in the late 1960s was accompanied by a downward trend in serious cerebral trauma.

3. The decision, in 1976, to outlaw by rule and ethic the use of the helmeted head as the initial point of contact in blocking and tackling was followed by both another drop in fatal cerebral injuries, and a substantial drop in cervical spinal cord injuries.

Moreover, these latter changes have not caused (to date) an anticipated increase in another neurologic type of injury, that to the brachial plexus.

In addition, analysis of recent epidemiologic data disconfirmed the possibility that a particular type or brand of helmet or playing surface was a determinant in cerebral or spinal injuries in football.

Further, continuous use of the facemask during the period of evaluation was not associated with any trends that would suggest its involvement as a determinant in serious neck injuries. This is corroborated by Torg's clinical analysis of each case reported to his Registry, and by

TABLE 2-17. Trends in Significant Collegiate Women's Gymnastic Injuries by Event[8]

	1975-76		1977-78	
	R*	%	R*	%
Free Exercise	12.1	59	12.1	33
Balance Beam	3.0	15	8.3	23
Unevens	2.4	12	9.1	25
Vault	3.0	15	6.1	17
Trampoline	0.0	0	0.8	2

* R = Cases/100 Athletes.

Shield's analysis of the 16 patients with football quadriplegia who were admitted to Rancho Los Amigos Hospital from 1964 through 1973. Of these, 15 were flexion injuries.[13,16]

In football, as in gymnastics, and probably in wrestling and other sports in which reliable data are not available, the problem of neurotrauma is principally a matter of player technique and conditioning (conditioning should be considered part of "technique"). Education of coaches, athletes, and officials about the catastrophic hazards of improper techniques should continue to be emphasized in preventive efforts.

A catastrophic injury, however, is only one outcome on an injury spectrum of graded severity stemming from a particular etiologic mechanism. It is advisable to continuously monitor any injury pattern that is associated with the threat of permanent impairment. For example, a NAIRS examination of trends of significant injuries in women's collegiate gymnastics in 1975-77 (Table 2-17), suggested an upward trend associated with recent modifications of scoring criteria in that sport.[8] As a result of these more demanding criteria, these athletes may be attempting more "risk" routines than they are truly prepared to attempt. That an improperly executed gymnastic skill could result in severe neurotrauma instead of a less serious transient injury remains an epidemiologic concern.

REFERENCES

1. AMA Committee on the Medical Aspects of Sports: Spearing and Football. *In* Tips on Athletic Training. X. Chicago, Am. Med. Assoc., 1968.
2. Blyth, C., and Arnold, D.: The Forty-seventh Annual Football Fatality Report. Chapel Hill, N.C., The Am. Football Coaches Assoc., 1979.
3. Clarke, K.: Calculated risk of sports fatalities. J.A.M.A., *197*:894, 1966.
4. Clarke, K.: Premises and pitfalls of athletic injury surveillance. Am. J. Sports Med., *3*:292, 1975.
5. Clarke, K.: Survey of spinal cord injuries in schools and college sports, 1973-75. J. Safety Res., *9*:140, 1977.
6. Clarke, K., Alles, W., and Powell, J.: An epidemiological examination of the association of selected products with related injuries in football, 1975-77. Final Report, U.S. Consumer Product Safety Commission, Contract #CPSC-C-77-0039, 1978.
7. Clarke, K., and Braslow, A.: Football fatalities in actuarial perspective. Med. Sci. Sports, *10*:94, 1979.
8. Clarke, K., and Buckley, W.: Women's injuries in collegiate sport—a preliminary comparative overview of three seasons. Am. J. Sports Med., *8*:187, 1980.
9. Clarke, K., et al.: First Annual Gymnastics Catastrophic Injury Report. Washington, D.C., U.S. Gymnastics Safety Assoc., 1980.
10. Clarke, K., and Powell, J.: Football helmets and neurotrauma—an epidemiological overview of three seasons. Med. Sci. Sports, *11*:138, 1979.
11. Competitive sports and their hazards. Stat. Bull. Metropol. Life Ins. Co., *46*:1, 1965.
12. Schneider, R.: Serious and fatal neurosurgical football injuries. Clin. Neurosurg., *12*:226, 1965.
13. Shields, C., Fox, J., and Stauffer, E.: Cervical cord injuries in sports. Phys. and Sportsmed., *6*:21, 1978.
14. Shared Responsibility for Sports Safety. A statement of the Committee on Competitive Safeguards and Medical Aspects of Sports. Shawnee Mission, Kans., Nat. College Athletic Assoc., 1978.
15. The Use of Trampolines and Minitramps in Physical Education. A policy statement of the American Alliance for Health, Physical Education, Recreation, and Dance. Washington, D.C., 1978.
16. Torg, J.: Cervical neurotrauma in football. Unpublished presentation, Am. Orthop. Soc. Sports Med. Annual Meeting, July 1979, and subsequent personal communications.
17. Torg, J., et al.: The National Head and Neck Injury Registry—Report and Conclusions, 1978. J.A.M.A., *241*:1477, 1979.
18. Use of the Trampoline for the Development of Competitive Skills. A policy statement of the National Collegiate Athletic Association Committee on Competitive Safeguards and Medical Aspects of Sports. Shawnee Mission, Kans., 1978.

Chapter 3

A Standard for Protective Equipment

Voigt Hodgson

The ideal standard for athletic protective equipment should assure that participants in a sport will be minimizing their risk of injury by wearing gear that can meet the demands of the impact environment from the standpoint of structural integrity and shock attenuation. Such a standard should certify only those pieces of equipment that meet the criteria given without exposing other parts of the body or the opponent to risk of injury, and without impairing athletic performance.

Two basic approaches to the problem of developing a standard exist. One is an engineering approach in which the protective system is compressed by impact between two rigid surfaces, one of which may have a rudimentary shape of the part meant to be protected by the equipment. In this approach the protective equipment is the only part of the test system absorbing energy, and its performance is gauged on the basis of a kinematic or kinetic measurement that is not necessarily related to injury.

The proponents of the engineering approach believe that for a given input energy this is a more severe test, since there is a minimum of deflection or friction in the system to absorb energy. Therefore, the characteristics of the protective part can be more clearly judged relative to other designs and performance limits. Usually the motion of the test is translational and the instrumentation system is kept as simple as possible to make tests repeatable and reproducible among laboratories.

The other approach is biomechanical and seeks to combine: a humanoid surrogate of the body part; a limit level of response that is related to human tolerance; and worst case impact environment situations.

The proponents of the biomechanical approach seek to maintain biofidelity of the surrogate response so that it can be calibrated in terms of human-injury criteria. When placed in a field-simulating environment, the quantities of measurement are relevant to the injury threshold. (NOTE: It is usually necessary to sacrifice some fidelity in the surrogate by making it stronger and more durable than the real-life part of the body that it represents.)

The nature of the latter approach allows for a compromise between degree of protection and athletic performance required. For example, while comfort and size range may not appear as important as impact attenuation, they must be considered since they are important purchasing factors, and thus affect the injury incidence. In quality control standard tests to certify the quality of the product, some of the biomechanical fidelity may be relaxed in the interest of simplicity, speed, and reproducibility.

This chapter illustrates the development and utilization of an athletic equipment standard based on a biomechanical approach. The NOCSAE Football Helmet Standard is used as the illustration.[12]

METHODS

Impact Surface

Examination of rare films, which are clear enough to display injuries, reveals that the primary hazards to the head are impact with other heads, driving knees, or the turf. All three are relatively stiff, blunt surfaces. Impacts can occur to any part of the head, but head injuries are produced mainly by impacts against a relatively firm surface, with the major component of force aligned transverse to the superior-inferior axis. Unless the impact is anticipated and the neck muscles deliberately set, only the mass of the head is involved. If the muscles are not set, head accelerations and the risk of injury are higher. A flat, firm, rubber pad,* 1.3 mm (0.5 in.) thick, mounted on a rigid base is used to simulate these injury surfaces.

Impact Speed

The fastest football players can run an average of 36.6 m (40 yd) in 4.4 sec (8.2 m/sec or 27 ft/sec), evidently reaching maximum speeds of around 10.7 m/sec (35 ft/sec). If a player wearing a helmet runs into a brick wall with his head at this speed, serious injury or death would most likely result. Since it is impossible for a practical size helmet to protect under these extreme conditions, the standard test speed is less than this. A survey of the performance of representative helmets helped to arrive at a helmet drop height of 152 cm (60 in.), which produces an impact

speed of 5.5 m/sec (17.9 ft/sec).*

Football helmets must withstand countless numbers of impacts. For this application, resilient foams that revert to their original shape after impact are the most practical, although not as efficient as crushable foams. In comparison, crash helmets are designed primarily for one massive impact and can be fitted with a rigid foam that crushes at a certain load level.

Number of Impacts

Football is a multiple-impact sport in which impact is delivered anywhere on the helmet. Although it is highly unlikely, repetitive blows can occur at or near the same spot. Resilient materials recover their original shape at varying rates. Usually the stiffest and most efficient recover slowest of all, but at the same time cannot be compressed as much as softer materials. Consequently, to allow for degradation in performance due to only partial recovery, and thus to force design improvement in the material or geometry, two impacts on each of six locations are required at various ambient temperatures. These impacts are delivered at any one location within 75 ± 15 sec. On front and side locations, two additional incremental drops from lower levels are needed to determine the helmet performance, as it varies over a range of energy. It is not adequate for a helmet standard compliance performance to increase exponentially and score just under the limit of the minimum requirement. The least slip in quality control of material or construction, change in temperature, or odd-shaped head, and the margin of safety vanishes.

Weather Factors

It is essential for a standard to reject equipment that deteriorates seriously in impact performance due to the weather ex-

---

* Using the standard system of rating resiliency of rubber and rubber-like materials, the pad is 38 durometer on the Shore A scale.

* By comparison, the U.S. Government Motorcycle Helmet Standard[1] requires helmets of about the same size as those used in football to be dropped from 183 cm (72 in.), which produces an impact speed of 6.0 m/sec (19.6 ft/sec).

tremes of football. Heat is the primary environmental factor that degrades most helmets by softening liner materials. As a result, they bottom-out more easily and thus absorb less energy at high temperatures (e.g., 38°C [100°F]) than at the lower temperatures at which football is often played. Football helmet-liner materials vary widely and their performance deteriorates from heat; it is the purpose of the standard to eliminate those materials that deteriorate unsafely. Therefore, the helmet is dropped twice from a height of 152 cm (60 in.) on the right frontal boss at 49°C (120°F).

Generally, materials get stiffer, and performance improves, as the temperature drops. If helmets are tested at temperatures as low as −29°C (−20°F), the normally resilient materials suffer brittle failure; although in rupturing, energy is absorbed and acceleration is attenuated below normal values. This is not a realistic situation. Although the game is sometimes played in sub-freezing weather, head temperatures warm up the lining material enough to prevent it from becoming brittle. In addition, although some standards employ a moisture environmental condition, materials are either impervious to moisture, or if they absorb moisture, their ability to absorb energy improves.[6]

Head Model

The most important feature of the test system is the head model. Saczalski, et al. have shown how important it is that the surrogate match human response.[9] There is so much interplay between the mechanical properties of the helmet and those of the head, and so little room for error, that unless helmets are tested with a surrogate having the weight, shape, mass distribution, and deformation qualities similar to those of the head, the right matchup to the human head will not be effected. With an improper surrogate, adequate helmets may be eliminated, or helmets that are passed by the standard may not be of optimum stiffness, size, and comfort for the sport.

Because of cost, helmets are currently made in either two or three shell sizes with variations in liner thickness to accommodate a range of head sizes in each shell size. The largest size in each shell is critical since its liner is thinnest. The requirements of a size 8 helmet, which must decelerate a 5.4-kg (12-lb) head, are greater than those of a size 6⅝ helmet, which must protect a 3.6-kg (8-lb) head. The smaller head also tends to deform less than the larger one. Three sizes of head models, 6⅝, 7¼, and 7⅝, are used in the NOCSAE system.

Mechanical Test Setup

A test system must be repeatable within narrow limits to ensure that helmet compliance tests are conducted fairly. Also, if the same system is to be used for research, development, and quality control, reproducibility and ruggedness are desirable features to ensure that different laboratories are in reasonable agreement and the system is able to withstand a large number of impacts without mechanical breakdown. The essential mechanical parts of the NOCSAE test system are the head model mounted on a lightweight aluminum carriage, a position adjuster for controlling impact location, and stainless steel strand guidewires. The system is propelled by gravity (Fig. 3-1).

Performance Requirement

Figure 3-2 shows the 1500 Severity Index (SI)* concussion tolerance curve for distributed impact. This is superimposed on a kinematics chart that plots the relationship between displacement, pulse duration, and velocity change for uniform acceleration in discrete increments. Any impact experienced by the human-head

---

*$SI = \int_{0}^{T} A^{2.5}dt \leq 1500$, where A = acceleration in g's
2.5 = weighting factor
dt = time interval in seconds
T = pulse duration in seconds
$0.0025 < T < 0.050$

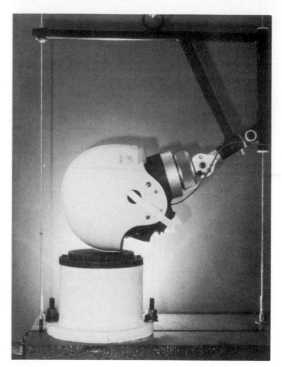

Fig. 3-1. NOCSAE Football Helmet Drop Test System featuring head models with near-human impact response.

surrogate that produces an acceleration- (or deceleration-) time history in which the effective (average) acceleration (area under the acceleration-time oscillogram divided by time) and time duration ordinate-abscissa combination, which when plotted lies below the curve, is expected to produce a concussion. When the acceleration and time are plotted, the corresponding velocity change and stopping distance can be compared to the impact velocity and helmet liner thickness, respectively, to evaluate the helmet effectiveness.

With the assumed ideal stopping (or starting) uniform acceleration (square wave), the stopping distance would equal the linear thickness and velocity change would equal impact velocity. Actually, the stopping distance for impact against a rigid surface is always less than liner thickness, and velocity change is always greater than impact velocity. Although in mechanical handling systems, uniform stopping is preferable for economy of time,

space, and materials, it may not be desirable for the head. The high-crush loads of nonresilient materials produce a steep onset of head acceleration that may be deleterious to the brain.[5]

Use of the SI as a compliance test gauge makes it more difficult to hold tight tolerances among several laboratories because of the weighting factor: i.e., a 15% change in acceleration can result in a 50% change in SI. However, it is justified because the exponent flies a warning flag that reveals undesirable rapid changes in helmet performance (approach of bottoming-out) more sensitively than measuring peak accelerations alone. Head injury is not something that gradually gets a little worse with each increment of acceleration. Rather, the threshold of concussion is sudden and usually reversible, but farther up the intensity scale, irreversible changes occur and a concussion is potentially lethal. Cerebrovascular accidents also occur suddenly at no known level of intensity and cause irreversible damage.

Acceleration-time pulses that integrate to an SI of 1000 equate to the original Wayne State University curve, which was based on its short duration and on results obtained from cadaver skull fractures due to rigid, flat-surface impact on the forehead.[7] Gadd, the originator of the SI,[2] has pointed out many instances of distributed (nonfracturing) impact in which volunteers experienced a much higher SI without concussion.[3] Accordingly, he has recommended, and the NOCSAE Standard has adopted, an SI of 1500 for distributed impacts in which the fracture hazard is absent. Since skull fractures in modern football have been virtually eliminated, football helmets fall into this category.

As Figure 3-2 illustrates, the use of a calibrated humanoid surrogate makes it possible to extrapolate from mechanical kinematics to human-tolerance criteria. This approach helps the designer to evaluate a helmet performance relative to an established injury level.

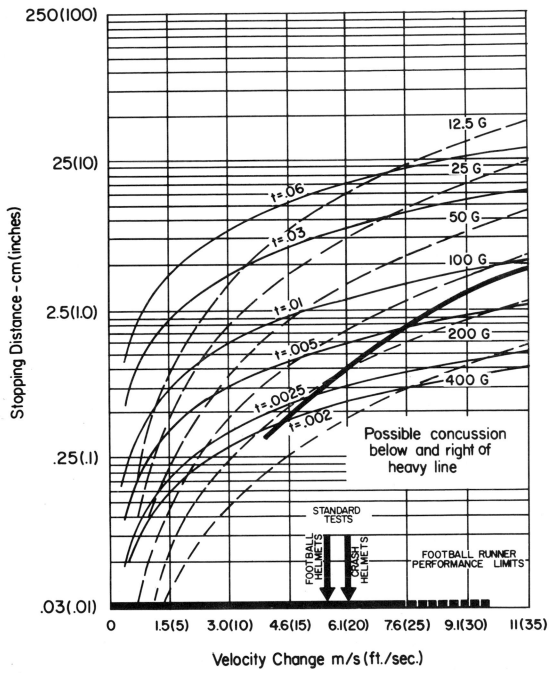

Fig. 3-2. Kinematics chart on which a cerebral concussion tolerance curve is superimposed, corresponding to a 1500 Severity Index for distributed impact (no fracture hazard).

The NOCSAE Standard was intended to force helmet designers to employ either slightly denser, stiffer resilient foams or slightly larger helmets than many of those on the market prior to the Standard. There is an emphasis on "slightly," because what may be good for preventing concussion at high levels of impact intensity may be too stiff for the head in lower intensity situations. Also, to be effective, helmets have to be worn as purchased and not tampered with for comfort's sake. There are practical constraints of size and comfort beyond which it is not fruitful to force the design of helmets.

RESULTS

Effect on Helmets

The immediate effect of the NOCSAE Standard was to prevent certification of 38% of the models presented. Of the 74 helmet models initially certified, the average performance for all locations was 812 SI and 154 g. The highest average score was on the front, being 1064 SI and 188 g for all models. Improvements were achieved through head size shifts; i.e., shifting a popular size like 7⅜ from the middle-shell size to the largest shell to provide more liner space. To provide the best performance at all impact intensity levels, a helmet should ideally be fitted with four or five layers of foam that increase in firmness toward the shell. Alternatively, a suspension system should be designed to do the same thing. For practical reasons, primarily space limitations, most models use two layers of foam and a few, three. In a group of ten models, the SI was reduced by a factor of two to one due to the 7⅜-size shift although at a sacrifice of stability, visibility, and perceived weight.[6]

After compliance testing improvements, the NOCSAE system began to be used for quality control of used helmets. Among the first large group of 849 noncertified helmets given a partial NOCSAE Standard test before reconditioning, 84% exceeded the SI limit.[7]* Improvements on SI in 143 precertified helmets ranged from 14% for liner replacements to 44% for shell and liner replacements. Also, depending on type, treatment, and position played, many types of certified helmets were found to

---

* Courtesy of D. Gleisner, All American Company, member of the National Athletic Equipment Reconditioners Association (NAERA), Elyria, Ohio, 1975.

degrade to various extents over one or several seasons. To maintain helmet improvements due to the Standard, the need for quality control in the reconditioning plants was recognized. Today, there is a nationwide network of test systems in manufacturing and reconditioning plants. The number of certified models has fallen from a high of 85 to the present 41. Part of this attrition can be attributed to the Standard, but some certified helmets have been taken off the market because of the high risk of litigation.

Effect on Injuries

In the laboratory, variables can be controlled one at a time to determine their effect on a process. This is more difficult in football because of other possible factors, such as rules changes, enforcement, teaching techniques, changes in other equipment, and improvements in treatment of injured players. Table 3-1 shows the trend of fatal head injuries in football since 1963. Comparing the pre-NOCSAE period, 1963-70 to the 1971-78 seasons in which NOCSAE research influenced helmet design, fatal head injuries decreased 54%. The big reductions in 1977-78 were probably due, in part, to a rules change in 1976 (which appeared to have little effect the first year) by NFSHSA, forbidding initial contact with the head in blocking and tackling. Also, many high schools were beginning to purchase new certified helmets, and more reconditioners were screening and recertifying helmets with NOCSAE test equipment, in preparation for the required 1980 compliance with the NOCSAE Standard for high schools. Several states play under NCAA rules, which required compliance with the NOCSAE Standard for the 1978 season.

It is difficult to ascertain whether changes in rules or equipment account for this greatly improved injury picture; their effects are really complementary. Along with other football authorities, NOCSAE

TABLE 3-1. Comparison of Junior High and High School Football Head Injury Deaths* in the Eight-Year Periods Preceding and During the NOCSAE Program†

	1963	1964	1965	1966	1967	1968	1969	1970	1971	1972	1973	1974	1975	1976‡	1977	1978
									NOCSAE Program Began September 1, 1970							
Head Injury Deaths	10	16	16	15	13	20	14	15	11	12	6	9	12	12	3	4
Average Deaths				14.9								8.6				
Percent Reduction								42								
Number of Players	850,000	← 1,000,000 →				1,100,000			→ 1,200,000 →				← 1,500,000			
Incidence of Deaths per 100,000 Players	1.2	1.9	1.6	1.5	1.3	2.0	1.3	1.3	1.0	1.0	0.5	0.8	1.0	0.8	0.2	0.3
Average Incidence				1.51								0.70				
Percent Reduction								54								

* Predominately subdural hematomas.

† 1963-70 number of players' figures revised from earlier published comparison to reflect both junior high and high school players.

‡ The rule change prohibiting initial contact of the facemask or helmet in blocking or tackling was in effect during 1976-78. NOCSAE certified helmets were required in several states, conforming to college rules in 1978, and were required in all states by 1980.

SOURCES: The 32nd through 47th Annual Surveys of Football Fatalities 1963-78; copyright 1979 by The American Football Coaches Association, Durham, N.C.; The National Collegiate Athletic Association, Shawnee Mission, Kans.; and The National Federation of State High School Associations, Elgin, Ill.

officials, knowing the aforementioned limitations imposed on helmet designs, made recommendations leading to the 1976 rules changes to take some of the burden off the helmet.

As evidenced by a comparison of the statistics published in 1958 by Gurdjian and Webster,[4] with those published in 1979 by Torg et al.,[13] the reduction in head injuries is evidently not due to treatment. Gurdjian and Webster found that among a group of 40 patients who underwent surgery for subdural hematoma, 14 of the 16 who underwent operation within 24 hours or less (acute), died, for a mortality rate of 81%. In a group of six who were operated on within 24 to 72 hours, three died, for a mortality rate of 50%. Of 18 operated on within 3 to 5 days, four died, for a mortality rate of 22%. Torg's study, which indicates that the major cause of death due to craniocerebral injuries is intracranial hemorrhages, showed that in a group of 72 injured players in 1971-75, 58 died, for a mortality rate of 81%. Overall, from 1971 through 1977 he found a mortality rate of 75% in 123 players. This study did not report the number of hours between the time of injury and time of surgery.

Effect on the Neck

The results of football neck injury surveys have recently been reported by Torg et al.,[13] and Mueller and Blyth.[8] The approximate 50% reduction in total neck injuries undoubtedly reflects the decreased use of the head as a result of the rules changes in 1976. Even with these dramatic reductions in neck injury, helmets have been blamed for causing neck injury, either because of the so-called "guillotining"* effect of the rear rim, in which the helmet is assumed to be forcefully rotated on the head under the facemask, or because the helmets do not absorb sufficient energy

in the crown.[10, 11] Until recently, it has not been possible to quantitatively study the effect of the helmet on the neck, and consequently, such charges could be leveled indiscriminately against the helmet on the basis of little or no evidence. Cures offered by individuals who do not have to accept responsibility for equipment performance put the manufacturers of helmets on the defensive.

Now that dummies with neck transducers are available, unpublished studies have shown that 15 to 30 cm (6 to 12 in.) of lining is required to attenuate axial loads to a level that may be tolerable under severe impact conditions. Before a standard requires added mass or leverage to the crown for axial protection, serious trade-offs must be considered. In general, impacts are not purely axial, and there is much evidence to indicate that neck tolerance to torsion and bending, which stress ligaments in shear, is much lower than to pure axial loading. Such axial loading is resisted by the compressive strength of the cervical vertebrae, intervertebral discs, and interconnecting ligaments in tension. Not enough can be done to the crown to protect the neck, and methods of bypassing the neck, while being investigated by NOCSAE, present practical difficulties.

Drop tests were performed on three intact cadavers with short and long necks and fitted with a conventional low-cut, rear-rimmed helmet and facemask. High-speed movies (500 frames/sec) have demonstrated that when blows are delivered to the facemask, the rear rim of the helmet impinges on the skin covering C7-T3 without causing injury. Although these results are based on only three cadaver tests, the original game evidence of rear-rim involvement is also meager.* Torg, et al. have reported on 209 cases of catastrophic neck injury occurring in football between 1971 and 1975 and analyzed them according to mechanism of injury. The facemask

---

* The term seems to have arisen either in court or in newspaper accounts of court cases.

---

* See cases 21, 22, and 24 in Schneider, R.C.[10]

acting as a lever was not implicated in any case.[13]

NOCSAE research is using cadavers and neck-load-indicating dummies to investigate the effects of such equipment factors as helmet crown design, chin straps, facemasks, rear rim, load transfer from helmet to the body, and other new features to develop a helmet standard for improved protection of both head and neck.

REFERENCES

1. Federal Safety Standard. MVSS 218, Motor Vehicle Safety Standard No. 218 Motorcycle Helmets—Helmets Designed for Use by Motorcyclists and Other Motor Vehicle Users, effective March 1, 1974.
2. Gadd, C.W.: Use of a weighted-impulse criterion for estimating injury hazard. *In* Tenth Stapp Car Crash Conference Proceedings. New York, Society of Automotive Engineers, November 1966.
3. Gadd, C.W.: Tolerable severity index in wholehead, nonmechanical impact. *In* Fifteenth Stapp Car Crash Conference Proceedings. New York, Society of Automotive Engineers, November 1971.
4. Gurdjian, E.S., and Webster, J.E.: Head Injuries, Mechanisms, Diagnosis and Management. Boston, Little, Brown and Co., 1958.
5. Hodgson, V.R.: Physical factors related to experimental concussion. *In* Impact and Crash Protection. Springfield, Charles C Thomas, 1970.
6. Hodgson, V.R.: National Operating Committee on Standard for Athletic Equipment Football Helmet Certification Program. Med. Sci. Sports, 7:225, 1975.
7. King, A.I.: Survey of the state of the art of human biodynamic response. *In* Aircraft Crashworthiness. Charlottesville, University of Virginia Press, 1975.
8. Mueller, F.O., and Blyth, C.: Catastrophic head and neck football injuries. Phys. and Sportsmed., 7:71, 1979.
9. Saczalski, K.J., et al.: A critical assessment of the use of non-human responding surrogates for safety system evaluation. *In* Twentieth Stapp Car Crash Conference Proceedings. New York, Society of Automotive Engineers, October 1976.
10. Schneider, R.C.: Head and Neck Injuries in Football, Mechanisms, Treatment, and Prevention. Baltimore, Williams & Wilkins, 1973.
11. Snively, G.G., and Chichester, C.O.: Impact survival levels of head acceleration in man. Aerospace Med., 32:316, 1961.
12. Standard Method of Impact Test and Performance Requirements for Football Helmets. National Operating Committee on Standards for Athletic Equipment, September 1972, revised September 1977.
13. Torg, J.S., et al.: The National Football Head and Neck Injury Registry. J.A.M.A., *241*:1477, 1979.

Section II

Head Injuries

Chapter 4

Field Evaluation of Head and Neck Injuries

Joseph J. Vegso
Michael H. Bryant
Joseph S. Torg

The purpose of this chapter is to present clear, concise guidelines for classification, evaluation, and emergency management of injuries that occur to the head and neck as a result of participation in competitive and recreational activities.

Of the variety of injuries that can occur to the athlete, those involving the head and neck are the most difficult to evaluate and manage on the field. There are several reasons for this phenomenon. Because of the actual or potential involvement of the nervous system, risks can be high, and consequently the margin for error is low. The initial clinical picture frequently may be misleading. Patients with significant intracranial hemorrhage may at first present with minimal symptoms, only to follow a precipitous downhill course. On the other hand, short-lived problems such as a neuropraxia of the brachial plexus may at first present with paresthesia and paralysis, raising the question of a significant spinal injury, only to resolve within minutes with the individual returning to his activity. Fortunately, the more severe injuries that can occur to the head and neck are infrequent; consequently, most team physicians and trainers have little, if any, experience in dealing with them.

There are several principles that should be considered by individuals responsible for athletes who may sustain injuries to the head and neck:

1. The team physician or trainer should be designated as the person responsible for supervising on-the-field management of the potentially serious injury. This person is the "captain" of the medical team.
2. Prior planning must insure the availability of all necessary emergency equipment at the site of potential injury. At a minimum, this should include a spineboard, stretcher, and equipment necessary for the initiation and maintenance of cardiopulmonary resuscitation (CPR).
3. Prior planning must insure the availability of a properly equipped ambulance, as well as a hospital equipped and staffed to handle emergency neurologic problems.
4. Prior planning must insure immediate availability of a telephone for communicating with the hospital emergency room, ambulance, and other responsible individuals in case of an emergency.

INTRACRANIAL INJURIES

Injuries to the brain that occur as a result of sports may be either focal or diffuse lesions. The athlete that sustains such an injury may be conscious and ambulatory, conscious and nonambulatory, or unconscious. The initial state of the patient is not necessarily a reliable indicator of either the pathologic diagnosis or the severity of the injury. Rather, other parameters must be used to determine the nature and severity of the insult, as well as to determine how the injured athlete should be managed.

The athlete who receives a blow to his head, or a sudden jolt to his body that results in a sudden acceleration-deceleration force to the head, should be carefully evaluated. In those instances where the individual is ambulatory and conscious, the entire spectrum of intracranial pathology, ranging from a grade I concussion to a more severe intracranial condition, must be considered. Initial on-field examination should include the following:

1. evaluation of facial expression;
2. determination of orientation to time, place, and person;
3. presence of post-traumatic amnesia;
4. presence of retrograde amnesia;
5. evaluation of gait.

An individual with a grade I concussion (Fig. 4-1) will be confused and have a dazed look on his face. There may also be mild unsteadiness of gait. However, post-traumatic and retrograde amnesia are not prominent features.[3] This clinical picture is best described by the athletes themselves who say, "I had my bell rung." Usually the state of confusion is short-lived, and the athlete is completely lucid in 5 to 15 minutes. When his mind is clear, he may return to the activity under the watchful supervision of the team physician or trainer. However, associated symptoms such as vertigo, headaches, photophobia, and labile emotions should preclude returning to the game.

A grade II concussion is characterized by confusion associated with post-traumatic amnesia. The signs and symptoms described for grade I concussion may be

GRADES OF CEREBRAL CONCUSSION

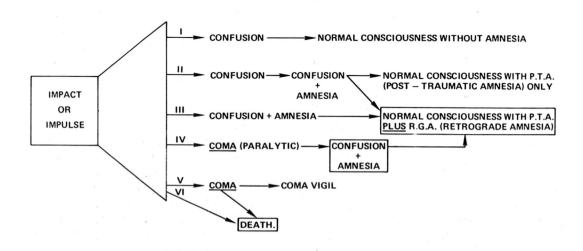

Fig. 4-1. Diagram of the six grades of cerebral concussion.

present.[3] Individuals manifesting post-traumatic amnesia, i.e., an inability to recall events that have occurred from the moment of injury, should not be permitted to return to play that day. These athletes require postinjury evaluation. They may develop the "postconcussion syndrome," which is characterized by persistent headaches, inability to concentrate, and irritability. In some instances, these symptoms may last for several weeks postinjury, and participation in the sport is precluded as long as symptoms are present.

In addition to the above symptoms grade III concussions are characterized by retrograde amnesia,[3] which is the inability of the individual to recall events prior to the injury. These athletes should not be permitted to return to the game, and the general rules for observation and follow-up care as given should be followed. When there is a traumatic intracranial lesion that produces a gradual increase in intracranial pressure, such as is seen in epidural and subdural hemorrhages, the individual may be conscious and ambulatory to the point of appearing capable of fulfilling his usual activity, and then suddenly collapses.

Frequently, a more severe grade II or III concussion may make the injured player disoriented and unable to ambulate because of vertigo or an ataxic gait. Essentially, the patient may be conscious but not able to ambulate independently. The all-too-common practice of having such an individual literally dragged off the playing area by two of his teammates leaves much to be desired, if only from an esthetic point of view. Since the player may have a serious intracranial injury, or in some instances, an associated cervical spine injury, an injured player who cannot walk unaided from the playing field after a reasonable period of time should be transported on a rigid stretcher or spineboard.

A grade IV concussion involves the "knocked out" player. This individual is in a paralytic coma, usually recovers after a few seconds or minutes, and then passes through states of stupor, confusion with or without delirium, and finally an almost lucid state with automatism before becoming fully alert.[3] This individual will most certainly have retrograde and post-traumatic amnesia. If the loss of consciousness lasts for more than several minutes or if there are other signs of a deteriorating neurologic state, the patient should be immediately transported to a hospital.

Initial evaluation of the athlete who has been rendered unconscious should involve the determination of whether or not he is breathing, whether he has a pulse, and the level of consciousness. If unobstructed respirations and an adequate pulse are present, there is no immediate need to do anything other than to keep in mind that head and neck injuries are frequently associated. Therefore, the player should be protected from injudicious manipulation or movement.

Such patients frequently remain semi-stuporous for more than several minutes. It should be emphasized that these individuals should be carried off the field on a spineboard or stretcher rather than be permitted to stagger off. An athlete who has been rendered unconscious for any period of time should not be allowed to return to contact activity, even if he is mentally clear. Overnight observation in a hospital should be seriously considered for these athletes.

Grade V concussions are those in which injury produces paralytic coma that may be associated with secondary cardiorespiratory collapse.[3] In those instances in which associated cardiorespiratory failure develops, CPR should be implemented immediately (see Appendix I).

Signs and symptoms that demand emergency action in an athlete who has sustained a blow to the head are: increasing headache, nausea and vomiting, inequality of pupils, disorientation, progressive or sudden impairment of consciousness, a gradual rise in blood pressure, and finally, a diminution of pulse rate. The development of any one or a combination of these may be indicative of increasing intracranial pressure.

An epidural hematoma may occur in the athlete who receives a severe blow to the head, e.g., a baseball player who has been struck by the ball. If a fracture occurs across the middle meningeal groove, severing the middle meningeal artery with subsequent formation of a "high pressure" hematoma, the player may do well for a short period of time; however, 10 to 20 minutes later he will develop one or more of the aforementioned danger signs. Such an individual should be transported immediately to a hospital.

A subdural hemorrhage occurs when the bridging veins between the brain and the cavernous sinus are torn as a result of a contrecoup or rotational accleration-deceleration. Low-pressure venous bleeding occurs, hematoma formation is slow, and the signs and symptoms of increasing intracranial pressure may not be evident for hours, days, or even weeks after the injury. In Schneider's series of 69 cases of acute subdural hematoma, 24 came to surgery or died within 6 hours of injury.[4] Thus, the physician and trainer should be suspicious of a blow to the head and watch the patient carefully. If an athlete develops any of the aforementioned danger signs and symptoms he should be transported immediately to a hospital for neurologic evaluation and treatment.

CERVICAL SPINE INJURIES

Athletic injuries to the neck and cervical spine can involve the bony elements, intervertebral discs, ligamentous and muscular supporting structures, elements of the brachial plexus, nerve roots, and the spinal cord itself. As in any trauma affecting the musculoskeletal or nervous system, appropriate management requires an understanding of both the severity of the injury and the anatomic structures involved. Fortunately, however, the more severe of these injuries are the least common.

The various athletic injuries to the cervical spine are:
1. nerve root-brachial plexus neurapraxia;
2. stable cervical sprain;
3. muscular strain;
4. brachial plexus axonotmesis;
5. intervertebral disc injury (narrowing-herniation) without neurologic deficit;
6. stable cervical fracture without neurologic deficit;
7. subluxations without neurologic deficit;
8. unstable fractures without neurologic deficit;
9. dislocations without neurologic deficit;
10. intervertebral disc herniation with neurologic deficit;
11. unstable fracture with neurologic deficit;
12. dislocation with neurologic deficit;
13. quadriplegia;
14. death.

Those responsible for on-the-field management of neck injuries should remember that only a small fraction of the total number of sports-incurred neck injuries result in permanent neurologic injury. However, it should be emphasized that if improperly handled, an unstable lesion without neurologic deficit can be converted to one with neurologic deficit.

Stable cervical sprains and strains eventually resolve with or without treatment. Initially, the presence of a serious injury should be ruled out by a thorough neurologic examination and determination of the range of cervical motion. Range of motion is evaluated by having the athlete actively nod his head, touch his chin to his chest, touch his chin to his left shoulder, touch his chin to his right shoulder, touch his left ear to his left shoulder, and touch his right ear to his right shoulder. If the patient is unwilling or unable to perform these maneuvers actively while standing erect, proceed no further. The athlete with less than a full pain-free range of cervical motion, persistent paresthesia, or weakness should be protected and excluded from further activity. Subsequent evaluation should include appropriate roentgenographic studies, including flexion and extension views to demonstrate fractures or instability.

The most common and most poorly understood cervical injuries are the pinch-stretch neurapraxias of the nerve root and brachial plexus. Clancy has reported a 49% incidence in college football players over their four-year exposure.[2] Typically, following contact with head, neck, or shoul-

der, a sharp burning pain is experienced in the neck on the involved side that may radiate into the shoulder and down the arm to the hand. There may be associated weakness and paresthesia in the involved extremity lasting from several seconds to several minutes. The key to the nature of this lesion is its short duration and the presence of a full, pain-free range of neck motion. Although the majority of these injuries are short-lived, they are worrisome because of the occasional plexus axonotmesis that occurs. However, the youngster whose paresthesia completely abates, who demonstrates full muscle strength in the intrinsic muscles of the shoulder and upper extremities, and who most importantly, has a full pain-free range of cervical motion, may return to his activity.

Persistence of paresthesia, weakness, or

TABLE 4-1. Field Decision Making—Head and Neck Injuries
(Unconscious Athlete)

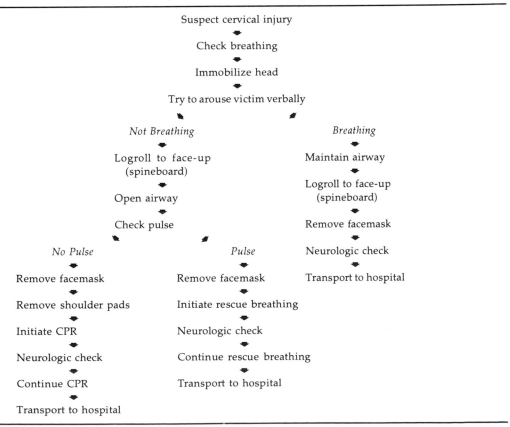

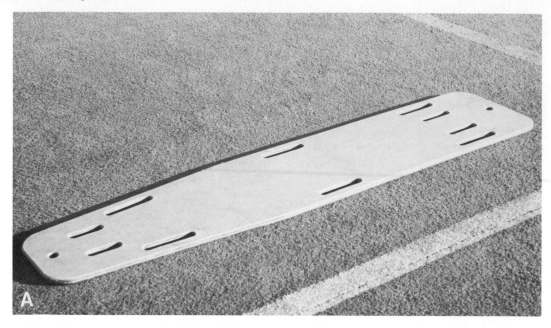

HALF SPINEBOARD

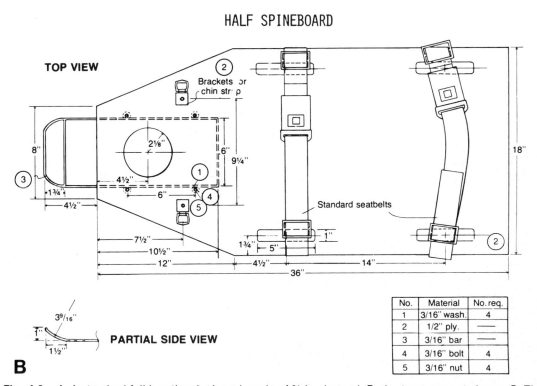

No.	Material	No. req.
1	3/16" wash.	4
2	1/2" ply.	——
3	3/16" bar	——
4	3/16" bolt	4
5	3/16" nut	4

Fig. 4-2. *A*, A standard full-length spineboard made of ¾ in plywood. Body straps are not shown. *B*, The Purdue University (West Lafayette, Indiana) spineboard can be constructed in any school wood shop. The board is made from ¾ in plywood. Body straps are standard seat belts or luggage straps that can be purchased at any Army-Navy surplus store. (Courtesy of William "Pinky" Newell.)

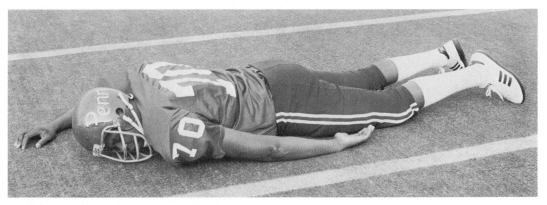

Fig. 4-3. Athlete with suspected cervical spine injury may or may not be unconscious. However, all who are unconscious should be managed as though they had a significant neck injury.

limitation of cervical motion requires that the individual be protected from further exposure and that he undergo neurologic and roentgenographic evaluation.

EMERGENCY MANAGEMENT

Managing the unconscious or spine-injured athlete is a process that should not be done hastily or haphazardly (Table 4-1). Being prepared to handle this situation is the best way to prevent actions that could convert a reparable injury into a catastrophe.

Have a "game plan." Be sure that all the necessary equipment is readily accessible, in good operating condition, and that all assisting personnel have been trained to use it properly. On-the-job training in an emergency situation is inefficient at best. Everyone should know what must be done beforehand, so that on a signal the game plan can be put into effect.

A means of transporting the athlete must be immediately available in a high-risk sport such as football and "on call" in other sports. The medical facility must be alerted to the athlete's condition and estimated time of arrival so that adequate preparation can be made.[5]

Having the proper equipment is an absolute must. A spineboard is essential (Fig. 4-2*A*, *B*), and is the best means of supporting the body in a rigid position. It is somewhat like a full body splint. By splinting the body, the risk of aggravating a spinal cord injury, which must always be suspected in the unconscious athlete, is re-

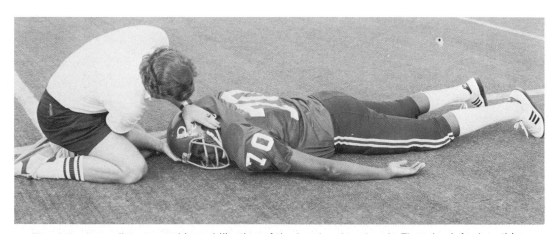

Fig. 4-4. Immediate manual immobilization of the head and neck unit. First check for breathing.

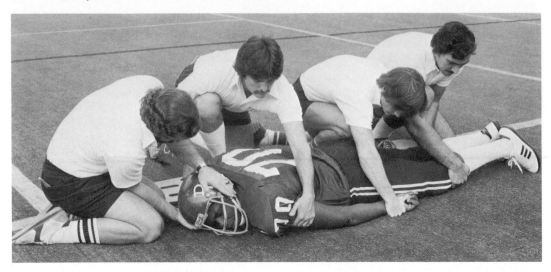

Fig. 4-5. Logroll to a spineboard. This maneuver requires four individuals: the leader to immobilize the head and neck and to command the medical-support team. The remaining three individuals are positioned at the shoulders, hips, and lower legs.

duced. In football, bolt cutters and a sharp knife or scalpel are also essential if it becomes necessary to remove the facemask. A telephone must be available to call for assistance and to notify the medical facility. Oxygen should be available and is usually carried by ambulance and rescue squads although it is rarely required in an athletic setting. Rigid cervical collars and other external immobilization devices can be helpful if properly used. However, manual stabilization of the head and neck is recommended even if other means are available.

Properly trained personnel must know, first of all, who is in charge. Everyone should know how to perform CPR and how to move and transport the athlete. They should know where emergency equipment is located and how to use it, and know the

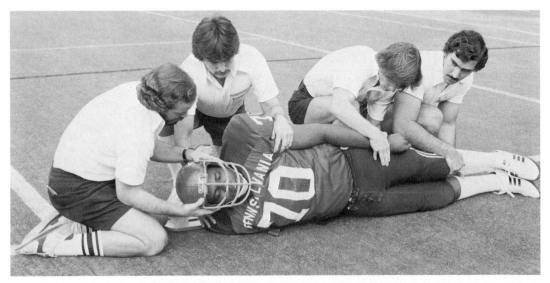

Fig. 4-6. Logroll. The leader uses the crossed-arm technique to immobilize the head. This technique allows the leader's arms to "unwind" as the three assistants roll the athlete onto the spineboard.

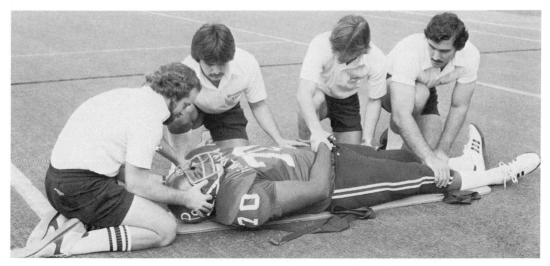

Fig. 4-7. Logroll. The three assistants maintain body alignment during the roll.

procedure for activating the emergency-support system. Individuals should be assigned specific tasks beforehand, if possible, so that duplication of effort is eliminated. Being well prepared helps to alleviate indecisiveness and second-guessing.

The single most important point to remember is: *prevent further injury.* Be sure that whatever action is taken does not

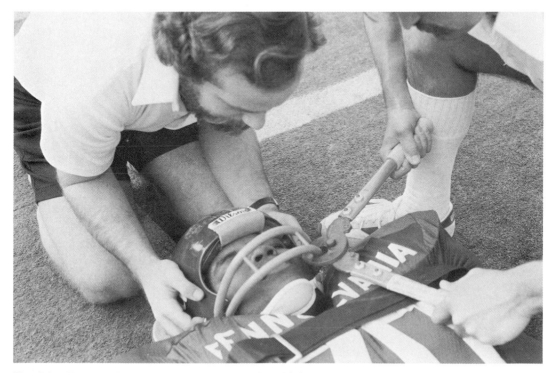

Fig. 4-8. Remove double- and single-bar masks with bolt cutters. Head and helmet must be securely immobilized.

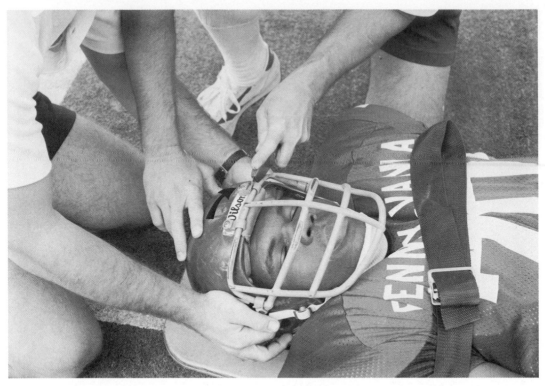

Fig. 4-9. Remove "cage"-type masks by cutting the plastic loops with a utility knife. Make the cut on the side of the loop away from the face.

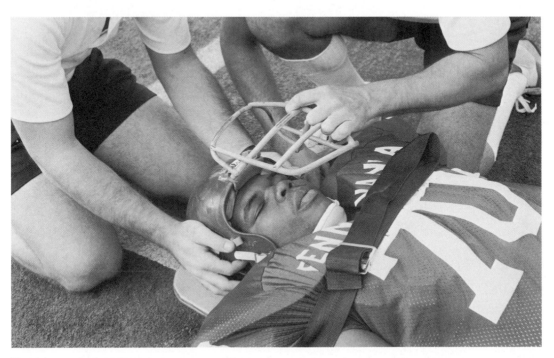

Fig. 4-10. Remove the entire mask from the helmet so it does not interfere with further resuscitation efforts.

cause further harm.[6] Therefore, immediately immobilize the head and neck by holding them in the neutral position (Figs. 4-3 and 4-4). Check first for breathing, then for pulse, and then for level of consciousness.

If the victim is breathing, simply remove the mouthguard, if present, and maintain the airway. It is necessary to remove the facemask only if the respiratory situation is threatened or unstable, or if the athlete remains unconscious for a prolonged period. Leave the chinstrap on.[6]

Once it is established that the athlete is breathing and has a pulse, evaluate the neurologic status. The level of consciousness, response to pain, pupillary response, and unusual posturing, flaccidity, rigidity, or weakness should be noted.

At this point, simply maintain the situation until transportation is available, or until the athlete regains consciousness. If the athlete is face down when the ambulance arrives, change his position to face up by logrolling him onto a spineboard. Make no attempt to move him except to transport him or to perform CPR if it becomes necessary.

If the athlete is not breathing or stops breathing, the airway must be established. If he is face down, he must be brought to a face-up position. The safest and easiest way to accomplish this is to logroll the athlete into a face-up position. In an ideal situation your medical-support team is made up of five members: the leader, who controls the head and gives commands only; three members to roll; and a fourth to help lift and carry when it becomes necessary.[6] If time permits and the spineboard is on the scene, the athlete should be rolled directly onto it. However, breathing and circulation are much more important at this point.

With all medical-support team members in position, the athlete is rolled toward the assistants: one at the shoulders, one at the hips, and one at the knees. They must maintain the body in line with the head and spine during the roll. The leader main-

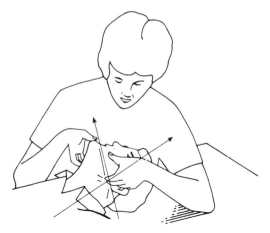

Fig. 4-11. Jaw-thrust maneuver for opening the airway of a victim with a suspected cervical spine injury. (© Reprinted with permission, American Heart Association.)

tains immobilization of the head by applying slight traction and by using the crossed-arm technique. This technique allows the arms to unwind during the roll (Fig. 4-5—4-7).

The facemask must be removed from the helmet before rescue breathing can be initiated. The type of mask that is attached to the helmet determines the method of removal. Bolt cutters are used with the older single- and double-bar masks. The newer masks that are attached with plastic loops should be removed by cutting the loops with a sharp knife or scalpel. Cut the loops on the side away from the face. Remove the entire mask so that it does not interfere with further rescue efforts (Figs. 4-8—4-10).

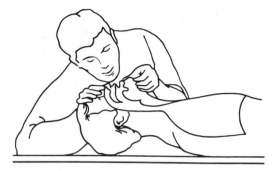

Fig. 4-12. Head tilt—jaw lift maneuver for opening the airway. Used if jaw thrust is inadequate or if a helmet is being worn. (© Reprinted with permission, American Heart Association.)

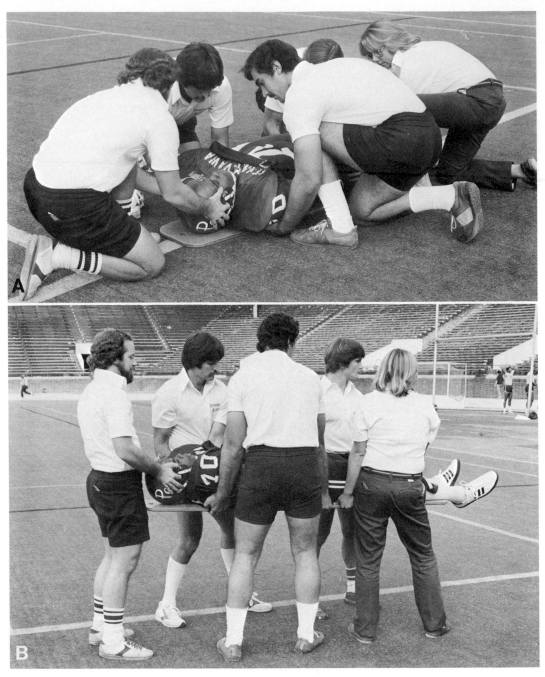

Fig. 4-13. *A* and *B*, Four members of the medical-support team lift the athlete on the command of the leader. The leader maintains manual immobilization of the head. The spineboard is not recommended as a stretcher. An additional stretcher should be used for transporting over long distances.

Once the mask has been removed, initiate rescue breathing following the current standards of the American Heart Association (see Appendix II).

Once the athlete has been moved to a face-up position, quickly evaluate breathing and pulse. If there is still no breathing, or if breathing has stopped, the airway

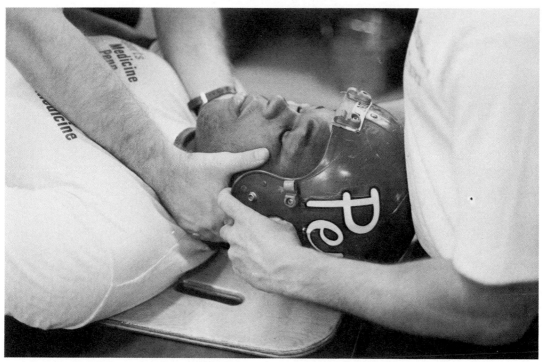

Fig. 4-14. The helmet should be removed only when permanent immobilization can be instituted. The helmet may be removed by detaching the chinstrap, spreading the earflaps, and gently pulling the helmet off in a straight line with the cervical spine.

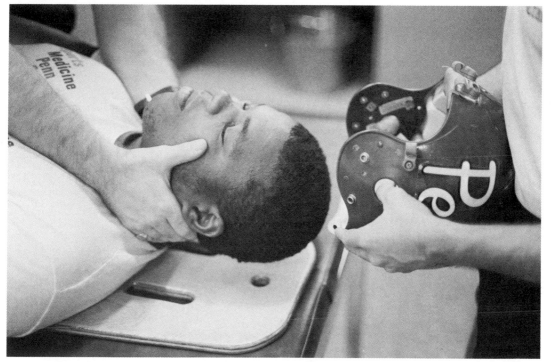

Fig. 4-15. The head must be supported under the occiput during and after removing the helmet.

must be established. "The jawthrust technique is the safest first approach to opening the airway of a victim who has a suspected neck injury, because in most cases it can be accomplished by the rescuer grasping the angles of the victim's lower jaw and lifting with both hands, one on each side, displacing the mandible forward while tilting the head backward. The rescuer's elbows should rest on the surface on which the victim is lying."[1] (See Fig. 4-11.)

If the jaw thrust is not adequate the head tilt-jaw lift should be substituted. Care must be exercised not to overextend the neck. "The fingers of one hand are placed under the lower jaw on the bony part near the chin and lifted to bring the chin forward, supporting the jaw and helping to tilt the head back. The fingers must not compress the soft tissue under the chin, which might obstruct the airway. The other hand presses on the victim's forehead to tilt the head back."[1] (See Fig. 4-12.)

The transportation team should be familiar with handling a victim with a cervical spine injury. They should be receptive to taking orders from the "leader." It is extremely important not to lose control of the care of the athlete; therefore, be familiar with the transportation crew that is used. In an athletic situation, prior arrangements with an ambulance service should be made.

Lifting and carrying the athlete requires five individuals: four to lift, and the leader to maintain immobilization of the head. The leader initiates all actions with clear, loud verbal commands (Fig. 4-13*A*, *B*).

The same guidelines apply to the choice of a medical facility as to the choice of an ambulance: be sure it is equipped and staffed to handle an emergency head or neck injury. There should be a neurosurgeon and an orthopedic surgeon to meet the athlete upon arrival. Roentgenographic facilities should be standing by.

Once the athlete is in a medical facility and permanent immobilization measures are instituted, the helmet is removed. The chinstrap may now be unfastened and discarded. The athlete's head is supported at the occiput by one person while the leader spreads the earflaps and pulls the helmet off in a straight line with the spine (Figs. 4-14 and 4-15).

REFERENCES

1. A Manual for Instructors of Basic Cardiac Life Support. Dallas, Am. Heart Assoc., 1977.
2. Clancy, W.G., Brand, R.L., and Bergfeld, J.A.: Upper trunk brachial plexus injuries in contact sports. Am. J. Sports Med., 5:209, 1977.
3. Ommaya, A.K., and Gennarelli, T.A.: Cerebral concussion and traumatic unconsciousness. Correlation of experimental and clinical observations on blunt head injuries. Brain, 97:638, 1974.
4. Schneider, R.C.: Head and Neck Injuries in Football. Mechanisms, Treatment, and Prevention. Baltimore, Williams & Wilkins, 1972.
5. Schneider, R.C., and Kriss, F.C.: Decisions concerning cerebral concussions in football players. Med. Sci. Sports, 1:115, 1969.
6. Torg, J.S., Quedenfeld, T.C., and Newell, W.: When the athlete's life is threatened. Phys. and Sportsmed., 3:54, 1975.

Chapter 5

Anatomy of the Brain and Its Coverings

Robert J. Johnson

THE SCALP

The scalp is the first tissue that receives the trauma of blows or impacts to the head. It may be described as consisting of five layers. The first is the skin, which consists of epidermis and corium. We may include the hair, which under certain circumstances may have some protective value. Second, we have the superficial fascia, or subcutaneous layer, which consists of dense fatty areolar tissue tightly bound to both the skin above and to the next layer below it (galea aponeurotica). Because the subcutaneous layer is well vascularized, blows are prone to rupture its small vessels and lead to sharply localized hemorrhages trapped within this layer (Fig. 5-1).

The third layer is a muscular one consisting of the epicranius muscle with its two bellies at the front and two at the rear of the scalp, and the expansive galea aponeurotica between them. The galea is, in reality, a flat intermediate tendon between the bellies of this anteroposteriorly oriented digastric muscle. The right and left occipitalis muscles originate from the superior nuchal lines of the skull, and the right and left frontalis muscles insert anteriorly into the skin at the two eyebrows. Because the fibrofatty subcutaneous layer is densely bound to the galea, blood or

fluid within the former cannot disperse readily from its site of origin.

The fourth layer is loose areolar tissue which intervenes everywhere between the galea aponeurotica (or the epicranius) and the underlying periosteum of the skull. This loose aerolar layer permits the scalp to move freely upon the skull and also allows blood or pus to spread easily within its substance. These may pass forward and into the tissues of the upper eyelid and deep to the orbicularis oculi. Scalping injuries involve the separation of the scalp from the skull along this weak connective tissue plane. Last, the fifth layer of the scalp is the pericranium or periosteum of the skull bones.

THE CRANIUM

The primary duty of the cranial portion of the skull is to support and protect the brain. To this end the cranium and the contained dural folds are configured so as to offer internal compartments that provide several weight-supporting surfaces. These private loges for the several parts of the brain can prevent it from becoming displaced, and the tendency to roll and rotate that it would otherwise suffer if the brain were contained inside a single sphere.

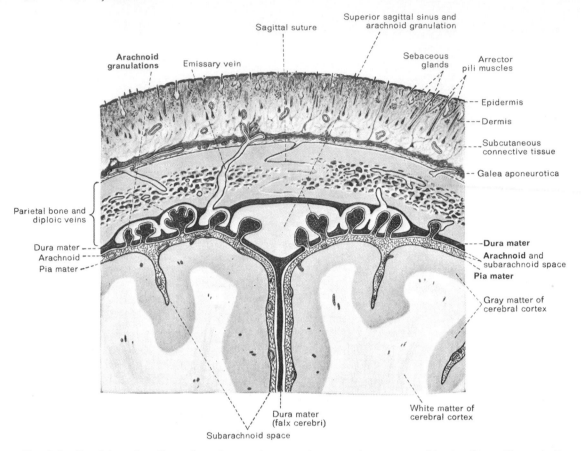

Fig. 5-1. Frontal section through scalp, cranium, meninges, and upperpart of brain. (From Clemente.[4])

The cranium is somewhat spheroidal, and this allows it—like a true sphere—to provide maximum protection against the indentations produced by external impacts with the minimum of structural mass or substance; however, because of variations in the shapes of skulls, some are more spheroidal than others. The short brachycephalic skull more closely approximates a sphere, while the elongated dolichocephalic skull is not as spherical. If a brachycephalic skull is compressed from any direction, its volume decreases, thereby compressing the brain inside. However, if a dolichocephalic skull is compressed along its anteroposterior axis, its internal volume increases slightly.[3] Thus, the shape of the cranium, as well as the thickness of the cranial bones, modify the effects of blows.

Because of the foramen magnum and the tentorial incisure, any compressive force applied to the brain has a component of elongation distortion downward through these two apertures. Thus, longitudinal tensions may be set up within the diencephalon and the brain stem.

At certain sites, the bones of the cranial vault are reinforced to receive the forces delivered upward from the facial skeleton via the heavier buttresses of bone present. Thus, the forces of mastication, as well as the forces of blows to the face, are ultimately transferred to the cranium via the facial buttresses of bone that are prolonged into the cranium. These strengthened lines of bone in the cranium modify or determine lines of stress, and therefore, lines of fracture.

Foramina or other apertures of the skull

may modify fracture lines, because they offer zones of weakness. However, some of the margins of these apertures may be so thickened that they actually become zones of strength. Fractures that pass through foramina may involve the contents of those foramina. Nerves and vessels in foramina may tear, and the hemorrhage, in turn, may damage the nerves piercing the foramen.

THE CRANIAL CAVITY

The floor of the cranial cavity is arranged in three fossae: anterior, middle, and posterior. The floors of these fossae resemble three steps, each with tread and riser, which descend from anterior to posterior. The lateral floor of the anterior cranial fossa is the orbital plate of the frontal bone, which also serves as the roof of the orbital cavity. Frequently this plate of bone is pneumatized by the horizontal extension of the frontal sinus. In the event a fracture occurs here the risk of meningitis is increased. More medially, the floor is formed by the cribriform plate of the ethmoid, which may communicate with the nasal cavity in case of fracture. The orbital surfaces of the frontal lobes of the brain rest upon the floor of the anterior cranial fossa.

The middle cranial fossa is divided into right and left depressions by the higher-standing body of the sphenoid bone, which is indented by the fossa hypophyseos for the pituitary gland. Thus, the middle cranial fossa is shaped somewhat like a butterfly with wings spread. The fossa for the hypophysis represents the body of the butterfly, and the lateral parts of the fossa, upon which the temporal lobes of the brain rest, are positioned like the spread wings. The riser between the right and left wings of this fossa and the anterior fossa is that part of the orbital plate of the great wing of the sphenoid that separates the middle fossa from the orbital cavity. On its other side, this orbital plate serves as the posterior half of the lateral wall of the orbit. Because this orbital plate fails to meet the lesser wing of the sphenoid, a space between them (the superior orbital fissure) permits communication between the middle cranial fossa and the orbital cavity.

The posterior cranial fossa supports the cerebellum and houses the pons and medulla in its anterior median region. Its floor is formed by the occipital bone, with the foramen magnum in its center anteriorly. The riser between it and the middle fossa is formed laterally by the posterior (or cerebellar) surfaces of the petrous portions of the right and left temporal bones. In the median area, the riser or anterior wall of this fossa is formed by the basilar portion of the occipital bone and the posterior surface of the body of the sphenoid bone, including the dorsum sellae.

The posterior cranial fossa is roofed in by the tentorium cerebelli (Figs. 5-2 and 5-3). Since the tentorium has a U-shaped central defect anteriorly (the tentorial incisure), the mesencephalon or upper part of the brain stem ascends through this defect or space, and is continuous with the right and left diencephalons of their respective cerebral hemispheres. As it passes through the tentorial incisure, the mesencephalon has about 1 to 4 mm of free space between it and the edge of the tentorium cerebelli on either side. This limited tolerance should be remembered, because lateral shifts of the brain stem due to supratentorial hematoma or other expanding lesions force the cerebral peduncle of the opposite side to impinge against the firm, unyielding edge of the tentorium. This produces a "Kernohan's notch or groove" in the peduncle, with consequent hemiplegia, which is contralateral to the notch. Thus, hemiplegia develops on the same side as the original lesion (the hematoma). If supratentorial pressure increases, the uncus of the parahippocampal gyrus may herniate downward through this same available space between the cerebral peduncle and the margin of the tentorium cerebelli. The

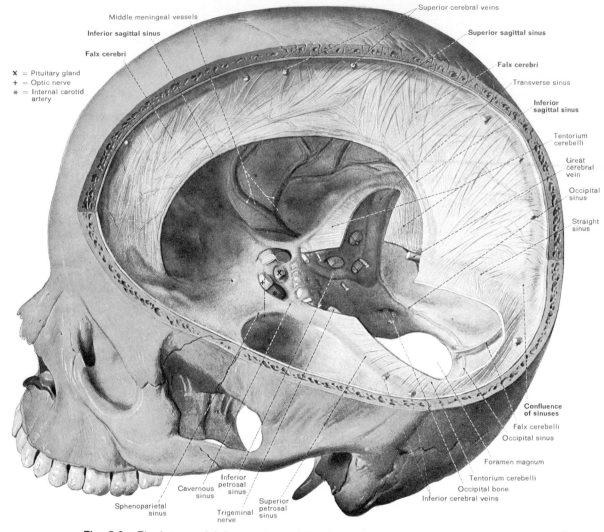

Middle meningeal vessels

Inferior sagittal sinus

Falx cerebri

X = Pituitary gland
+ = Optic nerve
* = Internal carotid
      artery

Superior cerebral veins

Superior sagittal sinus

Falx cerebri

Transverse sinus

Inferior
sagittal sinus

Tentorium
cerebelli

Great
cerebral
vein

Occipital
sinus

Straight
sinus

Confluence
of sinuses

Falx cerebelli

Occipital sinus

Foramen magnum

Tentorium cerebelli

Occipital bone

Inferior cerebral veins

Inferior
petrosal
sinus

Cavernous
sinus

Superior
petrosal
sinus

Sphenoparietal
sinus

Trigeminal
nerve

Fig. 5-2.   The intracranial dura mater and the dural venous sinuses. (From Clemente.[4])

herniating uncus may produce a force that causes a lateral shift of the mesencephalon with a Kernohan's groove as a possible result.

The downward-herniating uncus can also impinge upon the oculomotor nerve below it, and damage it by stretching or compressing it against the dural fold known as the clivus ridge. When the mesencephalon shifts laterally, the oculomotor nerves may be damaged by yet another mechanism. Since the oculomotor nerves not only descend at a 45° angle, but also diverge at a 45° angle, it is apparent

that a shift to one side or the other soon stretches the nerves on the side opposite to the direction of mesencephalon displacement.

Another possible mode of damage to the oculomotor nerve occurs with descent of the brain stem. Such descent carries the basilar artery downward along with its terminal branches, the posterior cerebral arteries. The posterior cerebral artery on either side lies directly above the oculomotor nerve and crosses it at approximately a right angle. Descent of the posterior cerebral artery may drag downward on

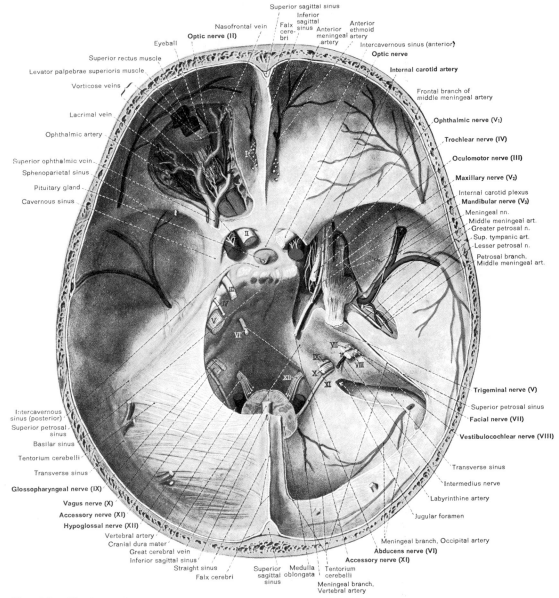

Fig. 5-3. The base of the cranial cavity showing dura mater and vessels and nerves. (From Clemente.[4])

the oculomotor nerve, and either stretch it or compress it against the clivus ridge (Fig. 5-3). The adjacent trochlear nerve escapes comparable injuries because it is shielded by its position laterally under the protection of the free edge of the tentorium cerebelli. Any downward displacement of the brain stem immediately stretches the abducens nerve causing a lateral rectus muscle paresis.

THE MENINGES

The cranial cavity is lined everywhere with the dura mater. The dura consists of two layers. Where the dura is apposed to the skull, the two layers are the meningeal and the periosteal (or endosteal) layers. The latter lies directly against the bone. Although their fibers run in different directions in any given area, and thus maintain some individual identity, the two layers cannot be separated by dissection. However, at the sites of the superior sagittal sinus and the lateral dural venous sinuses, these two layers are fully separated by the presence of these sinuses. The endothelial walls of the sinuses fit against the separated surfaces of the two dural layers. It thus appears that the dural venous sinuses run within the dura mater. There are three major sites where the meningeal layer alone is drawn inward as a double-layered fold, thereby creating the falx cerebri, the tentorium cerebelli, and the inconspicuous falx cerebelli.

In the midsagittal plane of the cranial cavity, the meningeal layer is drawn downward in a double-layered fold, in the lower-free margin of which is the inferior sagittal sinus (Fig. 5-2). This median sagittal fold is the falx cerebri, and it stands as a firm plate between the cerebral hemispheres. Its lower border falls short of reaching the corpus callosum, a massive commissural bundle, which links the two hemispheres. In unilateral expanding masses a portion of the hemisphere on the involved side may be forced under the lower margin of the falx cerebri to herniate toward the opposite side with consequent local damage to brain tissue.

The tentorium cerebelli is a fold of dura that forms a roof over the posterior cranial fossa below, and at the same time serves as the floor for supporting the posterior part of the supratentorial brain. It is chiefly the occipital lobes of the brain, which rest upon the upper aspect of the tentorium cerebelli, and which are thus separated from the cerebellum. The tentorium cerebelli is not horizontal, but peaks upward centrally to somewhat resemble a conical tent. And, like an Indian teepee, it has an anterior opening through which the mesencephalon ascends. This opening, the tentorial notch or incisure, has already been discussed. The tentorium cerebelli has, therefore, an attached margin, like the base of the tent, and a free margin which

forms the edges of the tentorial incisure (Fig. 5-3). The attached margin is anchored to the cranium along a nearly horizontal curved line where it houses the right and left lateral dural venous sinuses. This attached margin extends forward and medially on either side along the petrosal crest and finally bridges the short gap between the apex of the petrosa and the posterior clinoid process. These last few millimeters of the attached margin create the clivus ridge, mentioned previously in connection with compression of the oculomotor nerve.

In the midline, the extensive falx cerebri separates the two cerebral hemispheres, while posteriorly the tentorium cerebelli separates the cerebellum from the inferior aspect of the occipital lobes and serves as a support for the latter. The smaller falx cerebelli projects along the midline in the floor and posterior part of the posterior cranial fossa. It forms a small partition separating the right and left posteriormost portions (arciform lobes) of the cerebellum. These three dural folds thus extend into the interior of the cranial cavity like baffle plates and create separate loges for the several parts of the brain. As previously mentioned, these separate compartments have a protective value since they prevent a tendency for the brain to roll and rotate (or twist) with the various motions of the head.

The dural folds also house the dural venous sinuses, which receive all of the venous drainage from the brain. The superior sagittal sinus, running in the attached margin, and the inferior sagittal sinus, in the lower-free margin of the falx cerebri, both receive superficial cerebral veins from the hemispheres. The lateral dural venous sinuses (right and left) run in the attached margin of the tentorium cerebelli and receive the veins draining the cerebellum below, as well as superficial cerebral veins from the occipital lobes. All of these veins coming from brain tissue must pass through the subarachnoid space, pierce the arachnoid, and enter the dural sinuses. As they pass from the arachnoid to the dura they cross the potential subdural space. If displacements of the brain stretch these bridging veins and the veins tear while in this interval, they bleed into the subdural space. Several bridging veins leave the sylvian fissure (superficial middle cerebral veins) to pass to the small sphenoparietal venous sinus that runs along the posterior free border of the lesser wing of the sphenoid bone. Posterior displacements of the brain put these bridging veins in jeopardy, and may cause subdural hematoma.

THE MENINGEAL ARTERIES

On the external surface of the dura, and intimately and firmly attached to it, are a number of so-called meningeal arteries with their accompanying venae comitantes. These vessels lie between dura and bone and branch to both the dura subjacent to them and to the overlying bone. As stated, they are firmly attached to the dura when the dura is stripped away from the bone. What is not usually obvious is that their many small osseous branches, which supply the overlying bone, are broken by such dural stripping, even though the main trunk of the artery remains intact. By far the greater part of the blood flowing in these meningeal vessels is actually destined for the overlying bone of the skull. Not only does bone itself have a higher metabolic demand than dura, but the diploë between the inner and outer tables of cranial bone is filled throughout life with hematopoietic tissue for the production of red blood cells.

Breaking the osseous branches of the meningeal arteries is the primary source of bleeding in epidural or extradural hematomata. Note that this bleeding occurs at arterial pressure. Obviously the venae comitantes, as well as the occasionally torn dural venous sinus, can also be sources of bleeding. The mere stripping of dura from the overlying bone, which has been indented by impact and has snapped back to a normal configuration without fracturing, is sufficient to rupture the osseous branches. At certain places the main trunks of the meningeal arteries may lie in bony canals, or be so deeply embedded in bone that they are likely to be torn in any fracture that occurs here. However, this is clearly not the only mechanism that causes bleeding.

The middle meningeal artery, which runs across the floor of the middle cranial fossa and spreads its branches widely up the side of the skull, is by far the largest of the meningeal arteries. Smaller meningeal arteries, derived from the ophthalmic artery, supply the dura and bone of the floor and walls of the anterior cranial fossa. Several equally small meningeal arteries, derived from the external carotid system, supply the dura and bone of the floor and walls of the posterior cranial fossa. Thus, epidural hematomata are more common in the middle cranial fossa and over the dorsolateral aspect of the brain, but they can also occur in the anterior and posterior cranial fossae.

The leptomeninges consist of the arachnoid and the pia mater. Between these two membranes lies the subarachnoid space, which is filled with about 150 ml of cerebrospinal fluid. The arachnoid is applied to the inner aspect of the dura but does not adhere to it except at certain sites, such as at arachnoid granulations and the places where veins pierce it to enter the dural venous sinuses. The pia mater is a thin layer of connective tissue intimately adherent to the surface of the brain and spinal cord. It must be penetrated by all the branches of the cerebral arteries and veins that enter the neural substance. A forest of trabeculae, composed of arachnoidal cells, extends from the inner aspect of the arachnoid membrane across the subarachnoid space to spread upon and fuse with the pia mater. Thus, the subarachnoid space is actually an extensive cleft in the meshwork of arachnoid cells. Arteries and veins on the surface of the brain, if ruptured or torn, bleed into the subarachnoid space.

ARTERIES OF THE BRAIN

The blood supply of the brain is derived from four arteries, the right and left internal carotid arteries, and the right and left vertebral arteries (Fig. 5-4). Each of these can be damaged by cervical, as well as intracranial trauma. Such trauma may result in laceration, contusion with thrombosis, and vasospasm.

In the neck, the internal carotid artery together with the internal jugular vein and vagus nerve, is embedded in the carotid sheath. This artery enters the carotid canal in the petrous part of the temporal bone and makes its way into the cranial cavity via the upper aspect of the foramen lacerum. It is immediately contained within the cavernous sinus on the lateral aspect of the body of the sphenoid. In the event of fractures here, small branches of the internal carotid may establish arteriovenous aneurysmal connections with the venous network within the cavernous sinus. Passing through the roof of the cavernous sinus, each internal carotid establishes communications with the other and with the right and left posterior cerebral arteries, which are derived from the vertebrobasilar system. Thus, the circle of Willis forms in which the four arteries that supply the brain communicate with one another by means of anastomoses. However, this anastomotic system varies in effectiveness or completeness from one person to another.

The three cerebral arteries are the anterior, middle, and posterior. The anterior and middle cerebral arteries are derived from the internal carotid artery, while the posterior cerebral artery is derived from the vertebrobasilar system. However, occasionally one or the other posterior cerebral artery arises, as they do in the embryo, from the internal carotid artery.

The right and left vertebral arteries ascend in the neck through the foramina transversaria of the cervical vertebrae (Fig. 5-4). Typically, each artery skips the foramen of the seventh cervical vertebra and enters that of the sixth. Thereafter, it passes successively through each of the foramina to finally exit from the transverse foramen of the first cervical vertebra or atlas. The artery then turns sharply posteriorly to pass around the lateral and posterior aspects of the lateral mass of the atlas. Next it crosses the posterior arch of the atlas, pierces the atlanto-occipital membrane, and enters the neural or vertebral canal. It then penetrates the dura and the arachnoid, ascends in the subarachnoid space through the foramen magnum, and enters the posterior cranial fossa. The right and left vertebral arteries now incline toward one another as they ascend in front of the medulla. They meet and fuse to form the basilar artery at the level of the junction of the pons and medulla (inferior pontine sulcus). The basilar artery continues to ascend within the subarachnoid space, remaining in the midline between the pons and the clivus. At the junction of the pons and the mesencephalon (superior pontine sulcus), the basilar artery divides into the right and left posterior cerebral arteries. These leave the posterior cranial fossa by passing onto the superior aspect of the tentorium, and thereafter supply the right and left occipital lobes (Fig. 5-4).

Several sites of the vertebrobasilar system are in particular jeopardy from athletic trauma. As the vertebral artery ascends through the foramina transversaria, it may be damaged by fractures or dislocations. Osteophytic protrusions at the uncovertebral joints, a late sequel of degenerative disc disease and past trauma, may compress the vertebral artery and lead to vertebrobasilar insufficiency. Because of stiffening of the arterial wall and a reduction in the caliber of the lumen, there is increased likelihood of even minor cervical spine trauma causing critical vascular impairment in the older individual with atherosclerotic changes in the vertebral

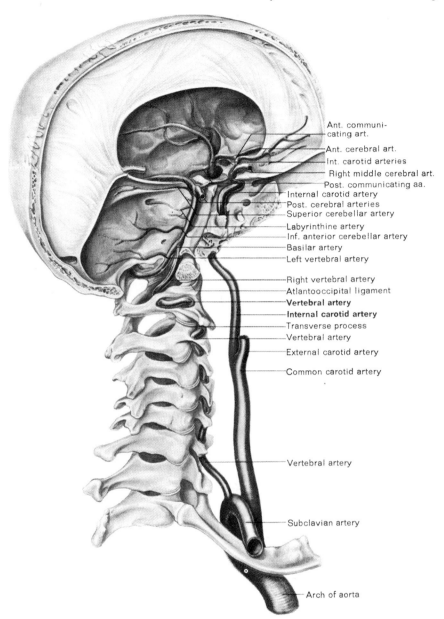

Ant. communi-
cating art.

Ant. cerebral art.

Int. carotid arteries

Right middle cerebral art.

Post. communicating aa.

Internal carotid artery

Post. cerebral arteries

Superior cerebellar artery

Labyrinthine artery

Inf. anterior cerebellar artery

Basilar artery

Left vertebral artery

Right vertebral artery

Atlantooccipital ligament

Vertebral artery

Internal carotid artery

Transverse process

Vertebral artery

External carotid artery

Common carotid artery

Vertebral artery

Subclavian artery

Arch of aorta

Fig. 5-4. The vertebral and internal carotid arteries shown in the neck and in the cranial cavity. In this specimen ossification in the atlanto-occipital membrane immediately adjacent to the aperture for the vertebral artery has created the posticulus posterior. This, with the posterior arch of the atlas, creates a bony foramen for the vertebral artery, which is a variation occasionally found. (From Clemente.[4])

artery. This is particularly true at the atlanto-axial joint level. Turning the head to one side or the other while looking upward may stretch and angulate the artery so much that these motions result in abrupt reductions of arterial flow to the brain stem and occipital lobes (transient ischemic at-

tacks). As the right and left vertebral arteries cross the posterior arch of the first cervical vertebra and pierce the atlanto-occipital membrane, they may be subject to hazardous compression between the arch of the atlas and the occipital bone, in severe and forcible hyperextension of the head and cervical spine.[2] Such traumatic compression may be more than a mere momentary occlusion, for it may cause intimal contusion, laceration, and thrombosis with consequent prolonged occlusion. Arterial wall trauma may also precipitate vasospasm in the arterial distribution beyond the site of trauma. At a higher level, the basilar artery may be involved in fractures through the clivus.

During their ascent in relation to the brain stem, the vertebral and basilar arteries give off a series of innumerable branches to the medulla, the pons, and the mesencephalon. These branches penetrate the brain stem as paramedian and short and long circumferential branches. In general, all such branches pass into and irrigate brain stem tissue in the horizontal plane. Since the brain stem is essentially vertical when the head is erect, we can compare the penetrating branches to the teeth of a comb when the comb is held vertically. Not to be forgotten is the origin of the uppermost part of the anterior spinal artery, which supplies central branches to the cervical cord as well as to the medulla. This anterior spinal artery originates by the fusion of two short trunks from the right and the left vertebral arteries. Therefore, the upper cervical cord may also be endangered in trauma to the vertebral arteries.

A series of branches arise from the proximal parts of the anterior, middle, and posterior cerebral arteries and penetrate into the basal surface of the brain to supply the basal ganglia (basal or ganglionic arteries)

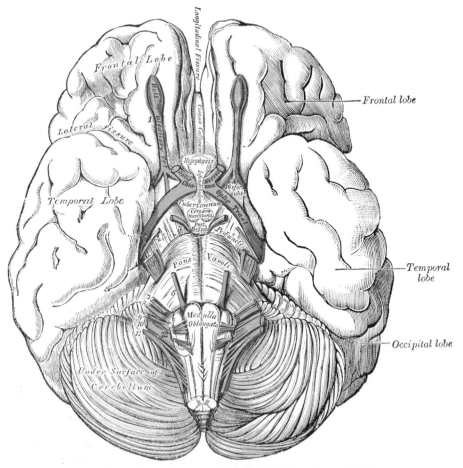

Fig. 5-5.   Inferior surface of the brain. (From Goss.[5])

and the thalamus (thalamogeniculate arteries). Lateral shifts of the cerebral tissue due to hematomata may angulate these small, but often long, basal arteries and thus impede their blood flow. Cerebral contusions and lacerations may damage the branches of the three great cerebral arteries (anterior, middle, and posterior), which spread over the surface of the hemispheres. Their many penetrating branches irrigate the cortex and the subjacent white matter, and extend to the walls of the ventricular cavities.

THE BRAIN

The cerebral hemispheres (Figs. 5-5 and 5-6) reside within the right and left sides of the supratentorial portion of the cranial cavity. The hemispheres are partially separated from each other in the midline by the falx cerebri. On the other hand, they are connected to each other by the tethering band of commissural fibers known as the corpus callosum. Displacement of the hemispheres may contuse the medial surface of the hemispheres (particularly at the cingulate gyrus) against the resistant falx cerebri. This displacement may produce internal stress and strain within the corpus callosum and cause focal lesions of some length anteroposteriorly.

Although the cerebrum is protected and buffered everywhere by cerebrospinal fluid within the subarachnoid space, this space allows a certain amount of cerebral displacement before impact against the cranial wall or the dural folds. This displacement, plus further deformity from indentation of the skull or from inertial loading of the brain, can lead to contusions against not only the dural folds (falx cerebelli and tentorium cerebelli), but also the basal and polar areas of bony contact.

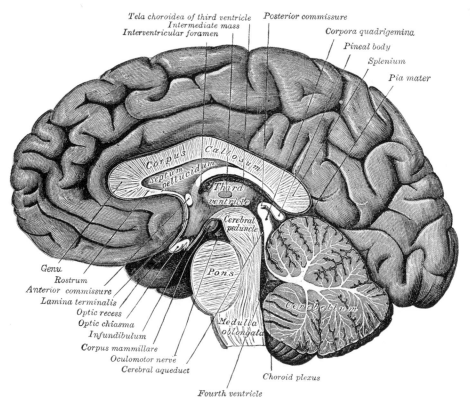

Fig. 5-6. Medial surface of the brain demonstrating the major divisions visible in the sagittal section. (From Goss.[5])

Thus, contusions are prone to develop at the frontal pole of the brain; in the adjacent surfaces of the frontal and temporal lobes, from impingement against the sphenoidal ridges (free margins of the lesser wings of the sphenoid bone); on the orbital surface of the frontal lobe; and on the inferolateral surface of the occipital lobes. The uncus of the parahippocampal gyrus may be contused against the margin of the tentorium, as well as herniated downward through the tentorial incisure by forces of long duration, such as cerebral swelling and intracerebral hematoma. The inferior surface of the cerebellum may be contused against the floor of the posterior cranial fossa. As previously mentioned, the cerebral peduncles may impinge against the free margins of the tentorium cerebelli during lateral displacements. Since the brain stem may also be displaced downward and even undergo slight torsion, it is apparent that it can be subjected to internal stresses as well as those which may occur in the cerebral hemispheres. Such internal stress may produce minute and diffuse neuronal and microglial damage, as well as vascular damage at the capillary level.

Internal shear stress, as well as cortical and surface vascular damage, may lead to degeneration and atrophy of long-fiber tracts in the cerebrum and in the brain stem. Thus, there may be diffuse atrophy of cerebral white matter, which leads to enlargement of the various parts of the ventricular system that it surrounds. Areas of long-tract degeneration likely seen in the brain stem include the brachium conjunctivum (the major outflow tract from the cerebellum), the corticospinal tracts, the medial lemnisci, and the central tegmental fasciculus (a multipurpose bundle best seen in the tegmentum of the pons).[1] Loss of cells in the hippocampus (Ammon's horn) and the presubiculum, as well as reduction of Purkinje cells in the inferior part of the cerebellum have been noted, particularly in boxers.

REFERENCES

1. Adams, J.H.: The neuropathology of head injuries. *In* Handbook of Clinical Neurology. Vol. 23, Part 1. Edited by P.J. Vinken, and G.W. Bruyn. New York, American Elsevier, 1975.
2. Schneider, R.C., et al.: Vascular insufficiency and differential distortion of brain and cord caused by cervicomedullary football injuries. J. Neurosurg., 33:363, 1970.
3. Unterharnscheidt, F., and Sellier, K.: Mechanics and pathomorphology of closed brain injuries. *In* Head Injury. Edited by W.F. Caveness, and A.E. Walker. Philadelphia, J.B. Lippincott, 1966.
4. Clemente, C.C.: Anatomy, A Regional Atlas of the Human Body. ed. 1. Munich, Urban and Schwarzenberg, 1975.
5. Goss, C.M. (ed.): Gray's Anatomy of the Human Body. 29th American ed. Philadelphia, Lea & Febiger, 1973.

Chapter 6

Head Injury Mechanisms

Thomas A. Gennarelli

To determine how a particular mechanical input to the head results in a particular outcome requires an analysis of multiple factors. First the nature, the severity, and the site and direction of the input to the head are important. The primary mechanical damage, which that input causes, may then affect either the scalp, the skull, or the brain. Finally, the overall result of mechanical input produces a complex interaction of pathophysiologic events which results in temporary or permanent neurologic disability.

In general terms, head injuries include three distinct varieties. *Skull fracture* can occur with or without damage to the brain, but is not itself an important cause of neurologic death or disability. Instead, injuries to the neural substance of the brain cause neurologic dysfunction and can readily be divided into two categories. *Focal injuries*, which cause local damage and comprise such entities as cortical contusion, subdural hematoma, epidural hematoma, and intracerebral hematoma, account for approximately 50% of all hospital admissions for head injury and are responsible for two thirds of head-injury deaths. *Diffuse injuries*, which are not associated with localized damage, but rather with widespread disruption of either the structure or the function of the brain ac-

count for approximately 40% of head-injured patients admitted to the hospital. Although they are responsible for only one fourth of the deaths, diffuse injuries are the most serious cause of persisting neurologic disability in the survivors.

BIOMECHANICAL MECHANISMS OF INJURY

The types of mechanical input to the head are numerous and complex. Figure 6-1 provides a flow-chart analysis of known and proposed mechanisms of injury. Mechanical input to the head can either be slow (static loading), or as more commonly occurs, rapid (dynamic loading). Static loading of the head implies that forces are applied gradually, usually over 200 to 500 msec or longer. This is comparable to a slow squeezing effect on the skull and results in serious skull fracture. Only after multiple comminuted skull fractures is consciousness lost and the brain itself injured. Static loading is not common, particularly in sports injuries. The more common dynamic loading occurs over periods of less than 200 msec and usually involves two components. *Impact* to the head is the most common event of dynamic loading, but impulsive loading of the head can also occur. *Impulsive loading* occurs

65

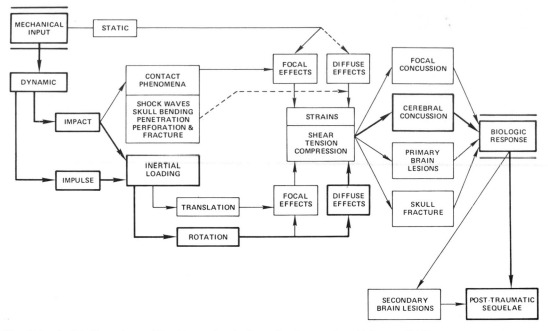

Fig. 6-1. In this flow-chart of the biomechanical mechanisms of head injury, solid lines represent the most important mechanism while dashed lines depict less important or unproved mechanisms.

when the head is not directly struck but is set into motion and is either accelerated or decelerated. Such loading results from impact to the thorax on which the head is freely movable. Impact produces the most frequent mechanical input to the head and usually causes acceleration of the head (inertial loading), as well as many regionalized effects known as contact phenomena. The contact phenomena are a complex group of mechanical phenomena that occur both locally and distant from the point of impact. The magnitude and importance of these contact phenomena vary with the size of the impacting device and with the magnitude of force of the impact. Immediately beneath the point of impact there is localized skull deformation with in-bending of the skull surrounded by a periphery of out-bending. If the degree of local skull deformation is significant, penetration of the skull, perforation, or fracture occur. Additionally, shock waves that travel with the speed of sound propagate throughout the skull from the point of impact, as well as directly through the

brain substance. The role of shock waves in causing local changes in brain tissue pressure and consequently brain injury has been a matter of debate. However, because of the extremely rapid transmission of these waves through the brain, shock waves are probably not the most important injury mechanism for the brain.

CONTACT PHENOMENA AND SKULL FRACTURE

Local contact phenomena, which result from impact, are the most important mechanisms of skull fracture. The occurrence of skull fracture depends upon the material properties of the skull, the magnitude and direction of impact, the size of the impact area, and the thickness of the skull in various areas. The material properties of the skull are similar to those of other bony structures in the body. In general, mechanical failure of the skull occurs in tensile stress more readily than in compression. Thus, when a patient falls and strikes his head on an object, or when an object strikes the patient's head at the point of in-bending, the inner table of the skull is subjected to tensile strain, whereas the outer table is compressed. If the impact is of sufficient magnitude, and the skull is sufficiently thin at the point of impact, a skull fracture begins in the area of tensile loading on the inner table of the skull. Alternately, if the region of impact is over a thick portion of the skull, local in-bending has no effect. However, the skull bends out around the impact zone, putting the outer table under tension and the inner table under compression. If this area of out-bending is in a thin area of the skull, a fracture may occur at some distance from the point of impact in the outer table. A skull fracture is propagated from its origin along lines of least resistance; therefore, it is not surprising that not all skull fractures occur immediately beneath the impact area.

The common locations of skull fractures reflect to some degree the direction of impact forces. Low-frontal impacts, those on the forehead or supraorbital area, propagate fractures up the vault along the frontal bone as well as down along the base of the skull into the anterior cranial fossa. Most of the fracture line may develop along the thin cribriform plate at the base of the skull or along the orbital roofs, rather than on the surface of the skull. If the impact point is higher in the frontal area, vault fractures are more common than basilar fractures. A frontolateral impact propagates a fracture line through the thin inferolateral aspect of the skull, rather than over the thicker frontal bone. Thus, fractures occur in the squamous portion of the temporal bone and orbital roofs. High-lateral impacts, above and behind the ear, similarly tend to propagate fractures at a distance from the impact, again because of the thinness of the inferior portion of the temporal bone. These fractures propagate along the floor of the middle cranial fossa and upward toward the site of impact. Posterior impacts involving the occipital or posterior parietal areas cause fracture lines that travel downward through the occipital bone toward the foramen magnum.

Skull fractures can be viewed in the same light as fractures elsewhere in the body. Healing is anticipated within several weeks after fracture, and therefore the fracture itself is of no clinical importance. The exceptions to this rule include fractures of the skull base, fractures that cross meningeal vessels, and fractures that are compound or open.

Depressed skull fractures may be clinically important if they result in brain contusion, laceration, or compression. These fractures result from impacts from a small-diameter object that perforates the skull. Because the skull fails in tension sooner than in compression, fracturing of the inner table is always more serious than that of the outer table. In-driven bone fragments can then perforate or lacerate the dura or brain and cause local brain damage. This cortical injury is associated with a serious risk of infection and seizures. Thus, while linear skull fractures, with the exceptions noted above, are usually of limited clinical significance depressed skull fractures can cause long-standing neurologic problems.

INERTIAL (ACCELERATION) EFFECTS

Inertial loading of the head, whether caused by impact or by impulsive loading, accelerates or decelerates the head. From the mechanical point of view, acceleration and deceleration are the same physical input and differ only in direction. Acceleration of the head may be translational (movement in a straight line, Fig. 6-2*A*) or angular (rotational head and neck movement, Fig. 6-2*B*).

A controversy, which will not be entered here, exists regarding which of these two types of inertial loading is *the* cause of brain injury. This has been compounded by considering brain injury as a unitary

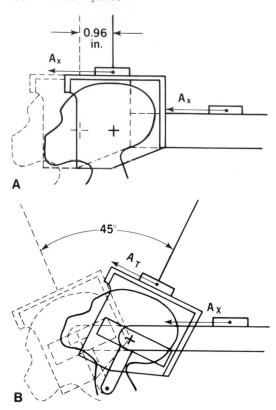

Fig. 6-2. Types of inertial loading of the head. Acceleration can be either translational (*A*) in which the center of gravity (+) moves in a straight line, or angular (*B*) in which the center of gravity travels in an arc. Pure acceleration loads are delivered to experimental animals by placing their heads within helmets so that no impact occurs during head movement.[2]

concept and little attention has been focused on the mechanisms which cause the individual varieties of brain injury (see Chaps. 7 and 8). As shown in Figure 6-1, the common denomination of injury is the type, magnitude, and distribution of *strain* that occurs in the brain. Strain of differing type and in differing proportions is generated by either acceleration mode and depending on whether acceleration maximizes pressure gradients,[5] cavitation,[4] or shearing,[8] various theories can be championed to support both translational and angular acceleration as injurious. Detailed reviews of these theories are available for the interested reader.[3, 6, 7, 10]

In fact, both types of acceleration are in-

jurious, but there is mounting evidence that the effects of translational and angular acceleration on the brain differ markedly. This was tested directly by me in a series of experimental head injuries in primates. In these tests, the effects of impact were eliminated by encasing the head in a special helmet, which diffused loading over the entire skull. Two groups of animals were then subjected to pure acceleration loads. The first group was subjected to pure translational acceleration in a posteroanterior direction with the axis of acceleration along the sagittal plane (Fig. 6-2*A*). The second group of animals was subjected to angular acceleration by rotating the head and neck through a 45 to 60° arc with the center of rotation in the cervical spine (Fig. 6-2*B*).

The physiologic and pathologic results in these two groups differed markedly. At the maximum accelerations it was impossible to induce a cerebral concussion in monkeys undergoing translational acceleration, yet it was easy to induce concussion from rotational acceleration. It is therefore evident that the type of acceleration delivered to the head had a profound influence on the type of resulting neurologic dysfunction. Furthermore, it was apparent from these experiments that *focal structural lesions commonly resulted from translational acceleration, and diffuse injuries of the brain primarily from rotational acceleration.*

The initial experiments were followed by a series of 100 primate head injuries produced by a nonimpact angular acceleration mechanism.[1] In this series, the animal's head was placed within a helmet so that the input forces were diffused over the head to avoid contact forces associated with impact. As angular acceleration increased, changes in heart rate and blood pressure occurred before consciousness was lost. Brief periods of apnea followed by respiratory irregularities occurred if angular acceleration increased further. Only at substantial acceleration levels did concussion develop. Thus, a continuum of events was defined and was related to the level of acceleration input into the head.

It is evident from these experiments that considerable physiologic dysfunction can occur with subconcussive injuries, and that impact is not necessary for cerebral concussion. Furthermore, at high levels of acceleration the subdural bridging veins were torn and large acute subdural hematomas caused death. In fact, detailed neuropathologic examination of the animal brains disclosed virtually every type of head injury that occurs in humans.

Therefore, many of the physiologic and pathologic consequences of head injury can be produced by a single injury mechanism, i.e., acceleration. This is an important concept because of the frequent occurrence of subdural hematoma in sports (particularly in football and boxing). It must be understood that the mechanism of hematoma production is not related to the contact forces of impact, but rather results from acceleration of the head. This must be taken into account in designing safety equipment for sports. In a contact sports environment, it is almost impossible to protect against the effects of head acceleration, but protective headgear can decrease the local effects of impact. Thus, sports helmets could be expected to decrease skull fracture, but not to substantially influence the production of acceleration-related injuries such as concussion and acute subdural hematoma.

PATHOPHYSIOLOGIC MECHANISMS OF HEAD INJURY

The response of the brain to mechanical input is a complex series of events. Although the specific result of the brain's response varies with the magnitude of mechanical input, as well as with the direction and type of input, the pathophysiologic events that occur in the brain can be viewed as either primary or secondary. The primary brain injury depends entirely on the mechanical brain damage caused by mechanical input. Fortunately, in most instances, mechanical brain damage is not overwhelming. Usually secondary events such as ischemia-hypoxia, hemorrhage, edema, and the liberation of neurotoxic substances injure the brain more than primary mechanical damage. Primary mechanical damage can affect either the brain fibers themselves, as seen in cerebral contusions, white matter axons, or cerebral, dural, or meningeal blood vessels. Disruptions of arteries or veins within or around the brain can lead to subsequent hemorrhaging. It is often the degree of hemorrhaging rather than the disruption of the arterial and venous structures that causes the brain damage. Hemorrhage into the extradural, subdural, or intracerebral areas is, therefore, a secondary event, which if treated appropriately can result in a favorable outcome. However, if hemorrhage is massive or if treatment cannot reverse the effect of hemorrhaging, then the outcome is not favorable.

Another secondary event that occurs after the primary mechanical damage is cerebral ischemia or hypoxia. These events can be caused by inadequate ventilation resulting in systemic, whole-body hypoxia. The cerebral vascular reaction to injury may be such that the cerebral blood flow is insufficient to meet the metabolic demands of the brain. This then results in ischemia, localized to the brain or to part of the brain, and not in whole-body hypoxia. If inadequate blood flow, or inadequate oxygen delivery to the brain persists long enough, cerebral necrosis or infarction occurs. This is a secondary complication of head injury that should be preventable; if it is not, there is permanent damage to the brain caused by the mechanical input. The importance of cerebral edema is still being debated, but recent evidence suggests that cerebral edema causes cerebral dysfunction only if it is severe enough to increase intracranial pressure.

Even less is known about the secondary effects of toxic substances released at the time of mechanical input. In areas of cerebral ischemia, increased tissue acidosis and lactic acid accumulation occur and further embarrass cerebral function. If synaptic or axonal damage occurs, intracellular contents of neuroactive peptides or neurotransmitters are released. The action of these neurotransmitters may further impair cerebral function, but this postulate remains to be proven.

The combination of these injury factors causes one of two series of events to predominate. *Focal injuries* result from primary mechanical damage in a localized area of the brain. Local hemorrhaging, edema, or ischemia cause localized swelling around primary mechanical damage and result in a local mass effect. The local mass effect increases local tissue pressure and pressure gradients within the brain. These increases rapidly result in shifts of the brain and herniations of brain tissue beneath the falx, through the tentorial incisura, and through the foramen magnum. The herniations, if of sufficient magnitude, compress the brain stem, and if they act long enough cause secondary hemorrhaging into the brain stem. At this point, vital centers controlling consciousness and respiratory and cardiac functions are permanently damaged. Thus, a cascade of events can result from focal injuries, which cause localized damage that affects remote areas in the brain stem. It is, therefore, not the primary mechanical event, nor the primary mechanical brain damage that is most injurious, but rather the consequences of this damage. Therapy for focal injuries is therefore aimed at stopping the potential progression of this series of events.

Diffuse injuries to the brain have a different pathophysiologic mechanism. In these injuries, damage throughout the cerebral hemispheres is widespread. This damage can be physiologic and cause only temporary neurologic dysfunction. In this instance, if the secondary factors of ischemia, hemorrhage, and edema are controlled, the patient should have a good quality survival. If the injury is more severe, the anatomic disruption of axons in the white matter of both hemispheres can occur and is irreversible. Widespread cerebral dysfunction is usually associated with diffuse swelling of the brain, which at first is a vascular event. Diffuse swelling can result from massive vasodilatation and an increase in intravascular cerebral blood. This condition, if it exists, then causes true edema or increased tissue water, with a consequent rise in intracranial pressure. Even if these factors are controlled with therapy, the end result will depend on the amount of primary disruption that occurred at the moment of injury.

The end result of either focal or diffuse injuries depends on the severity of secondary factors and how adequately these are controllable. When these secondary factors are adequately controlled, the final result is related to the extent of primary mechanical damage. In focal injuries, the final result depends on the location and size of the focal damage. If this damage, such as from a contusion, is in a "silent" area of the brain, no abnormality may be detectable. If, however, the focal damage is in the speech, sensory, motor, or visual areas of the brain, then a focal neurologic deficit results. In diffuse injuries, the final result depends on the number of axons physically disrupted. If little disruption occurs, the outcome will be good, but if the number of axons disrupted is large, global injury to the brain will result. This is often manifested as personality changes, memory disorders, cognitive deficiencies, or intellectual dysfunction.

SUMMARY

The most common type of sports injury to the head results from a rapidly applied mechanical input to the head. Most often this is an impact or a direct blow to the head. An impact causes two phenomena to be set in motion. First, local factors beneath the site of impact (contact phenomena) cause deformation of the skull and shock wave propagation through the skull and brain. The magnitude, direction of impact, and size of the impacting device are the factors that produce mechanical damage. Damage is maximized by high-magnitude forces, which are applied to thin areas of the skull, and impact with small objects. Resulting skull deformation can cause skull fracture and underlying cerebral contusion. The events resulting from contact phenomena of impact can be minimized by decreasing the magnitude of impact forces, and by diffusing the size of the impact over the head. Protective headgear should be designed to achieve these goals.

Head injury is also caused by acceleration or deceleration of the head, regardless of whether an impact to the head has occurred, or whether the head is set in motion by impacts elsewhere on the body. Acceleration forces cause shear, tensile, and compression strains to develop within the brain, with shear being most injurious. Injuries that result from acceleration cause contusions at a distance from the site of impact, diffuse injuries to the brain, and subdural hematoma. Head protective devices are less able to keep the head from accelerating or decelerating and thus less likely to eliminate the type of injuries caused by acceleration forces.

The response of the brain to mechanical input and the ultimate biologic result of the input relate to several pathophysiologic mechanisms. The primary mechanical damage occurs at the time of head injury, is irreversible, and is maximal at the time of injury. If other factors are controlled, this primary mechanical damage is the sole determinant of the outcome. However, secondary factors such as ischemia, hypoxia, hemorrhaging around or within the brain, cerebral swelling, and the possible effects of toxic substances can all complicate the primary mechanical damage. Potentially, however, these events should be controllable. If these factors cannot be controlled, they add more dysfunction to the primary mechanical damage. If control of these problems is successful, no further damage occurs and the ultimate outcome then depends on the primary mechanical damage.

REFERENCES

1. Abel, J., Gennarelli, T.A., and Segawa, H.: Incidence and severity of cerebral concussion in the rhesus monkey following sagittal plane angular acceleration. *In* Twenty-Second Stapp Car Crash Conference Proceedings. New York, Society of Automotive Engineers, 1978.
2. Gennarelli, T.A., Thibault, L.E., and Ommaya, A.K.: Pathophysiologic responses to rotational and translational acceleration of the head. *In* Sixteenth Stapp Car Crash Conference Proceedings. New York, Society of Automotive Engineers, 1972.
3. Goldsmith, W.: Physical processes producing head injuries. *In* Head Injuries. Edited by W. Caveness and A.E. Walker. Philadelphia, J.B. Lippincott, 1966.
4. Gross, A.G.: A new theory on the dynamics of brain concussion and brain injury. J. Neurosurg., XV:552, 1958.
5. Gurdjian, E.S., Webster, J.E., and Lissner, H.R.: Observations on the mechanisms of brain concussion, contusion, and laceration. Surg. Gynecol. Obstet., 101:684, 1955.
6. Gurdjian, E.S.: Impact Injury and Crash Protection. Springfield, Charles C Thomas, 1970.
7. Gurdjian, E.S.: Impact Head Injury. Springfield, Charles C Thomas, 1975.
8. Holbourn, A.H.S.: Mechanics of head injuries. Lancet, II:440, 1943.
9. Ommaya, A.K., and Gennarelli, T.A.: Cerebral concussion and traumatic unconsciousness. Correlation of experimental and clinical observations on blunt head injuries. Brain, 97:633, 1974.
10. Ommaya, A.K., and Hirsch, A.E.: Tolerance for cerebral concussion from head impact and whiplash in primates. J. Biomech., 4:13, 1971.

EDITOR'S NOTE

Gennarelli and Ommaya are to be credited with demonstrating the effect of sagittal plane angular (rotational) acceleration in causing diffuse injuries of the brain. For purposes of completeness, the preceding work in this area is briefly reviewed.

The mechanisms of head injury were described under three general hypotheses by Hirsch[7]: (1) a pressure gradient hypothesis, whereby acceleration impacts set up pressure gradients causing shear stresses in primarily the craniospinal junction, or set up cavitation-induced lesions in the antepole, that is, the contrecoup injuries; (2) bending or stretching of the upper cervical cord due to head-neck motion; (3) skull deformation together with sudden rotation of the head causing shear primarily at the interface of the soft contents with the hard shell.

In this first hypothesis, Gurdjian was an early proponent of linear accleration causing shear in the brain stem.[2] His work spawned a number of injury indices based on linear accleration as graphically represented in the Wayne Curve.[6] The most notable of these linear accleration-based indices were those of Gadd,[3] Slattenschek and Tauffkirchen,[10] Brinn and Staffeld,[1] and the work of Stalnaker, McElhaney, and Roberts.[11] Chapter 3 by Hodgson, entitled "A Standard for Protective Equipment" details the National Operating Committee on Standards for Athletic Equipment's (NOCSAE) development of its Standard for football helmets based on the Wayne Curve as well. Although it is only this last citation of Hodgson's that is sports-related, an historical perspective places the greatest effort to understand head injuries in the automotive setting where all of these other citations are found.

The latter part of the first hypothesis dealing with cavitation was a theory espoused by Gross, whereby damage results from the "violent collapse of cavities formed within the brain."[4] Both coup- and contrecoup injuries were explained by cavitation theory.[5]

In the second hypothesis, the investigators used cats as the experimental model, and induced cervical stretch to evoke a concussive state. Corneal reflex was the basis of assessing concussion. Both the choice of the model, owing to its anatomic relationship of cranium to spine,

and the reflex assessment sign, have been critically negated by Thomas.[12]

In the third hypothesis, Holbourn appeared to be one of the earliest proponents of angular acceleration being the key to the relationship. He related concussion to a rotational acceleration injury,[9] with this view further developed by Hirsch.[8]

REFERENCES

1. Brinn, J., and Staffeld, S.E.: Evaluation of Impact Test Acceleration. *In* Fourteenth Stapp Car Crash Conference Proceedings. New York, Society of Automotive Engineers, 1970, p. 188.
2. Bibliography of Elisha S. Gurdjian, M.D. (Through 1971). Clin. Neurosurg., *19*:20, 1972.
3. Gadd, C.W.: Use of Weighted Impulse Criterion for Estimating Injury Hazard. *In* Tenth Stapp Car Crash Conference Proceedings. New York, Society of Automotive Engineers, 1966, p. 168.
4. Gross, A.G.: A new theory on the dynamics of brain concussion and brain injury. J. Neurosurg. XV:552, 1958.
5. Gross, A.G.: Impact thresholds of brain concussion. Aviation Med., *29*:725, 1958.
6. Gurdjian, E.S., Webster, J.E., and Lissner, H.R.: Observations on the mechanism of brain concussion, contusion, and laceration. Surg. Gynecol. Obstet., *101*:684, 1955.
7. Hirsch, A.E., Ommaya, A.K., and Mahone, R.H.: Tolerance of subhuman primate brain to cerebral concussion. *In* Impact Injury and Crash Protection. Edited by E.S. Gurdjian. Springfield, Charles C Thomas Publishers, 1970, p. 352.
8. Hirsch, A.E., Ommaya, A.K., and Mahone, R.H.: Tolerance of subhuman primate brain to cerebral concussion. *In* Impact Injury and Crash Protection. Edited by E.S. Gurdjian. Springfield, Charles C Thomas Publishers, 1970, p. 364.
9. Holbourn, A.H.S.: Mechanics of head injuries. Lancet, *II*:440, 1943.
10. Slattenschek, A., and Tauffkirchen, W.: Critical evaluation of assessment—methods for head impact applied in appraisal of brain injury hazard, in particular in head impact on windshields. International Automobile Safety Conference Compendium. New York, Society of Automotive Engineers, 1970, p. 1103.
11. Stalnaker, R.L., McElhaney, J.H., and Roberts, V.R.: M.S.C. tolerance curve for head impacts. Transactions of the A.S.M.E. Paper No. $\mu 1 =$ WA/BHT = 10. New York, The American Society of Mechanical Engineers, 1971, p. 4.
12. Thomas, M.L.: Mechanisms of Head Injury. *In* Impact Injury and Crash Protection. Edited by E.S. Gurdjian. Springfield, Charles C Thomas Publishers, 1970, p. 300.

Chapter 7

Radiographic Evaluation of the Head and Facial Bones

Helene Pavlov

RADIOGRAPHIC TECHNIQUES AND ANATOMY

The radiographic examination of the cervical spine, skull, facial bones, and central nervous system is difficult to obtain and interpret, and is especially challenging in the acutely injured patient who is confused, semiconscious, or in pain. Diagnosing head and cervical spine injuries in the acutely traumatized patient requires trained technicians and the cooperative effort of the orthopedic and radiologic personnel in order that the correct radiographic examinations are obtained, and additional injury to the patient is avoided.

Skull and Facial Bones

Because of the spacial relationship of the skull and facial bones there is always superimposition; therefore, radiographic projections can be confusing. The number of projections in a skull series differs in every radiographic department, but includes at least four films—one anteroposterior (AP) view, both lateral views, and one posteroanterior (PA) view. In addition, there are special views performed or monitored by a radiologist that enhance the detail of specific areas.

Plain Films

The most utilized plain films for a trauma series are the AP and lateral views taken to evaluate the skull, and the Waters' view taken to evaluate the facial bones.

The *straight AP view* is obtained with the person's head lying on a grid cassette and the central ray perpendicular to the cassette. This view is essential in the unconscious patient with possible cervical spine fractures because it can be obtained while the patient is still on the litter. The orbitomeatal line (OM), i.e., the line between the outer canthus of the eye and the external auditory meatus is perpendicular to the cassette.[16, 23, 24, 28] This view demonstrates the orbits, ethmoid, frontal and maxillary sinuses, the nasopharynx, the internal auditory canal, and a calcified pineal gland.[22]

The *inclined AP view* is obtained with the same patient position but the central ray is angled 15° cephalad to the OM line. This view demonstrates the frontal, maxillary and ethmoid sinuses, the nasopharynx, mandible, and orbits (Fig. 7-1*A*).

The *AP (half-axial) Towne view* uses the same patient position but the central ray is angled 30° caudad to the OM line. This view demonstrates the occipital bone including the foramen magnum, petrous

73

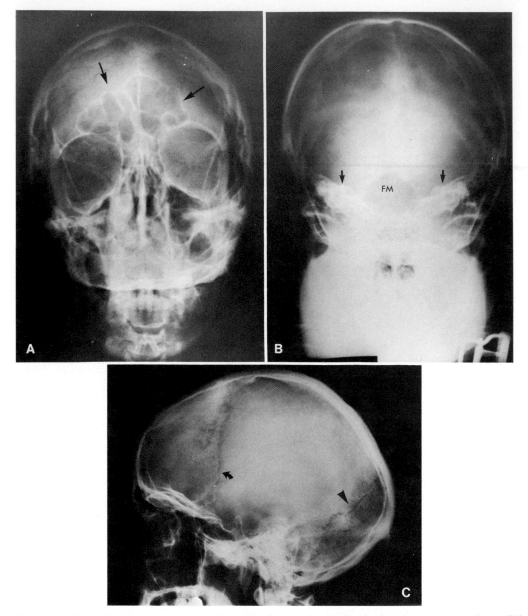

Fig. 7-1. *A,* Inclined AP view demonstrating the orbits, frontal sinuses (arrows), nasopharynx, and mandible. *B,* Towne view demonstrating the occipital bone, foramen magnum (FM), and petrous ridges (arrows). *C,* Laterial view of the skull demonstrating the nasopharynx, the multiple sinusoidal vascular channels (arrow), and the interdigitating cranial sutures (arrowhead).

pyramids, and mastoid air cells (Fig. 7-1*B*).

For the *lateral views,* the side closest to the cassette distinguishes right or left. Both laterals should be obtained. Initially this view can be obtained with the patient supine on the litter using a horizontal central ray. Lateral views demonstrate the nasopharynx, the maxillary, ethmoid, sphenoid and frontal sinuses, the mastoid air cells, external auditory canal, and the temporal and parietal bones (Fig. 7-1*C*).

The *straight PA view* is obtained with the patient's face against the cassette and

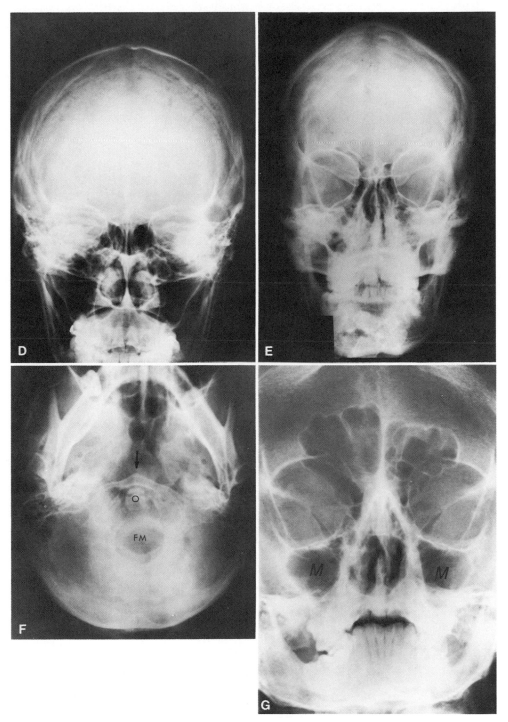

Fig. 7-1 (Cont'd).   *D,* A straight PA view in which the petrous ridges project through the orbits. The frontal, sphenoid and maxillary sinuses, and the nasopharynx are demonstrated. *E,* On a Caldwell inclined PA view, the orbits are projected above the petrous ridges. *F,* The submentovertical or axial view demonstrating the mandible, foramen magnum (FM), the odontoid (O), and the anterior arch of C1 (arrow). *G,* A Waters' view is specific for the facial bones, including the orbits, and frontal and maxillary sinuses (M).

the OM line and the central ray perpendicular to the cassette. In this view the petrous ridge projects through the orbits. The ethmoid, frontal and maxillary sinuses, nasopharynx, and mandible are also demonstrated (Fig. 7-1D).

The *inclined PA-Caldwell view* is obtained with the same patient position but the central ray angled 15° caudad to the OM line. This view demonstrates the orbits unobstructed by the petrous ridges, the superior orbital fissure, and frontal and ethmoid sinuses (Fig. 7-1E).

The *submentovertical* view, axial, or base view is obtained only when it is certain that the neck can safely be hyperextended. The cassette is placed under the vertex of the head. The central ray is perpendicular to the cassette and the OM line is parallel to the cassette. This view demonstrates the base of the skull, mandible,

foramen magnum, and nasal cavity and may identify a basilar skull fracture in a patient with pneumocephalus and normal routine skull radiographs (Fig. 7-1F).

The *Waters' view* is specific for examination of the sinuses and facial bones. It is obtained with the patient's nose and chin positioned against the cassette and the central ray angled approximately 37° caudad to the OM line. This view demonstrates the orbits, maxillary, frontal and ethmoid sinuses, and the nasopharynx (Fig. 7-1G).

Additional facial bone views are the specific AP, lateral, and oblique views that best delineate the individual facial bones such as the orbits, sinuses, nose, zygomatic arches, or the mandible. Simply ordering a "facial bone" examination is improper as the request should be specific, i.e., nose, mandible, orbits, or sinuses (Fig. 7-2A, B).

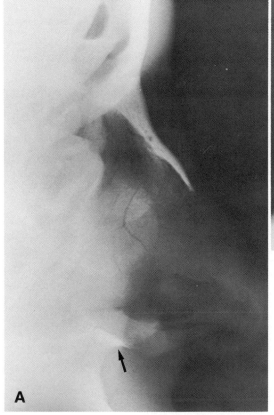

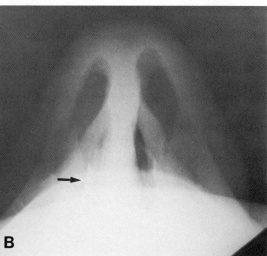

Fig. 7-2. *A,* A lateral view of the nose demonstrating the nasal bone, soft tissues, and maxillary spines (arrow). *B,* An occlusal view is specific for showing the maxillary spines. The right-maxillary spine is medially displaced and fractured (arrow).

Special Views

Coned down, oblique, stereoscopic, and tomographic views are performed or monitored by a radiologist, and should be obtained when a specific area is not clearly seen on the routine views.

Coned-down views center the central ray on the specific area of interest, and narrow the area exposed in order to increase detail. This technique is particularly useful in examining the orbit and sinuses.

Oblique views are obtained by rotating the skull so that the abnormal area is in tangent to the radiographic beam. This is especially useful in evaluating a depressed skull fracture to determine the depth of the fracture fragments.

Stereoscopic views are obtained by taking two exposures, each with a slight change in the tube angle while the patient remains stationary. These two radiographs provide evaluation of the special relationships. These views are useful to locate intracranial fracture fragments and radiopaque debris and to identify facial bone fractures.

Tomographic views blur the structures outside the plane of interest in order to increase detail in the plane of interest. Tomography is useful in examining the orbit, maxillary sinuses, and internal ear, and should be used when a facial bone fracture is suggested on the initial plain films, but is not definite.

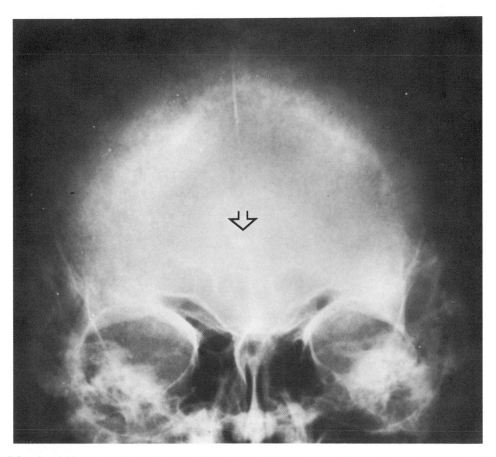

Fig. 7-3. A calcified pineal gland (arrow) should be midline on the frontal views. A displacement of over 2 mm from midline results from increased intracerebral pressure in one hemisphere displacing the pineal toward the opposite side.

Brain

When a brain injury is suspected because of either the trauma sustained or the patient's neurologic status, a computed tomogram (CT) is the most diagnostic study. In most emergency room situations, however, the radiographic examination of the brain starts with routine skull films. When a CT head scan is not available and additional information is required, either an arteriogram, a radionuclide brain scan, or a pneumoencephalogram may be indicated.

Plain Films

The plain films of the skull suggest brain injury when there is a fracture, especially if there are depressed fracture fragments or radiopaque debris within the cranial vault. The demonstration of intracranial air indicates communication with a sinus or a fracture through the base of the skull, even though the fracture may not be documented on the routine films.

A displaced pineal on the plain film confirms intracranial and possible brain injury. The pineal is a small gland that can calcify by age six years and is calcified in 60% of adults.[22] The pineal is normally midline (Fig. 7-3).

Computed Tomography (CT)

The CT is the newest roentgen modality for evaluating the head and is the only radiographic method that directly examines the brain. The CT displays multiple cross-sectional slices of the skull and brain at different levels (Fig. 7-4A –D). The CT examination documents the location and size of an intracranial injury. The examination is noninvasive; however, occasionally an intravenous contrast injection is used to enhance an abnormality.[17]

Cerebral Arteriography

Cerebral arteriography is the intra-arterial injection of contrast to delineate the arterial, capillary, and venous blood flow of the brain.[14, 25] Although the CT head scan has replaced arteriography as an emergency procedure, an arteriogram is still often necessary to demonstrate a subdural hematoma, a post-traumatic aneurysm, an arteriovenous shunt, or the site of a bleeding vessel.

Nuclear Medicine

Radionuclide studies involve injecting an isotope and then scanning the patient with a gamma camera to detect the radiation. The intravenous injection of $Tc99^m$ pertechnetate can be traced by dynamic and static brain scanning. Dynamic scanning, obtaining multiple scans at two second intervals, demonstrates the gross vas-

Fig. 7-4. Normal CT brain scan in which sections of the brain are viewed in cross section. These slices proceed caudally. *A,* The sulci markings can be identified as well as the central linear falx. *B,* This section is through the occipital horns of the lateral ventricles (arrows) containing calcified-choroid plexus. The brain tissue is uniform. *C,* This section demonstrates the frontal horns of the lateral ventricle, the choroid plexuses, and the centrally located calcified pineal gland. *D,* The frontal horns of the lateral ventricle and the midline third ventricle (arrow) are identified on this section. Courtesy of James C. Hirschy, M.D., New York, N.Y.

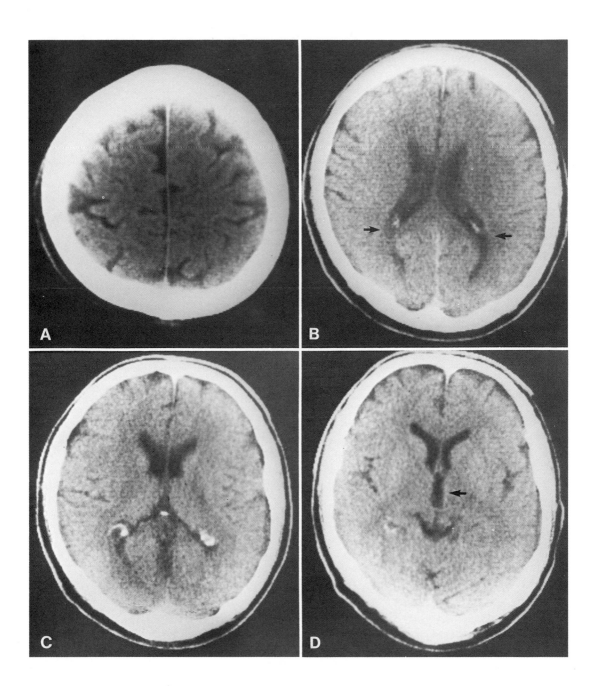

(Legend on facing page.)

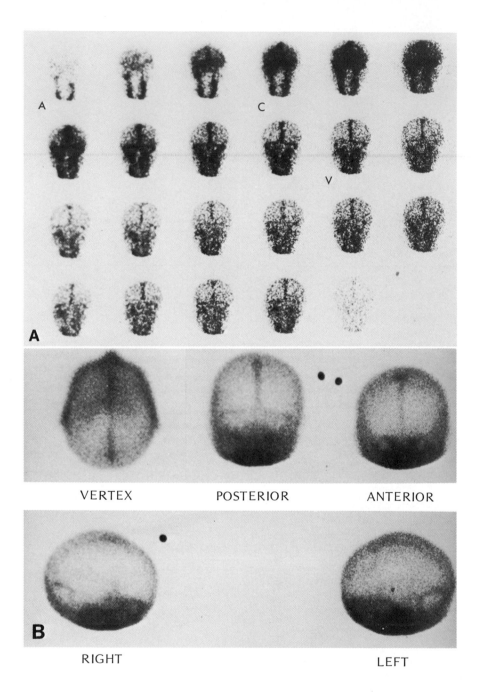

VERTEX   POSTERIOR   ANTERIOR

RIGHT   LEFT

Fig. 7-5. Radionuclide brain scan as seen on the gamma camera following the intravenous isotope injection. *A,* A dynamic brain scan in sequential 2 second displays. Each row is read from left to right. The blood flow can be followed by the isotope augmentation. The arterial (A) phase, the capillary (C) phase in which the entire brain is perfused, and the venous (V) phases are demonstrated. *B,* A normal static brain scan includes an anterior, posterior, and both lateral and submentovertical vertex views. These views are obtained by placing that portion of the head against the gamma camera for radiation detection and display. The normal isotope uptake should be uniform and symmetric. (Courtesy of Jay W. MacMoran, M.D., Director, Department of Radiology, Germantown Hospital, Philadelphia, Pa.)

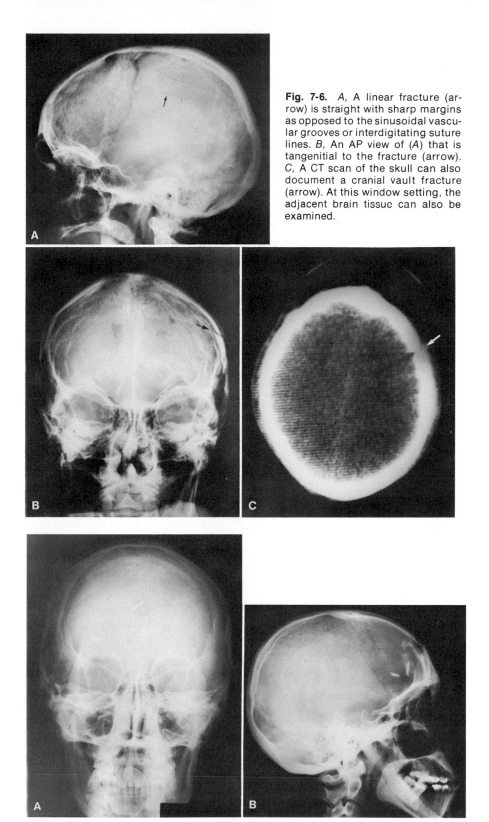

Fig. 7-6. *A*, A linear fracture (arrow) is straight with sharp margins as opposed to the sinusoidal vascular grooves or interdigitating suture lines. *B*, An AP view of (*A*) that is tangenitial to the fracture (arrow). *C*, A CT scan of the skull can also document a cranial vault fracture (arrow). At this window setting, the adjacent brain tissue can also be examined.

Fig. 7-7. *A*, On the PA view of the skull, multiple osseous fragments are seen in the midline. *B*, Lateral view of (*A*) confirming the frontal location of a comminuted depressed skull fracture.

cular flow to the brain (Fig. 7-5*A*). The static scan, obtained minutes after the injection, and the dynamic scan demonstrate the integrity of the skull and the blood-brain barrier (Fig. 7-5*B*).

The intrathecal injection of Tc99^m or In111 DTPA (diethylenetriamine pentaacetic acid) is used to evaluate the ventricular system in cases of post-traumatic hydrocephalus, and is most useful in cases of persistent post-traumatic cerebral spinal fluid rhinorrhea or otorrhea.

Pneumoencephography

Pneumoencephography is the injection of air into the ventricular system. It is dangerous and painful and has been largely replaced by the CT examination. On the rare occasion of an intraventricular lesion, however, a pneumoencephalogram may be required prior to surgery for more exact evaluation and localization.

FRACTURES

Skull Fractures

Skull fractures can be linear or depressed and either can be associated with underlying brain injury. Linear fractures are occasionally complicated by extension into a sinus or across a blood vessel. Depressed fractures are often complicated by

Fig. 7-7 (Cont'd). *C*, Lateral view of a different patient demonstrating a confluence of linear lucencies in the posteroparietal area. *D*, Frontal view of (*C*) demonstrating a depressed fracture. *E*, A CT scan at the bone-window setting demonstrating a depressed skull fracture. Scan performed at window for brain tissue revealed no injury.

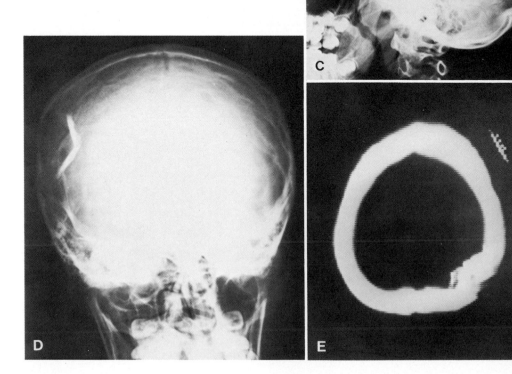

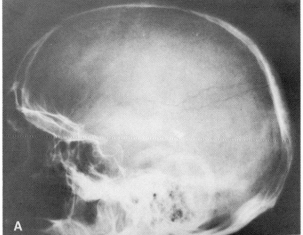

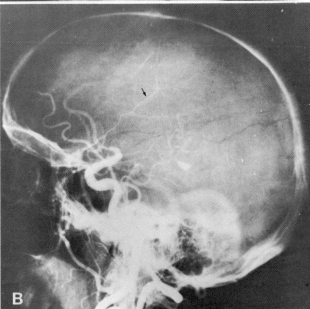

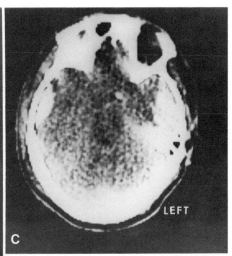

Fig. 7-8. *A,* Bilateral linear fractures through the temporoparietal bones. Pineal is calcified. *B,* A retrograde brachial arteriogram demonstrating the "tram track" sign (arrow) indicating arteriovenous communication and confirming that the temporoparietal fracture extends through the middle meningeal artery. *C,* Cerebral contusion and hematoma in the left temporo-occipital area. There are bilateral asymmetric epidural hematomas in the mid- to anterior-temporal areas, and a localized area of edema medial to the left epidural hematoma.

brain injury and subsequent infection or abscess.

Identification of a linear skull fracture on plain films, especially when bilateral, can be difficult because of the normal vascular grooves and sutures. In addition, scalp lacerations, dirt, foreign bodies, and hair produce multiple artifacts that can simulate fractures.[1,27] A linear skull fracture is a straight linear lucency with sharp edges. Because of the occasionally confusing shadows, demonstration on more than one view, or on a CT scan, may be necessary (Fig. 7-6*A*–*C*). Linear fractures are not

always associated with brain damage, but a CT head scan is indicated whenever there is a clinical suspicion of neurologic impairment.

A depressed skull fracture is evaluated best on tangential plain films or on a CT head scan in which the depth and location of the bony fragments can be determined (Fig. 7-7*A*–*E*).

A fracture in the temporoparietal region is frequently associated with rupture of the middle meningeal artery and an epidural hematoma. An arteriogram documents an arterial injury. A CT examination is also

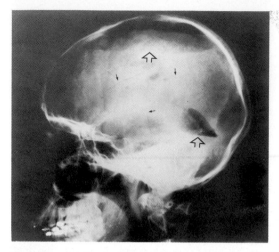

Fig. 7-9. A lateral view of this patient reveals a comminuted linear fracture (small arrows), but more importantly, a large pneumocephalus. There are air fluid levels (open arrows) because the patient was sitting and a horizontal radiographic beam was used. (Courtesy of Jay W. MacMoran, M.D., Director, Department of Radiology, Germantown Hospital, Philadelphia, Pa.)

A pneumocephalus is air around the brain and is associated with a fracture through a sinus or base of the skull (Fig. 7-9).[8, 12] Occasionally, the fracture may be demonstrated only with tomography or on the submentovertical view.

Persistent bloody or clear discharge from the nose (rhinorrhea) or the ear (otorrhea) following trauma is associated with a fracture through a sinus or the temporal bone, respectively. Because the actual fracture cannot always be demonstrated, the origin of the fluid may not be obvious, and a nuclear medicine examination may be helpful. The intrathecal isotope is injected and a cotton plug is placed in the nose or ear; this is measured for isotope collection 6 to 24 hours later.[7] The presence of the isotope on the cotton confirms that the discharge is cerebrospinal fluid.

usually necessary to determine the size of the hematoma and its involvement of the ventricles and midline structures (Fig. 7-8A–C).

Facial Bone Fractures

Facial bone fractures are easy to overlook radiographically, and the best way to

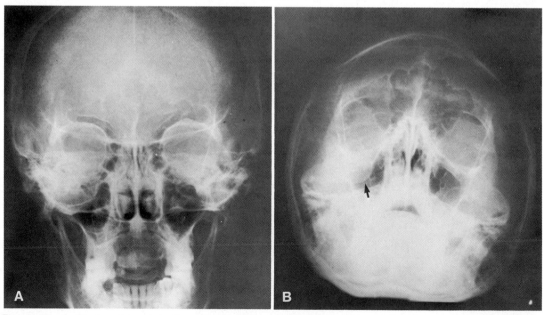

Fig. 7-10. *A,* PA view demonstrating asymmetry in the infraorbital areas. *B,* Waters' view demonstrating a depressed fracture of the floor of the right orbit showing the orbital contents (arrow) extending into the superior portion of the maxillary sinus.

examine the radiographs for possible fractures is to note asymmetry.

Orbital fractures may involve the floor, rim, roof, or walls of the orbit. Specific orbital views and a Waters' view should be obtained whenever an orbital fracture is suspected. A fracture of the orbital floor is a blow-out fracture and the eye may descend into the maxillary sinus (Fig. 7-10A,B).[8,11] A blow-out fracture is best demonstrated on the Waters' view; however, tomography and stereoscopic views always should be employed when the diagnosis is uncertain.

Comparison of one side of the face to the other is also useful in identifying maxillary sinus fractures (Fig. 7-11A). Tomography, both routine and CT, is important and further delineates the number and position of the fractures, as well as the associated soft tissue swelling and hematoma (Fig. 7-11B–D).

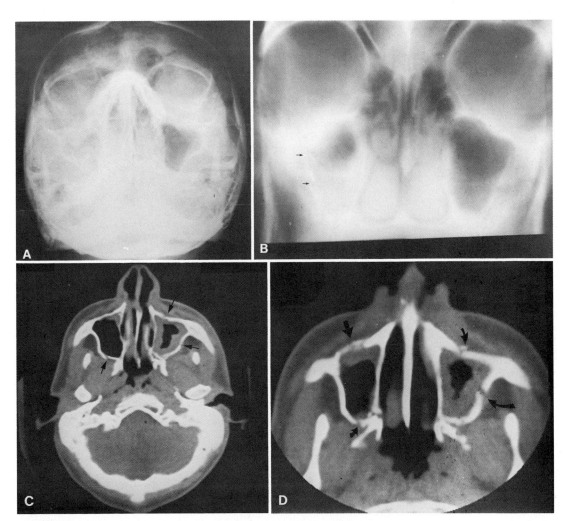

Fig. 7-11. *A*, Water's view demonstrating asymmetry. The right side of the face is more dense than the left. A definite fracture is not seen. *B*, A tomogram of both maxillary sinuses demonstrating fractures of the lateral wall of the right maxillary sinus (arrows). The increased density in the inferior portion of the sinus represents blood. *C*, A CT scan of a different patient demonstrating comminuted bilateral maxillary sinus fractures. (arrows). *D*, A close-up CT view clearly delineating the maxillary sinus fractures and the location of the fragments (arrows). The edematous lining of the maxillary sinuses is also evident. (Fig. 7-11 *C, D* courtesy of James C. Hirschy, M.D., New York, N.Y.)

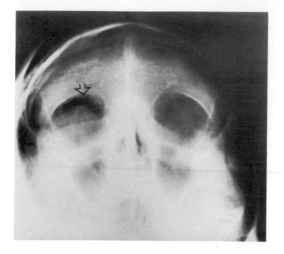

Fig. 7-12. Waters' view demonstrating asymmetry. The right orbit is too lucent due to periorbital air (arrow), which usually indicates an ethmoid sinus fracture.

Subcutaneous air, especially intraorbital air, is an indication of an ethmoid or paranasal sinus fracture, even without demonstrating the fracture (Fig. 7-12).

Fractures of the zygomatic arch are suspected by asymmetry on the Waters' view, but are best demonstrated on an underpenetrated submentovertical view in which the arch is projected in tangent (Fig.

7-13*A, B*). The position of the fracture fragments of a mandible fracture is demonstrated on oblique views or on a submentovertical view of the skull (Fig. 7-14*A, B*). Fracture through the condyles of the mandible is best seen on the Caldwell view (Fig. 7-14*C*). Faciomaxillary fractures, as described by LeFort,[8, 26] are best demonstrated in the Caldwell and Waters' views.

BRAIN INJURY

Brain injury should be expected whenever plain films of the skull reveal a skull fracture, intracranial osseous fragments, radiopaque foreign debris, a pneumocephalus, or a shift of a calcified pineal gland over 2 mm to one side of midline. Unfortunately, a midline pineal gland does not exclude bilateral brain injury or generalized cerebral edema.

Brain injury following acute trauma includes cerebral edema, contusion, and hematoma. Subsequent brain damage includes hydrocephalus and atrophy. The CT brain scan is the most useful radiographic modality for evaluating brain injury.[5, 9, 13, 15] It analyzes the displayed structures by their relative densities. The

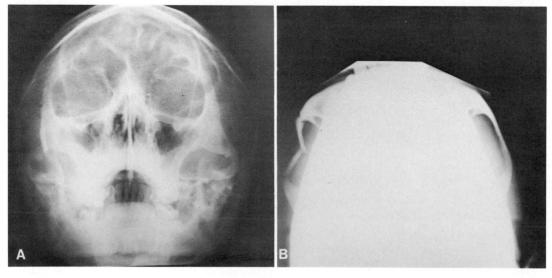

Fig. 7-13. *A,* Asymmetry of the face is noted with increased density on the right, and irregularity of the right zygoma. *B,* An underpenetrated submentovertical view demonstrating a comminuted fracture of the right zygomatic arch.

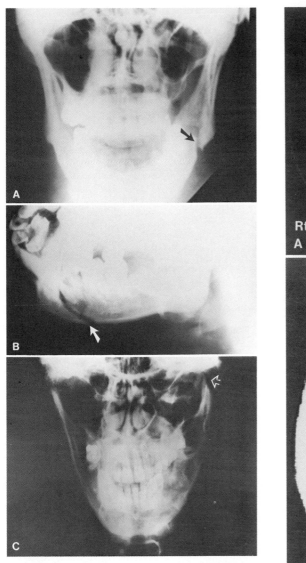

Fig. 7-14. *A,* A mandible fracture on the PA view (arrow); demonstrated clearly on the oblique view (*B*). *C,* A fracture through the mandibular condyle seen on a Caldwell view (arrow).

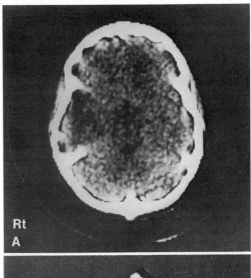

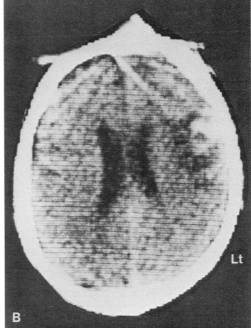

Fig. 7-15. *A,* Cerebral edema on the CT display is hypodense or blacker than brain tissue. There is a localized area of edema in the right temporal lobe. *B,* Blood is hyperdense or whiter than brain tissue. In this patient, there is a cortical hemorrhage in the left temporal lobe with medial edema and compression of the ipsilateral ventricle. There is no shift of the midline structures.

density of a lesion on the CT display is proportional to the hemoglobin content; the more hemoglobin in a lesion, the greater the density. The density of a vascular lesion can be increased by the intravenous injection of positive contrast materials.[9, 17, 21]

Cerebral Edema

Cerebral edema may occur 12 to 24 hours postinjury. On the CT display, edema is hypodense, i.e., less dense than the surrounding tissue. It may exist alone or surrounding an area of hemorrhage (Fig. 7-15*A*).[2, 3, 15, 20] Rarely, edema may be isodense, the same density as brain tissue,

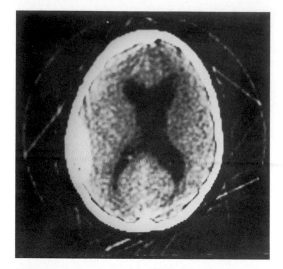

Fig. 7-16. An epidural hematoma is a contained lenticular-shaped collection of blood at the periphery of the brain. The epidural hematoma in this patient is associated with compression of the ipsilateral ventricle.

and identified only if there is associated ventricular compression. The cerebral edema associated with a subdural

hematoma contributes to the neurologic symptoms and must be considered prior to the evacuation of a subdural collection, as that may not improve the neurologic status.

Cerebral Contusion

Cerebral contusion or laceration is common as a contrecoup injury, i.e., the patient is hit on the front of the head and the brain shifts within the skull tearing the cerebral vessels in the temporal or occipital area. Cerebral contusion has a mixed density pattern of hypodense and hyperdense patches, and the amount of density depends on the size of the hemorrhagic areas (Fig. 7-15*B*).[5, 13]

Hematoma

A hematoma is an organized hemorrhage, which can be epidural, subdural, intracerebral, or intraventricular.

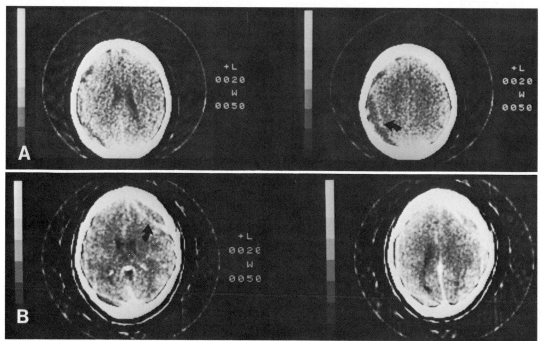

Fig. 7-17. *A,* The crescent-shaped isodense area along the convexity of the right hemisphere (arrow) represents a subacute subdural hematoma in which the blood has been reabsorbed and replaced with cerebrospinal fluid. *B,* A chronic subdural hematoma in the left frontal area. The ring enhancement (arrow) is produced after contrast infusion.

An *epidural hematoma* is a localized biconvex or lenticular high density area at the brain-skull interface. Almost every epidural hematoma is associated with a skull fracture. A small one may resolve without sequelae, but a large one may be associated with rapid neurologic deterioration requiring immediate evacuation (Fig. 7-16).

A *subdural hematoma* is a crescent-shaped collection of blood along the convexity of the brain (Fig. 7-17A). Initially, a subdural hematoma is dense on the CT examination because there is fresh blood present, but as the hemoglobin is reabsorbed, approximately 10-days postinjury, it is replaced by cerebral spinal fluid and becomes isodense or hypodense. During the subacute stage, a unilateral subdural hematoma may be indicated on the CT only by a shift of the midline structures or ventricular compression. A subacute bilateral subdural hematoma may have a nor-

mal CT study.[6] A chronic subdural hematoma may have a dense capsule, which with contrast infusion may be more dense (Fig. 7-17B).

A cerebral arteriogram or a radionuclide brain scan should be performed when a subdural hematoma is clinically suspected and the CT brain scan is inconclusive.

On a cerebral arteriogram, a subdural hematoma is diagnosed by a displacement of the adjacent vessels. An acute subdural hematoma spreads along the convexity of the brain and is crescent-shaped, while in the more chronic stages, the hematoma becomes encapsulated and biconvex or lenticular-shaped (Fig. 7-18A, B).[25] The presence of a subdural hematoma on one side without comparable midline shift, requires evaluation of the opposite side to document either bilateral subdural collections or cerebral edema of the opposite hemisphere.

A dynamic and static radionuclide brain

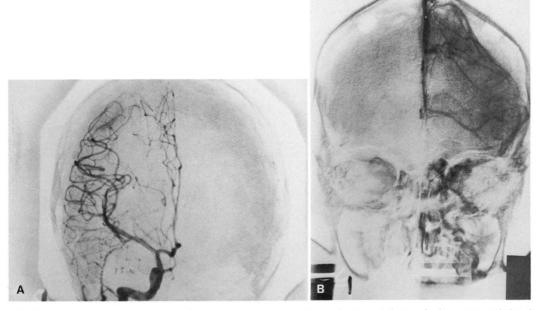

Fig. 7-18. Arteriographic demonstrations of subdural hematoma in two patients. *A,* An acute subdural hematoma demonstrated on an arteriogram as a crescent-shaped displacement of the vessels from the periphery. *B,* An arteriogram demonstrating a lenticular displacement of the vessels from the periphery, representing a chronic subdural hematoma. The lack of a shift of the midline structures toward the opposite side suggests a space-taking lesion in the opposite hemisphere of similar size. (Courtesy of Jay W. MacMoran, M.D., Director, Department of Radiology, Germantown Hospital, Philadelphia, Pa.)

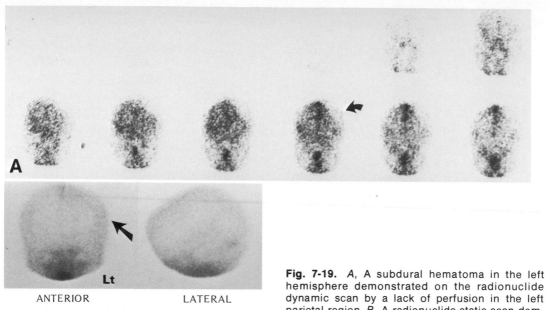

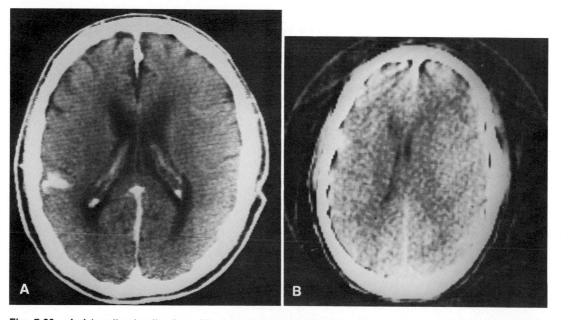

ANTERIOR   LATERAL

LATERAL   POSTERIOR

Fig. 7-19. *A,* A subdural hematoma in the left hemisphere demonstrated on the radionuclide dynamic scan by a lack of perfusion in the left parietal region. *B,* A radionuclide static scan demonstrating increased uptake in the periphery of the left hemisphere (arrows) indicating a defect in the blood-brain barrier, consistent with a subdural hematoma. (Courtesy of Jay W. MacMoran, M.D., Director, Department of Radiology, Germantown Hospital, Philadelphia, Pa.)

Fig. 7-20. *A,* A localized collection of blood in the right hemisphere. The ventricles are not displaced. This is an intracerebral hematoma. *B,* An isodense area in the left hemisphere. The blood from a large intracerebral hematoma is being reabsorbed; however, there is persistent ventricular compression and shift of the midline structures.

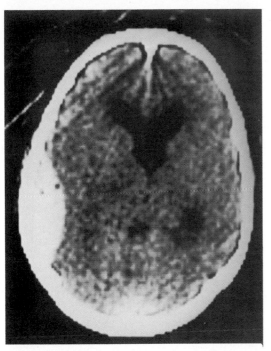

Fig. 7-21. Ventricular dilatation consistent with post-traumatic hydrocephalus. There is also an epidural hematoma.

scan is useful to evaluate a subdural hematoma, and is most positive in the subacute stage when the neovasculature in the capsule of the subdural hematoma is well developed (Fig. 7-19A, B). Immediately following trauma, augmented isotope uptake along the convexity of the brain may be due to a scalp or skull lesion, or a subdural hematoma. Serial scans, every four or five days, however, differentiate these entities because the uptake decreases with a skull or scalp lesion and increases with a subdural hematoma. Unfortunately, small bilateral subdural hematomas may be misinterpreted as negative brain scans.[10]

An *intracerebral hematoma* on the CT brain scan is a homogeneous area of increased density within the brain substance that may be surrounded by a low-density edematous halo (Fig. 7-20A). Before the availability of the CT examination, the incidence of intracerebral hematomas was underestimated and the entity overlooked. Intracerebral hematomas can occur even 2

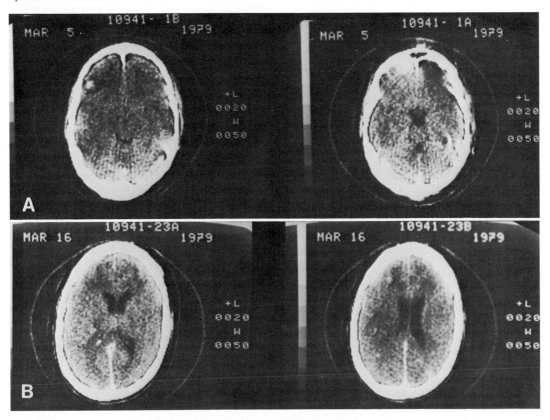

Fig. 7-22. Serial CT scans demonstrating post-traumatic atrophy. *A,* Hematoma in the right frontal lobe. *B,* Eleven days later the blood has been resorbed. There is a low-density area in the right frontal lobe and associated ventricular enlargement. These findings indicate atrophy of the brain in this area.

weeks following traumatic injury.[4, 19] On serial CT examinations, a decrease in density does not signify resolution or healing (Fig. 7-20B). The change in density only indicates a decrease in the hemoglobin content. A decrease in the mass effect, the reexpansion of the ventricles, and the return of the central structures to midline are the important indicators of resolution.[9, 18]

An *intraventricular hematoma* following trauma is more common than was previously expected, because prior to CT this entity was diagnosed only by an intraventricular puncture or autopsy. With early diagnosis the hemorrhage may be treated by drainage, although cases have resolved without treatment and without sequelae.

POST-TRAUMATIC HYDROCEPHALUS AND ATROPHY

Post-traumatic hydrocephalus usually results from intraventricular hemorrhage; however, regardless of cause, hydrocephalus is demonstrated on CT as ventricular dilatation (Fig. 7-21). Serial CT brain scans establish the change in the ventricular pattern. The ventricles usually return to normal after the blood is reabsorbed.[15]

Post-traumatic atrophy is similar to brain atrophy from any cause. Brain atrophy on the CT brain scan is seen as a focal low-density area with associated local ventricle enlargement (Fig. 7-22A, B).

REFERENCES

1. Allen, W.E., Knir, E.L., and Rothman, S.L.G.: Pitfalls in evaluation of skull trauma—A review. Radiol. Clin. North Am., *11*:479, 1973.
2. Ambrose, J.: Computerized transverse axial scanning (tomography): Part 2. Clinical application. Br. J. Radiol., *46*:1023, 1973.
3. Ambrose, J.: Computerized x-ray scanning of brain. J. Neurosurg., *40*:679, 1974.
4. Baratham, G., and Dennyson, W.G.: Delayed traumatic intracerebral hemorrhage. J. Neurol., Neurosurg. Psychiatry, *35*:698, 1972.
5. Davis, K.R., et al.: Computed tomography in head trauma. Semin. Roentgenol., *12*:53, 1977.
6. Davis, K.R., et al.: Some limitations of CT in diagnosis of neurological disease. Am. J. Roentgenol., *127*:111, 1977.
7. DiChiro, G., and Reames, P.M.: Isotopic localizations of cranionasal cerebrospinal fluid leaks. J. Nucl. Med., *5*:376, 1964.
8. Dolan, K.D., and Jacoby, C.G.: Facial fractures. Semin. Roentgenol., *13*:37, 1978.
9. Dublin, A.B., French, B.N., and Rennick, J.M.: Computed tomography in head trauma. Radiology, *122*:365, 1977.
10. Freedman, G.S.: Radionuclide imaging of the injured patient. Radiol. Clin. North Am., *11*:461, 1973.
11. Fueger, G.F., Milauskas, A.T., and Britton, W.: The roentgenologic evaluation of orbital blowout injuries. Am. J. Roentgenol., *97*:614, 1966.
12. Greenfield, J.G., and Russell, D.S.: Traumatic lesions of the central and peripheral nervous system. *In* Neuropathology. Edited by M. Greenfield. Baltimore, Williams & Wilkins, 1963.
13. Koo, A.H., and LaRoque, R.L.: Evaluation of head trauma by computed tomography. Radiology, *123*:345, 1977.
14. Lee, T.P.: Techniques of cerebral angiography. Radiol. Clin. North Am., *12*:223, 1974.
15. Merino-de Villasante, J., and Taveras, J.M.: Computerized tomography (CT) in acute head trauma. Am. J. Roentgenol., *126*:765, 1976.
16. Merrill, V.: Atlas of Roentgenographic Positions. St. Louis, C.V. Mosby, 1967.
17. Messina, A.V.: Computed tomography: contrast media within subdural hematomas. A preliminary report. Radiology, *119*:725, 1976.
18. Messina, A.V., and Chernick, N.L.: CT: the "resolving" intracerebral hemorrhage. Radiology, *118*:609, 1975.
19. Morin, M.A., and Pitts, F.W.: Delayed apoplexy following head injury (traumatische Spat-Apoplexie). J. Neurosurg., *33*:542, 1970.
20. New, P.F.J., et al.: Computerized axial tomography with EMI scanner. Radiology, *110*:109, 1974.
21. Norman, D.: Current status of computerized tomographic brain scanning. *In* Diagnostic Radiology. Edited by A.R. Margulis, and C.A. Gooding. San Francisco, University of California Press, 1976.
22. Ozonoff, M.B., and Burrows, E.H.: Intracranial calcification. *In* Radiology of the Skull and Brain. Vol. I. Edited by T.H. Newton, and D.G. Potts. St. Louis, C.V. Mosby, 1971.
23. Potts, D.G.: A system of skull radiolgoy. Radiology, *94*:25, 1970.
24. Rumbaugh, C.L., and Davis, D.O.: The normal skull: techniques and indications. Semin. Roentgenol., *9*:91, 1974.
25. Taveras, J.M., and Wood, J.H.: Diagnostic neuroradiology. *In* Golden's Diagnostic Radiology. 2nd ed. Vol. II. Edited by L.L. Robins. Baltimore, Williams & Wilkins, 1976.
26. Tilson, H.B., McFee, A.S., and Soudah, H.P.: The Maxillofacial Works of Rene LeFort. Houston, University of Texas Press, 1972.
27. Tomsick, T.A., Chambers, A.A., and Lukin, R.R.: Skull fractures. Semin. Roentgenol., *13*:27, 1978.
28. Weathers, R.M., and Lee, A.: Radiologic examination of the skull. Radiol. Clin. North Am., *12*:215, 1974.

Chapter 8

Cerebral Concussion and Diffuse Brain Injuries

Thomas A. Gennarelli

Traumatic injuries to the brain can be classified into focal brain injuries and diffuse brain injuries. *Focal brain injuries* are those in which a lesion large enough to be visualized with the naked eye has occurred and comprise cortical contusion, subdural hematoma, epidural hematoma, and intracerebral hematoma. These lesions cause neurologic problems, not only because of local brain damage, but also because of masses that develop within the cranium and lead to brain shift, herniation, and ultimately brain stem compression. *Diffuse brain injuries* are associated with more widespread or global disruption of neurologic function, and are not usually associated with macroscopically visible brain lesions. Diffuse brain injuries result from the shaking of the brain within the skull, and are thus lesions that are caused by the inertial or acceleration effects of the mechanical input to the head. Both theoretic[9] and experimental[7] evidence point to rotational acceleration as the primary injury mechanism for diffuse brain injuries.

Since diffuse brain injuries, for the most part, are not associated with visible macroscopic lesions, they have historically been lumped together to include all injuries not associated with focal lesions. Recently, however, diagnostic information has been gained from CT scanning, as well as from neurophysiologic studies, which enables us to more clearly define several categories within this broad group of diffuse brain injuries. These injuries are discussed in detail.

Four categories of diffuse brain injury are now recognized.

1. *Mild concussion.* Several specific concussion syndromes exist that involve temporary disturbance of neurologic function without loss of consciousness.
2. *Classic cerebral concussion.* Classic cerebral concussion is a temporary, reversible neurologic deficiency caused by trauma that results in temporary loss of consciousness.
3. *Diffuse injury.* Diffuse injury is a traumatic brain injury with prolonged loss of consciousness (more than 24 hours). Residual neurologic, psychologic, or personality deficits often result.
4. *Diffuse white matter shearing injury* (shearing injury). Shearing injuries are an extreme form of diffuse brain injury with considerable anatomic disruption of white matter fibers throughout both hemispheres. This lesion has long been recognized by neuropathologists and only recently diagnosed clinically.[3, 13, 15]

MECHANISMS OF CONSCIOUSNESS

Since most diffuse brain injuries involve a disturbance of consciousness, a brief review of the mechanisms that subserve the consciousness state is in order. Consciousness, though difficult to define, is that easily recognized state in which a person can meaningfully interact with his environment. The neuroanatomic substrate of the awake state is a complex interaction involving the cerebral cortex, subcortical structures including the hypothalamus, and numerous brain stem centers. Disconnection of one of these functions from the other two results in an altered state of consciousness. In general terms, the awake state requires the neural activity of the ascending reticular activating system of the brain stem to be projected to the cerebral cortex of both cerebral hemispheres. This projection may be either direct or indirect via hypothalamic-diencephalic centers. Similarly, feedback from the cerebral cortex of both hemispheres onto both the diencephalon and the reticular activating system of the brain stem is necessary for awakeness.

In more general terms, unconsciousness can be produced either by dysfunction of the diencephalon-brain stem or by dysfunction of both cerebral hemispheres. Head injuries cause loss of consciousness in the former instance by compression or by hemorrhage into the brain stem from supratentorial mass lesions produced by focal injuries. Diffuse cerebral injuries, on the other hand, cause widespread dysfunction of both cerebral hemispheres, and thereby alter consciousness by disconnecting the diencephalon or brain stem activation centers from hemispheric activity. Extremely severe diffuse brain injuries, such as those that occur in the shearing injury, can cause not only bilateral cerebral hemisphere dysfunction but also direct anatomic damage within the brain stem itself.

THE SPECTRUM OF DIFFUSE BRAIN INJURIES
(TABLE 8-1)

Diffuse brain injuries form a continuum of progressively more severe brain dysfunction that is caused by increasing amounts of acceleration damage to the brain. Since normal brain function is a delicately balanced electrochemical series of events occurring in billions of cells at any one moment, it is easy to understand how mechanical forces can alter brain function. At low levels of input, this function can be disrupted, at least temporarily, without

TABLE 8-1. Diffuse Brain Injuries

	Mild Concussion	Cerebral Concussion	Diffuse Injury	Shearing Injury
Loss of consciousness	none	immediate	immediate	immediate
Length of unconsciousness	none	<24 hours	>24 hours	days-weeks
Decerebrate posturing	none	none	occasional	present
Post-traumatic amnesia	min	min-hours	days	weeks
Memory deficit	none	min	mild-mod	severe
Motor deficits	none	none	mild	severe
Outcome at 1 month			%	
Good recovery	100	95	21	0
Moderate deficit	0	2	21	0
Severe deficit	0	2	29	9
Vegetative	0	0	21	36
Death	0	0	7	55

causing any structural disruption of the tissue. Thus *physiologic dysfunction can occur in the absence of structural or anatomic disruption*. This concept is the basis for understanding the concussion syndromes, which by their definition are transient, reversible events. It is also easy to imagine that if profound mechanical input is delivered to the brain, structures within the brain can become physically and anatomically disrupted. In this instance, permanent sequelae would occur in those structures that are anatomically disrupted. Therefore, as the magnitude of mechanical input increases, function is first interrupted. Later, when anatomic disruption occurs, both function and structure are disrupted. *The degree of functional disruption, since it precedes anatomic disruption, is always greater than the degree of anatomic disruption.*

To illustrate this concept, one can envision a set of ten axons, each of which participates to an equal degree in a particular neurologic function. Each of the ten axons is stronger and more resistant to mechanical strain than the one that precedes it. If a mild mechanical stress is applied to the ten axons, none is disrupted, but the first axon (the most sensitive one) will have a temporary loss of function. The overall result may not be noticeable, because the other nine axons are still functioning normally. Greater mechanical stress may cause dysfunction of the first five axons, and at this point, a decrease in overall neurologic function is apparent. However, since none of the axons is structurally damaged, function soon returns. A still larger mechanical input now causes physical disruption of the first three axons and physiologic dysfunction of the remaining seven axons. Now all ten axons have had an anatomic or physical disruption so that the neurologic function is totally abolished. However, seven of the axons recover their function, so that little, if any, neurologic deficit is identified. This example should clarify the concept that physiologic disruption is more sensitive to mechanical input than anatomic disruption.

Mild Cerebral Concussion Syndromes

The syndromes of mild cerebral concussion are included in the continuum of diffuse brain injuries because they represent the mildest form of injury in this spectrum. Mild concussion syndromes are those in which consciousness is preserved, but with some degree of noticeable temporary neurologic dysfunction. These injuries are exceedingly common, and because of their mild degree, are often not brought to medical attention; however, they are the most common brain injuries encountered in sports medicine.

The mildest form of head injury results in confusion and disorientation unaccompanied by amnesia. This temporary confusion, without loss of consciousness, lasts only momentarily after the injury, and is so commonplace that it needs no further description. This concussion syndrome is completely reversible and is associated with no sequelae.

Slightly more severe head injury causes confusion with amnesia that develops after 5 or 10 minutes. Again, this is an extremely frequent event, particularly in sports medicine. Athletes may experience such a "ding," and although confused, continue coordinated sensorimotor activities after the accident. If examined immediately after the accident, these players have total recall of the events immediately prior to impact. However, retrograde amnesia develops 5 or 10 minutes later, and thereafter the player does not remember the impact or events immediately before impact. The amnesia usually covers only several minutes before the injury, and although it may diminish somewhat, the player always has some degree of permanent, though short, retrograde amnesia despite resumption of a completely normal consciousness. The confusion and disorientation completely resolve in a matter of moments.

As the mechanical stresses to the brain increase, confusion and amnesia are present from the time of impact. Athletes can usually continue to play while having no recollection of prior events. By this stage, some degree of post-traumatic amnesia (forgetting events after the injury) also occurs, in addition to retrograde amnesia (forgetting events before the injury). The patient's length of confusion may last many minutes, but then his level of consciousness returns to normal; usually with some permanent degree of retrograde and post-traumatic amnesia.

These three syndromes of mild cerebral concussion have been witnessed frequently and described in detail.[5, 14] Although consciousness is preserved, it is clear that some degree of cerebral dysfunction has occurred. The fact that memory mechanisms seem to be the most sensitive to trauma suggests that the cerebral hemispheres, rather than the brain stem, are the location of mild injury forces. The degree of cerebral cortical dysfunction, however, is not sufficient to disconnect the influence of the cerebral hemispheres from the brain stem activating system and therefore consciousness is preserved. No other cortical functions except memory seem at jeopardy, and the only residual deficits that patients with mild concussion syndromes have is the brief retrograde or post-traumatic amnesia. However, since definite alteration of brain function has occurred, athletes who sustain a mild cerebral concussion should not be permitted to participate in the remainder of the contest.

Classic Cerebral Concussion

Classic cerebral concussion is that post-traumatic state that results in loss of consciousness. This state is always accompanied by some degree of retrograde and post-traumatic amnesia. In fact, the length of post-traumatic amnesia is a good measure of the severity of cerebral concussion. Inherent in the usual concept of classic

cerebral concussion is the transient and reversible disturbance of consciousness. In clinical terms, this means that full consciousness has returned within 24 hours. It has also been stated frequently that classic cerebral concussion is associated with no pathologic damage to the brain. However, because of its transient and reversible nature, patients with cerebral concussion do not have neuropathologic examinations. Evidence from experimental cerebral concussion does suggest some mild degree of microscopic neuronal abnormalities.[8] However, in practical terms, classic cerebral concussion can be viewed as a phenomenon of physiologic-neurologic dysfunction with no anatomic disruption.

There is unconsciousness or coma from the moment of head impact in patients with classic cerebral concussion. Although systemic changes such as bradycardia, hypertension, and brief apnea, or neurologic signs such as decerebrate posturing, pupillary dilatation, or flaccidity may occur, they do so only fleetingly and disappear within several seconds. The patient then awakens and is temporarily confused before regaining full alertness and orientation. As in the mild concussion syndromes, classic cerebral concussion is always associated with both retrograde and post-traumatic amnesia. Although these states vary in length, they tend to be longer in cerebral concussion than in the mild concussion syndromes.

Insufficient attention has been placed on the precise events of recovery from classic cerebral concussion. Although, by definition, the loss of consciousness is transient and reversible, sequelae of concussion are commonplace. Certainly, some sequelae such as headache or tinnitus may reflect injuries to the head, inner ear, or other noncerebral structures. However, subtle changes in personality, and in psychologic or memory functioning have been documented and must be of cerebral cortical origin. Thus, although the majority of patients with classic cerebral concussion have no sequelae other than amnesia for the events of impact, some patients may in fact have other long lasting, though subtle, neurologic deficiencies, which must be investigated further.

The mechanisms that underlie classic cerebral concussion are an extension of those of the mild concussion syndromes. With classic cerebral concussion, not only have the mechanical stresses and strains on the brain caused dysfunction of those cortical functions involving memory, but in this instance have caused sufficient physiologic disturbance to temporarily cause diffuse cerebral hemispheric disconnection from the brain stem reticular activating system. Since this dysfunction is physiologic and not structural, when the electrochemical milieu of the brain returns to normal, the normal interaction between the cerebral hemispheres and brain stem is re-established and consciousness is resumed. When classic cerebral concussion occurs in athletic events, prompt medical consultation is required. If the physician determines symptoms or physical signs of extracranial or intracranial abnormality, all sport activity must cease until the abnormality disappears. If no problems are immediately apparent, the athlete may resume his full activity in one to two weeks.

Diffuse Injury

Diffuse injury is the term given to a specific type of diffuse brain injury. Although this term is commonly used for all diffuse brain injuries more severe than classic cerebral concussion, it should be distinguished from shearing injury, which is discussed in this chapter. Diffuse injury is evidenced by loss of consciousness from the time of injury and continuing beyond 24 hours. It is common for patients with diffuse injury to be unconscious for days or weeks before beginning a recovery period. Diffuse injury differs from shearing injury in that there are few signs of decerebrate

posturing and no signs of increased sympathetic activity (hypertension, hyperhidrosis). Thus, patients with diffuse injury are comatose, with either purposeful movements to pain or with withdrawal movements to pain, and only occasionally have brain stem reflexive decorticate or decerebrate posturing. These patients often appear to be restless and may display an increase in random motor movements.

The longer duration of unconsciousness in diffuse injury suggests a more profound disturbance of cerebral function than that which occurs in classic cerebral concussion. Since unconsciousness may last for weeks, it is likely that diffuse injury represents that transition between pure physiologic dysfunction and anatomic disruption. Therefore, it is not surprising that if some degree of anatomic disruption occurs, recovery is incomplete; this indeed is the case with diffuse injury. As patients awaken from coma, they are confused and have long periods of post-traumatic and retrograde amnesia. Deficits of intellectual, cognitive, memory, and personality functions may be mild to severe. Some patients, however, do make an adequate recovery and are capable of resuming all normal activities; thus, the degree of anatomic injury may be mild or marked.

It is postulated that diffuse injury results from the same types of mechanical strains in the brain that cause the mild concussion syndromes and classic cerebral concussion. Physiologic function is impaired in a widespread area throughout the cerebral cortex and diencephalon, and actual tearing (anatomic disruption) occurs in some weaker fibers in both hemispheres. The degree of recovery then depends on the amount and location of anatomic damage. Since the cerebral hemispheres are disconnected from the brain stem reticular activating system for a prolonged period, the resulting prolonged coma makes these patients prone to the numerous complications of the comatose state. Therefore, the recovery process can be curtailed by secondary complications, which can result in death.

Shearing Injury

The shearing injury, also called diffuse white matter shearing injury or diffuse impact injury, is the most severe form of all diffuse brain injuries. It is more severe than diffuse injury and is associated with severe mechanical disruption of many axons in both cerebral hemispheres. Additionally, axonal disruption extends into the diencephalon and brain stem to a greater or lesser degree.

Patients with shearing injury immediately become deeply unconscious and remain so for a prolonged period. They differ from patients with diffuse injury by the presence of abnormal brain stem signs, such as decorticate or decerebrate posturing. In addition, they usually exhibit evidence of immediate autonomic dysfunction, such as hypertension, hyperhidrosis, and hyperpyrexia. Although these patients were formerly diagnosed as having "primary brain-stem injury" or brain-stem contusion, there is now ample evidence that such injuries are exceedingly rare, and that shearing injury is present in most patients with this clinical picture.[2, 10]

The abnormal brain-stem signs of decortication or decerebration are often asymmetrical, and if the patient survives, decrease after several weeks and eventually disappear. The same is true for autonomic dysfunction. These events suggest that recovery from the physiologic dysfunction of brain-stem function is occurring; however, residual deficiencies are profound.

Three types of recovery suggest that there is indeed a continuum of injury within this category of shearing injury. Patients with the least anatomic damage, i.e., with fewer torn axons, can recover to a greater or lesser degree. However, recovery rarely is good, and severe intellectual or bilateral sensorimotor deficits occur. A second pattern of shearing injury commonly occurs in which the patient survives but does not recover. These patients remain in a vegetative state, and although their eyes are open, they have no cognitive connection or response to their environment. However, the most common pattern with shearing injury is death. This indeed is the most severe of all diffuse cerebral injuries and is associated with so much anatomic disruption that it is incompatible with life.

Pathologic evaluation of patients who die with shearing injury shows little macroscopic change. Careful examination, however, does disclose two lesions that are regularly associated with shearing injury. Hemorrhagic lesions in the superior cerebellar peduncle and corpus callosum are virtually always present in shearing injuries. These may be the only visible findings, but disruption of the fornix or hemorrhages in the periventricular regions may also be seen.

The principal findings in shearing injury are evident only on microscopic examination of the brain. The lack of such examinations has caused an inadequate appreciation of the frequency of this severe lesion in the past. However, careful microscopic examination discloses torn axons throughout the white matter of both cerebral hemispheres. Depending on the time from injury to death, this is manifested by axonal retraction balls or by microglial clusters. If the patient has survived many weeks, degeneration of the long white matter tracts extends into the brain stem.

Thus, pathologic information verifies the concept that at this end of the spectrum anatomic disruption of innumerable axons has occurred. It is postulated that the survivors who have recoverable or nonrecoverable shearing injuries have suffered slightly less anatomical damage. Both diffuse injury and shearing injury are major brain injuries and in no instance should an athlete sustaining such injuries return to any contact sporting activity.

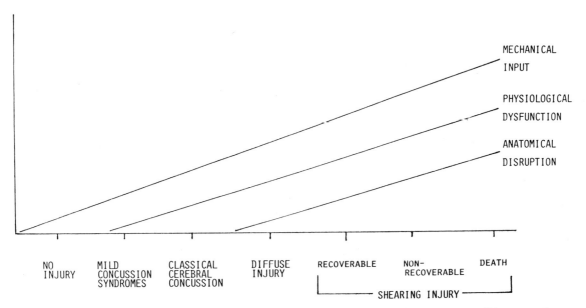

Fig. 8-1. The continuum of diffuse brain injuries. As mechanical strains increase, the mild concussion syndromes occur,[12] followed by classic cerebral concussion, diffuse injury, and shearing injury. Functional activity of the brain is always more disturbed than anatomic disruption.

THE SPECTRUM OF DIFFUSE CEREBRAL INJURIES

Diffuse cerebral injuries form a spectrum of severity, beginning with mild concussion syndromes on the one end and ending with shearing injury, which results in death, on the other end (Fig. 8-1). It is postulated that as mechanical input increases, brain acceleration causes progressively more shear, tensile, and compression strains to the brain substance. At first these strains are insufficient to cause any injury. As they increase, mild physiologic disruption of cortical processing causes the *mild concussion syndromes*. More severe input increases the strains in the brain. These are insufficient to cause disruption of axons, but are sufficient to cause temporary global dysfunction of cortical activity. This results in a temporary disconnection of the cerebral cortex from the reticular activating system necessary for consciousness, causing *classic cerebral concussion*. As mechanical strains increase further, the structurally weaker axons fail, and anatomic disruption begins. In *diffuse injury*, physiologic dysfunction is more prominent than mechanical disruption. As more and more axons break, the *shearing injury* is seen. By the time shearing injury occurs, sufficient physiologic dysfunction of brain-stem activity occurs, prolonged unconsciousness is produced, and depending on the amount of anatomic damage to axons, either partial recovery, nonrecovery, or death occur. Thus, a fatal shearing injury is a situation in which the mechanical input forces cause such large strains that an overwhelming number of nerve fibers are destroyed.

PHENOMENA RELATED TO DIFFUSE BRAIN INJURIES

Several events are related to diffuse brain injuries, which, because of different mechanisms of causation or because of different pathophysiologic effects, must be differentiated from diffuse brain injuries. These events include vasovagal phenomena and brain swelling.

Vasovagal syncope must be distinguished from the mild concussion syndromes and from classic cerebral concussion. This event is a fainting spell caused by intense, brief stimulation of the vagal parasympathetic nervous system. Activation of vagal centers commonly occurs from impacts or punches to the abdomen (the solar plexus punch of boxers), but may also be caused by head movements that stimulate the vagus nerve in or around the head. Blows to the face can cause sufficient head movement to activate the vagus. That this commonly occurs before the input forces are sufficient to cause classic cerebral concussion, is well-evidenced in experimental head injury.[1]

Whatever the cause, vagal hyperactivity results in profound bradycardia and hypotension. If mild, these may lead to lightheaded or swooning sensations. If severe, the bradycardia and hypotension can decrease cerebral blood flow sufficiently to result in loss of consciousness. Thus, a mild vasovagal episode may mimic one of the mild concussion syndromes, while a more severe event can cause fainting and loss of consciousness, and resemble a classic cerebral concussion. The true brain injury syndromes can usually be differentiated from vagal events by the absence of retrograde or post-traumatic amnesia, and by the presence of a slow, bounding pulse. Additionally, a momentary delay often occurs before the vasovagal syncope results in loss of consciousness. Thus, the patient may stagger for a few seconds before collapsing. Classic cerebral concussion occurs exactly at the time of impact and is always due to head, rather than body, impact.

Brain swelling is a poorly understood phenomenon that can accompany any type of head injury. Swelling is not synonymous with cerebral edema, which refers to a specific increase in extravascular brain water. Such an increase in water content may not occur in brain swelling, and current evidence favors the concept that brain swelling is due in part to increased intravascular blood within the brain. This is caused by a vascular reaction to head injury, which leads to vasodilatation and increased cerebral blood volume. If this increased cerebral blood volume continues for a long enough time, vascular permeability may increase and true edema may result.

Although brain swelling may occur in any type of head injury, the magnitude of the swelling does not correlate well with the severity of the injury. Thus, both severe and minor injuries may be complicated by the presence of brain swelling. The effects of brain swelling are thus additive to those of primary brain injury, and may in certain instances, be more severe than the primary injury itself.

Despite a lack of knowledge of the precise mechanism that causes brain swelling, it can be conceptualized in two general forms (Table 8-2). It should be remembered that many different types of brain swelling exist, and that acute and delayed brain swelling represent a phenomenologic, rather than a mechanistic approach.

Acute brain swelling occurs in several circumstances. Swelling that accompanies focal brain lesions tends to be localized, whereas diffuse brain injuries are as-

TABLE 8-2. Brain Swelling

I. Acute swelling
  A. Associated with focal lesions
    1. Acute subdural hematoma—hemispheric
    2. Contusions—focal
  B. Associated with diffuse lesions
    1. Diffuse injury—generalized
    2. Shearing injury—generalized

II. Delayed swelling
  A. Associated with lethargy
  B. Associated with light coma
  C. Associated with deep coma

---

sociated with generalized swelling. Focal swelling is usually present beneath contusions, but does not often contribute additional deleterious effects. On the other hand, the swelling that occurs with acute subdural hematomas, though principally hemispheric in distribution, may cause more mass effect than the hematoma itself. In such circumstances, the small amount of blood in the subdural space may not be the entire reason for the patient's neurologic state. If the hematoma is removed, the acute brain swelling may progress so rapidly that the brain protrudes through the craniotomy opening. Every neurosurgeon is all too familiar with external herniation of the brain, which when it occurs, is difficult to treat.

In an experimental model of acute subdural hematoma, this type of "malignant brain swelling" occurs regularly.[6] Shortly after the subdural blood is removed, the brain swells so massively that it protrudes well above the outer table of the skull (Fig. 8-2). Measurement of tissue water content, studies with labeled sucrose, and electron microscopic observations have failed to demonstrate cerebral edema in the swollen brain. This is indirect evidence that this variety of acute brain swelling is not due to cerebral edema, but rather to increased cerebral blood volume.

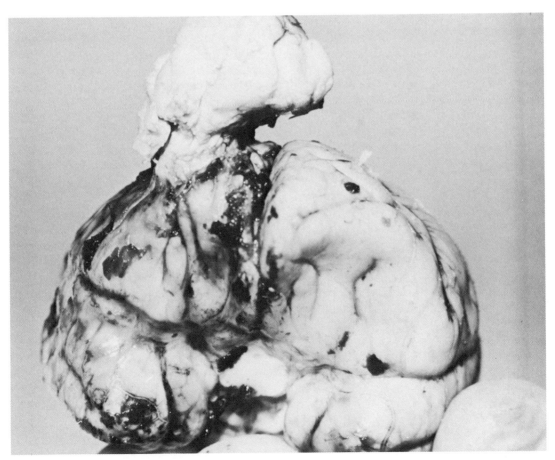

Fig. 8-2. This frontal view of a monkey brain demonstrates the massive amount of acute brain swelling that can occur after the removal of an acute subdural hematoma. The "mushroom" over the frontal lobe (viewer's left) is swollen brain that protruded through the craniotomy defect moments after a subdural hematoma was evacuated.

The more serious types of diffuse brain injuries are associated with generalized, rather than focal, acute brain swelling. Although not all patients with diffuse injury or shearing injury have brain swelling, the incidence of swelling is higher than in patients with either classic cerebral concussion or one of the mild concussion syndromes. Because of the serious nature of the underlying injury, it is difficult to determine the extent of swelling in these patients. The swelling, though widespread throughout the brain, may not cause a rise in intracranial pressure for several days. This late rise in pressure probably reflects the formation of true cerebral edema, and it may be that diffuse swelling associated with severe diffuse brain injuries is deleterious because it produces edema. In any event, this type of swelling is different from the type of swelling associated with acute subdural hematomas.

Delayed brain swelling may occur minutes to hours after head injury. It is usually diffuse and is often associated with the milder forms of diffuse brain injuries. Whether delayed swelling is the same or a different phenomenon than the acute swelling of the more serious diffuse injuries is unknown. However, in less severe diffuse injuries there is a distinct time interval before delayed swelling becomes manifest, thus confirming that the primary insult to the brain was not serious. Considering the high frequency of the mild concussion syndromes and of classic cerebral concussion, the incidence of delayed swelling must be low. However, when it occurs, delayed swelling can cause profound neurologic changes or even death.

In its most severe form, severe delayed swelling can cause deep coma. The usual history is that of an injury associated with a mild concussion or a classic cerebral concussion from which the patient recovers. Minutes to hours later the patient becomes lethargic, then stuporous, and finally lapses into a coma. The coma may either be a light coma with appropriate motor responses to painful stimuli, or a deep coma associated with decorticate or decerebrate posturing.

The key difference between these patients and those with diffuse injury or shearing injury, is that in the latter cases the coma and abnormal motor signs are present from the moment of injury, whereas with delayed cerebral swelling there is a time interval without these signs. This distinction is significant, however, since with diffuse injury or shearing injury a certain amount of primary structural damage has occurred at the moment of impact but is not present in delayed swelling. Therefore, the deleterious effects of delayed swelling should be potentially reversible, and if these effects are controlled, the outcome should be good. However, control of the effects of brain swelling may be difficult. Vigorous monitoring of, and attention to, intracranial pressure is necessary, and prompt and vigorous treatment of raised intracranial pressure is required in order to control brain swelling. If this is successfully accomplished, the mortality rate from increased intracranial pressure associated with diffuse brain swelling should be low.[4]

The severe form of delayed brain swelling often appears in a stereotypical fashion, primarily in children between 4 and 10 years of age. It may result from a variety of head injuries and is usually characterized by a more or less completely lucid interval immediately after injury. The children then become lethargic and lapse into coma, often in association with an early post-traumatic seizure. A dynamic sequence of events occurs over the next several months. First, brain swelling is manifest on CT scans by the absence of cerebral ventricles and subarachnoid spaces. If intracranial pressure is adequately controlled, a week or more after the injury brain swelling begins to diminish, often to the point that extracerebral collections occur. By one month after injury these collections disappear spontaneously and the brain, which had been swollen, begins to shrink. Thus, the ventricular system becomes enlarged, often in association with enlargement of the sulci around the brain, giving a computed tomographic appearance of cerebral atrophy. By this time some degree of neurologic recovery from the deep coma has occurred. Still later, approximately six to nine months after injury, the computerized tomographic appearance of cerebral atrophy disappears, and the brain resumes its normal configuration. The exact mechanisms that cause this prolonged series of events is unknown, but the final outcome in these patients, if their intracranial pressure is controlled, is good with no residual neurologic deficit.

Less severe delayed cerebral swelling may also occur with the mild concussion syndromes and with classic cerebral concussion. These often are not diagnosed because they are associated only with early post-traumatic lethargy, which soon disappears. However, these patients undergo the same type of early clinical course as those patients with more severe delayed cerebral swelling. Again, after a mild concussion or classic cerebral concussion, the patient awakens and is normal for some moments to hours. Thereafter, a degree of lethargy occurs that lasts for hours to days. This state is reasonably common and probably represents a mild degree of delayed brain swelling.

Whether mild or severe, delayed brain swelling is an epiphenomenon of diffuse brain injuries that is poorly understood. Since it does not occur in all patients with diffuse brain injuries, it can be viewed as a reaction to injury rather than as a primary injury. As with the immediate types of brain swelling, it is likely that delayed brain swelling initially represents a vascular reaction to injury in which the cerebral blood vessels lose their normal vascular control mechanisms and dilate widely. This results in increased cerebral blood flow and volume.[11] True edema formation may subsequently occur and result in increased intracranial pressure. Thus the effects of brain swelling, whether immediate or delayed, are added to the effects of the primary brain injury, and in the milder forms of diffuse brain injury, may represent the most serious threat to survival.

SUMMARY

Diffuse brain injuries are consequences of shaking of the brain. They result from acceleration effects of head trauma and have little if anything to do with localized phenomena of the impact. Acceleration causes shear, tensile, and compression strains to be generated throughout the brain, and these strains are the primary injurious factors. Since the brain is weakest in the shearing mode, rotational acceleration is more injurious than other types of acceleration because of the high shear strains it induces. The primary injuries to the brain caused by acceleration form a continuum of injuries, the severity increasing as acceleration of the brain increases. Low strains, caused by low levels of acceleration, may cause no injury. As acceleration increases, the mild concussion syndromes result, but these are not associated with loss of consciousness. Classic cerebral concussion is caused by a further increase in acceleration, and is associated with transient reversible loss of consciousness. If further strains are induced in the brain by higher levels of acceleration, anatomic damage begins to occur and is associated with more severe functional changes of the brain. Diffuse injury is a primary injury associated with prolonged loss of consciousness and mild diffuse anatomic damage. Shearing injury is the most severe form of the diffuse brain injuries and is accompanied by deep coma, signs of decerebrate posturing, and autonomic dysfunction. It is associated with widespread disruption of axons throughout the white matter of both cerebral hemispheres. Though patients may recover from mild forms, most patients with shearing injury either die or remain in a nonrecoverable vegetative state.

The continuum of diffuse brain injuries is associated with both physiologic dysfunction, and at the most severe end of the spectrum, anatomic disruption. Although the individual primary diffuse brain injuries are distinct, they are a continuum, and one syndrome may merge indistinguishably into the next. This can pose difficulties in making a precise diagnosis in certain cases. Since the functional changes, in themselves, are reversible, the end result of the primary injury is dependent on the amount of anatomic disruption that occurs at the moment of injury.

Brain swelling may be superimposed on primary diffuse brain injuries. Although brain swelling does not occur in every case of diffuse brain injuries, it can add deleterious effects to the primary injury by causing increased intracranial pressure. Rapidly occurring brain swelling is associated with severe diffuse brain injuries, whereas delayed brain swelling appears in conjunction with the less severe varieties of diffuse brain injuries.

Diffuse brain injuries and brain swelling form a distinct group of head injuries, which have different mechanisms of causation, different pathophysiologic influences on the brain, and different outcomes than focal brain injuries.

REFERENCES

1. Abel, J., Gennarelli, T.A., and Segawa, H.: Incidence and severity of cerebral concussion in the rhesus monkey following sagittal plane angular acceleration. *In* Twenty-Second Stapp Car Crash Conference Proceedings. New York, Society of Automotive Engineers, 1978.
2. Adams, J.H.: The neuropathology of head injuries. *In* Handbook of Clinical Neurology. Vol. 23. Edited by P.J. Vinken, and G.W. Bruyn. Oxford, North-Holland Publishing, 1975.
3. Adams, J.H., et al.: Diffuse brain damage of immediate impact type. Brain, *100*:489, 1977.
4. Bruce, D.A., et al.: Outcome following severe head injuries in children. J. Neurosurg., *48*:679, 1978.
5. Fischer, C.M.: Concussion amnesia. Neurology, *16*:826, 1966.
6. Gennarelli, T.A., Dzernicki, Z., and Segawa, H.: Acute brain swelling in experimental head injury. Submitted to J. Neurosurg., 1980.
7. Gennarelli, T.A., Thibault, L.E., and Ommaya, A.K.: Pathophysiologic responses to rotational and translational acceleration of the head. *In* Sixteenth Stapp Car Crash Conference Proceedings. New York, Society of Automotive Engineers, 1972.
8. Groat, R.A., Windle, W.F., and Magoun, H.W.: Functional and structural changes in the monkey's brain during and after concussion. J. Neurosurg., *2*:26, 1945.
9. Holbourn, A.H.: Mechanics of head injury. Lancet, *2*:438, 1943.
10. Mitchell, D.E., and Adams, J.H.: Primary focal impact damage to the brain stem in blunt head injuries: does it exist? Lancet, *1*:215, 1973.
11. Obrist, W.D., et al.: Relation of cerebral blood flow to neurological status and outcome in head-injured patients. J. Neurosurg., *51*:292, 1979.
12. Ommaya, A.K., and Gennarelli, T.A.: Cerebral concussion and traumatic unconsciousness. Correlation of experimental and clinical observations on blunt head injuries. Brain, *97*:633, 1974.
13. Strich, S.J.: The pathology of brain damage due to blunt head injuries. *In* The Late Effects of Head Injury. Edited by A.E. Walker, W.F. Caveness, and M. Critchley. Springfield, Charles C Thomas, 1969.
14. Yarnell, P.R., and Lynch, S.: The "ding": amnestic states in football trauma. Neurology, *23*:186, 1973.
15. Zimmerman, R.A., Bilaniuk, L., and Gennarelli, T.A.: Computed tomography of shearing injuries of the cerebral white matter. Radiology, *127*:393, 1978.

Chapter 9

Focal Intracranial Hematoma

Leonard A. Bruno

In discussing the occurrence of intracranial hematoma as a result of athletic injury, two major points must be emphasized. First, due to recent developments in clinical evaluation of patients and animal research correlation, we have a satisfactory understanding of the mechanism of occurrence of focal intracranial hematoma, which is somewhat different from older concepts of head-injured patients. Second, management of head-injured patients has advanced rapidly and changed dramatically over the last decade from what was accepted medical practice in the past.

DIAGNOSIS

In general, athletic head injuries tend to be dynamic injuries that occur from impact with contact phenomena. These injuries tend to be focal in nature and are generally less severe than diffuse injuries resulting from acceleration and deceleration. In the unconscious patient, the task is to differentiate between the role played by focal and diffuse strains developed within the head as a result of trauma.

The biologic response to mechanical trauma consists of four basic components: focal concussion; generalized cerebral concussion; primary brain lesions, such as contusions or hematoma; or skull fracture.

It is important to realize that each of these four components of biologic response can occur in isolation. The severity of head injury is determined by the relative contributions of these four components plus the added deleterious effects of secondary responses and injury developing after the primary traumatic event. Secondary brain injury, caused by cerebral ischemia or hypoxia resulting from increased intracranial pressure from hemorrhage or brain swelling, or the indirect consequence of hypotension or respiratory compromise, has come to be recognized as the important problem in the care and treatment of head-injured patients.

In the 1960s, it was neurosurgical dogma that patients brought to the hospital unconscious as a result of head injury, who were either deeply comatose or showed signs of neurologic deterioration under observation, required burr hole surgery, often bilateral, as an emergency procedure to assess and treat the possibility of significant intracranial hematoma. Patients were assumed, for all intents and purposes, to have subdural hematoma or epidural hematoma until proven otherwise.

In the early 1970s, computerized tomography (CT) of the brain provided a distinct advance in the diagnostic evaluation of severely head-injured patients. Prior to the development of CT scanning, the procedures most often used in diagnosing the pathologic process in severe head injuries were carotid angiography and ventriculography. These procedures were time consuming, somewhat difficult to perform, and involved a certain intrinsic risk from the test procedure alone.

Since 1973, these procedures have been replaced by the CT scan. Computerized tomograms of head-injured patients can be performed quickly, are noninvasive, and carry essentially no risk.[1] In addition to these logistical advantages, CT scanning provides much information never before available for head-injured patients. Focal lesions such as acute subdural hematoma, epidural hematoma, contusion, and intracerebral hemorrhage are easily diagnosed and visualized. Their distribution and contribution to the overall mass effect of any brain injury can be assessed. Just as important, the large number of patients with diffuse lesions can be classified. Currently, the CT scan is the primary and often only neuroradiologic procedure performed on severely injured patients. To obtain adequate skull roentgenograms delays the time before the patient can be taken to the intensive care unit for monitoring necessary treatment. The most important information obtained from the plain skull roentgenogram is definition of depressed skull fractures and the presence of linear fractures over meningeal vessels or venous sinuses. The CT scan identifies not only depressed skull fractures, but the extent of depression, the presence or absence of an underlying clot, and the state of the underlying brain. Therefore, in this regard it is superior to skull roentgenograms. Linear fractures may not be demonstrated on CT scan. However, more importantly, the presence of epidural hematoma is easily identified. For these reasons, routine skull roentgenograms in comatose patients following head injury are no longer obtained. If the CT scan is not available, many patients may require angiography. These include those with focal neurologic deficit and coma, those who show progressive neurologic deterioration, and those deeply comatose patients in whom it is impossible to differentiate between the primary, diffuse cerebral injury, and the late effects of an expanding intracranial mass.

Whenever possible, a CT scan should be performed to avoid the use of exploratory burr holes as the primary treatment for patients in whom such surgery frequently results in negative findings. Following a normal CT scan, if progressive deterioration of the patient's level of consciousness occurs or if intracranial hypertension develops, a repeat CT scan insures that there has not been the delayed development of intracranial hematoma.[1]

An accurate picture exists of the frequency of intracranial mass lesions that occur following head injury of all types. As determined by CT scan in a series of 146 children and 171 adults, the incidence of acute epidural, subdural, and intracerebral hematoma, or hemorrhagic contusions total 24% in children and 51% in adults.[1] Thus, the majority of head-trauma patients admitted to the hospital do not have an acute intracranial hematoma as the major cause of coma.

The entire spectrum of traumatic intracranial hematomas occurs in sports injuries. These include cerebral contusions, intracerebral hematomas, epidural hematomas, and acute subdural hematomas. The presentation of athletic head-injured patients who have had serious trauma is similar in most instances. Management depends on definitive diagnosis and varies depending on the underying pathologic process.

Head injuries in sports occur in a variety of ways. Many of these injuries involve significant impact to the skull or cranium by a bat, racquet, or club. Other injuries have components of impulse because athletes are often hurling themselves through space or moving at velocities significant enough to cause sizable impulse inertial loading of the brain to occur with rapid deceleration. Even in athletic contests such as baseball, basketball, or soccer in which head contact or injury is unlikely, serious brain injury can result from a slip, a fall, accidental collision, or contact with playing equipment.

Head injuries in the athletic setting tend to be of the impact type with translational or unidirectional application of force and minimal amounts of rotation. In these situations, it is not unusual for patients to suffer significant head injury without loss of consciousness. It is known from experimental work that the development of cerebral contusion or small intracerebral hematoma is related to head movement in an interesting manner.[2] If an athlete's head is stable and not moving at the time of impact, he most likely will develop cerebral contusion or a small hematoma under the site of contact. On the contrary, if the athlete is moving in space with a certain velocity and strikes an immovable object with his head, he will develop, in many instances, cerebral contusion or intracerebral hematoma on the side opposite to the area of contact. This is the present explanation of the cause for coup versus contrecoup contusion and hematoma. By their very nature, these types of impact or minimal impulse injuries rarely cause significant unconsciousness.

As outlined by Ommaya and Gennarelli,[2] the degree of alteration of consciousness is directly related to the amount of inertial loading and the rotational component induced at the time of injury, which then cause shear strains in the brain. In precise animal experiments carried out on rhesus monkeys, researchers have clearly demonstrated that the same degree of accleration, deceleration, and inertial loading, when applied to animals in a purely translational mode versus the same inertial loading applied to animals permitted to rotate their heads through 45°, gave the startling but reproducible result that all animals in the rotated group exhibited neurologic evidence of cerebral concussion, defined as the sudden onset of paralytic coma or traumatic unconsciousness. In contrast, none of the translated group showed this effect. Thus, it was possible to produce cerebral concussion only when the moving head was allowed to angulate or rotate. When rotation was prevented and the head allowed to move in a straight line only, cerebral concussion did *not* occur.

Conversely, the only animals to develop intracerebral hematoma were those that had received inertial loading in a translational or straight line manner. Petechial hemorrhage of the gray-white interfaces in the brain was present in a bilaterally symmetric fashion in every member of the rotated group of animals, but in only two of the translated group in a sparse asymmetric fashion. These experimental analogs have a clinical analog in athletic head injuries. Most athletic injuries are caused by impact and translational loading. Loss of consciousness in this situation is unusual; whereas development of intracerebral hematoma or contusion without loss of consciousness and without severe neurologic deficit is likely to result from this mechanism of injury.

Intracerebral Hematoma and Contusion

Athletic injuries of this type occur in patients with impressive intracerebral pathology who have never suffered loss of consciousness or focal neurologic deficit, but who do have persistent headache or periods of post-head-injury confusion and post-traumatic amnesia. As with any head-injured patients, athletic head-injured patients with such symptoms should have a CT scan to permit early differentiation between solid intracerebral hematoma and hemorrhagic contusion with surrounding edema.

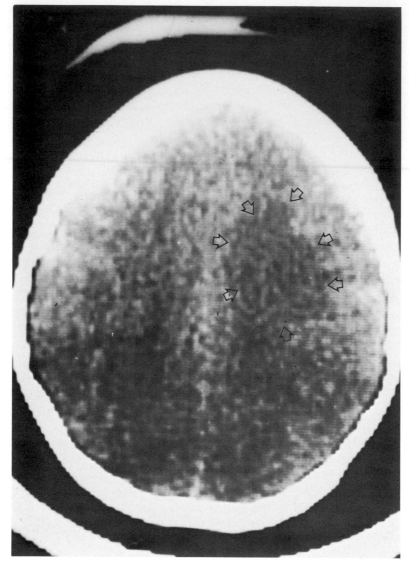

Fig. 9-1. *Case 1:* Arrows surround a focal area of cerebral edema, which on a CT display is hypodense or blacker than brain tissue. This localized area of edema in the right temporal lobe represents a small contusion.

Case 1: A 13-year-old boy was injured while playing ice hockey. At practice, he was struck with a hockey puck in the right temporal region. He fell to the ice, had a momentary episode of confusion, but recovered almost immediately except for complaints of shoulder pain. He was brought to the emergency room for evaluation of possible shoulder separation and was noted by the examining physician to be complaining of pain over the site where he was struck with the puck. Neurologic examination was completely within normal limits, but because of the location of the impact, skull roentgenograms were obtained, which demonstrated a linear fracture in the right temporal region. A CT scan (Fig. 9-1) showed an area of radiolucency or decreased density in the right temporal region indicative of edema, which most likely represents a small contusion with surrounding swelling.

Intracerebral hematoma and contusion can be caused by a combination of impact and impulse injury.

Case 2: While playing basketball on a macadam court at home, a 15-year-old youngster slipped, fell backwards, and struck the back of his head on the hard surface. The CT scan (Fig. 9-2) demonstrates diffuse bifrontal edema with multiple areas of small hemorrhagic contusion.

This is an example of a severe contrecoup type of injury. That is, his decelerating head struck the immovable court floor, causing his frontal lobes to strike the frontal bone of his skull. This type of injury occurs in sports in which the participant often has some type of induced body velocity. It happens to riders falling from horses, skiers, skaters, and occasionally boxers, basketball players, or hockey players falling onto the hard playing surface.

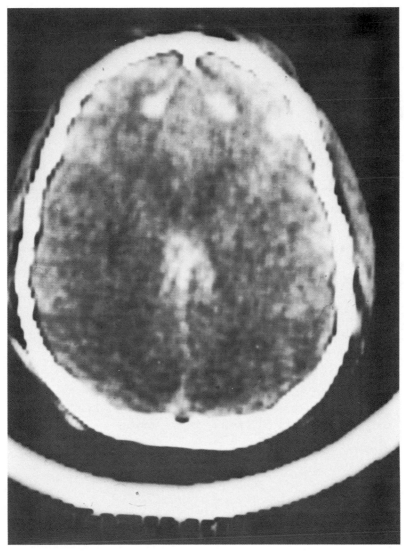

Fig. 9-2. *Case 2:* CT scan demonstrating diffuse bilateral frontal lobe edema with multiple areas of small hemorrhagic contusion. Blood is hypodense or whiter than brain tissue. This represents a severe contrecoup type injury.

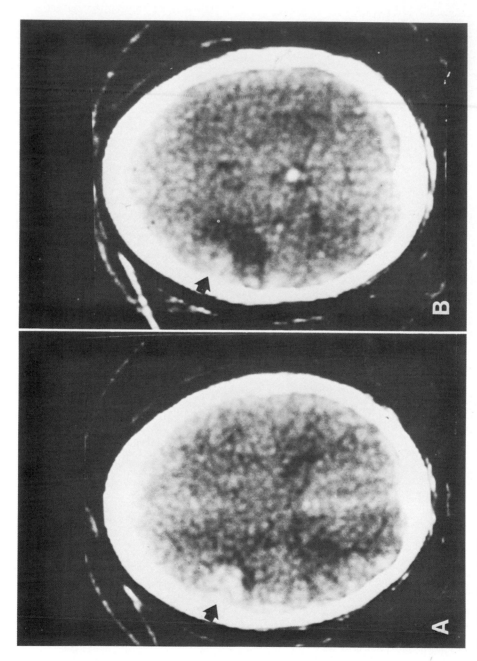

Fig. 9-3. *Case 3:* CT scan demonstrating a small left frontal intracerebral hematoma that is hypodense or whiter than brain tissue (arrow). *A.* CT display is the lesion immediately after initial injury. *B.* CT display taken 9 days postinjury. Postbeginning resolution of the hematoma.

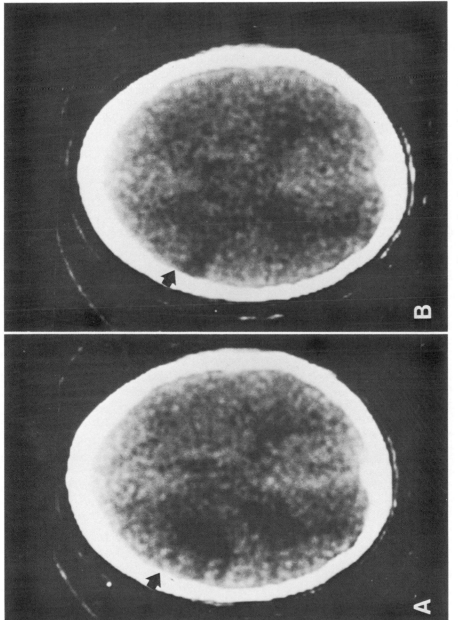

Fig. 9-4. *Case 3:* CT scan *A* taken 16 days postinjury, while the scan *B* was taken 3 months postinjury. Note the marked resolution of the intracerebral hematoma with appropriate conservative (nonoperative) management.

Case 3: A 16-year-old boy was struck in the left frontal region with a baseball. Following his injury he did not lose consciousness, had a fairly severe headache, was a bit lethargic and confused, but never went into coma and came to the hospital because of persistent headaches and nausea. The CT scan (Fig. 9-3) shows his initial picture (Fig. 9-3 *A*), and one obtained 9 days postinjury (Fig. 9-3 *B*). What can be seen is a small frontal intracerebral hematoma, which with appropriate conservative management proceeds to its natural history of resolution. A scan of the same patient at 16 days postinjury (Fig. 9-4 *A*) and again 3 months later (Fig. 9-4 *B*), shows that while the brain is somewhat slower than other organs to resolve such injuries, it does recover nicely. What would be anticipated if the scan were repeated a year later is that there would be no abnormalities whatsoever.

Case 4: A 14-year-old boy was allegedly struck with a soccer ball. He did not fall to the ground and had no loss of consciousness. He had no focal or easily recognizable neurologic deficit, and was brought to the hospital because of confusion, nausea, and headache. On neurologic examination, he had diffuse right-sided visual field deficit which could not be well defined. A CT scan (Fig. 9-5) demonstrated the intracerebral hematoma in the left occipital lobe. Because of the unusual location of the hematoma, the patient also underwent an arteriogram to determine if he had an underlying arteriovenous malformation or other predisposing condition. The study was negative. His CT scan from day 23 postinjury shows beginning resolution of the hematoma, and with administration of sufficient amounts of corticosteroids, no evidence of spreading cerebral edema or brain shift. By day 123, represented by the bottom series of scans, the hematoma had almost resolved. The patient made a complete recovery with no residual deficit.

Epidural Hematoma

Epidural hematomas are readily correctable lesions if they are identified and removed before secondary injury to the brain stem has occurred from increased intracranial pressure. A review of 300 head-injured patients in coma at the time of evaluation revealed epidural hematoma present in only 4 to 5%. Because they occur as a result of impact, epidural hematomas develop more often than usual in athletic head injuries although statistics on their incidence are not readily available.

The pathophysiology of epidural hematoma is that the middle meningeal or other meningeal arteries are often imbedded in bony grooves in the skull and skull fractures, crossing this bony groove, frequently tear the blood vessel at that site. Because bleeding in these instances is arterial, accumulation of clot continues under high pressure and will not tamponade early enough to prevent serious brain injury.

The classic picture of an epidural hematoma is that of loss of consciousness at the time of injury, followed by recovery of consciousness in a variable period, after which the patient is lucid. This is followed by the onset of increasingly severe headache, decreased level of consciousness, dilatation of one pupil (usually on the same side as the clot), and decerebrate posturing and weakness (usually on the side opposite the hematoma). In our experience, however, only one third of the patients with epidural hematoma present with this classic history. Another one third of patients do not become unconscious until late in their course, and the other third are unconscious from the time of injury and remain unconscious throughout their course.

The absence of a classic clinical picture of an epidural hematoma cannot be relied upon to rule out this diagnosis, and the best diagnostic test for evaluating these patients is CT scan (Fig. 9-6). If this is unavailable, angiography is necessary. Epidural hematoma can be a clinical diagnosis, however, and in a rapidly deteriorating patient, a plain skull roentgenogram is often adequate to plan surgery. Epidural hematoma is almost always associated with fracture, and since fracture is not uncommon in sports-related head injuries, should be considered as part of the differ-

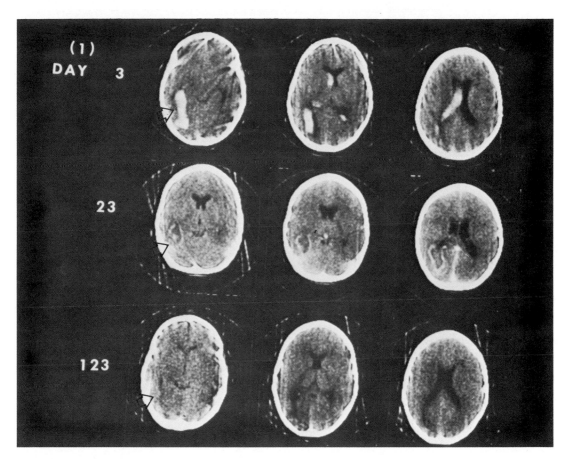

Fig. 9-5. *Case 4:* Serial CT scans taken at 3, 23, and 123 days postinjury demonstrating presence and subsequent resolution of a left occipital lobe intracerebral hematoma. Patient had been treated conservatively and made a complete recovery without neurologic deficit.

ential diagnosis in all instances. Despite the ready availability of CT scan in our institution, 15% of our patients, both adults and children with epidural hematomas, have been operated on with no special diagnostic tests. These patients had deteriorated so rapidly that immediate surgical decompression was necessary. The treatment of epidural hematoma is surgical removal of the clot.

Postoperatively, about 80% of epidural hematoma patients do not have elevated intracranial pressure. However, all patients should be monitored and treated expectantly. Therefore, an intracranial pressure monitor is inserted at the time of surgery.

Acute Subdural Hematoma

Athletic head injuries result from lower inertial loading than serious head injuries caused by vehicular accidents or falling from heights. Thus, an acute subdural hematoma also occurs much more frequently than epidural hematoma in athletes. In head-injured patients in general, approximately three times as many acute subdural hematomas occur as do epidural hematomas.

Acute subdural hematomas have been clearly identified as two main types: (1) those with a collection of blood in the subdural space, which are apparently not associated with underlying cerebral contu-

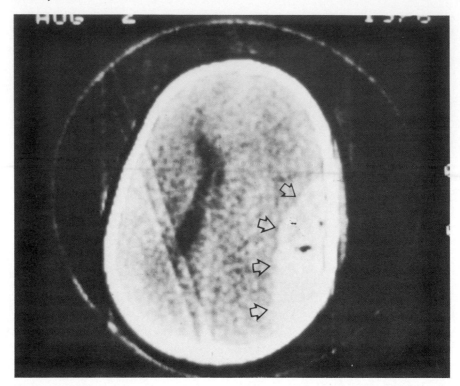

Fig. 9-6. Epidural hematoma is a contained lenticular-shaped collection of blood at the periphery of the brain. Also demonstrated is associated compression of the ipsilateral ventricle.

sion or edema (Fig. 9-7), and (2) those with collections of blood in the subdural space, but associated with an obvious contusion on the surface of the brain and hemispheric brain injury with swelling (Fig. 9-8). The mortality rate for simple subdural hematomas is approximately 20%, but this increases to more than 50% for subdural hematomas with an underlying brain injury.

Patients with an acute subdural hematoma are typically unconscious, they may or may not have a history of deterioration, and they frequently display focal neurologic findings. Patients with simple subdural hematomas are more likely to have a lucid interval following their injury, and are less likely to be unconscious at admission than those patients with hemispheric injury and brain swelling. It is necessary to obtain a CT scan or angiogram to diagnose an acute subdural hematoma. The size of the subdural clot relative to the size of the midline shift of the brain structures can be evaluated best by CT scan. Of patients with acute subdural hematoma, 84% also have an associated hemorrhagic contusion or intracerebral hematoma with associated brain swelling.

Case 5: A 21-year-old intercollegiate football player was admitted to the Hospital of the University of Pennsylvania on September 2, 1978, after collapsing during an intrasquad scrimmage. Upon arrival at the emergency room approximately 15 minutes after his collapse, he was unresponsive to painful stimuli, had a fixed dilated nonreactive left pupil, and showed episodic decerebrate rigidity. His vital signs were normal. Motion pictures of the contact activity during a live scrimmage the day before his admission showed that the player, an offensive guard, was kicked on the right side of his helmet by the knee of a linebacker. That evening and the following morning, he complained to his teammates of headaches and ringing in his ears, but he participated

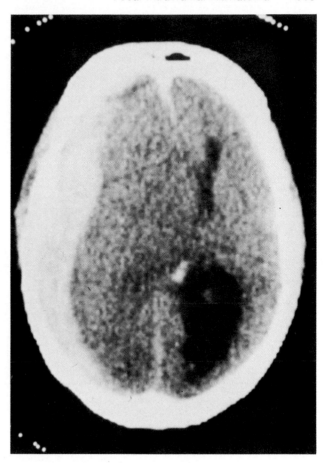

Fig. 9-7. CT scan of a large left subdural hematoma. There is compression of adjacent brain tissue and cerebral edema is not evident. Such a collection requires surgical decompression. The contrast between this lesion, which requires surgical intervention, and that demonstrated in Figure 9-8, which responded to conservative management, vividly illustrates the difference in the pathomechanics of an acute subdural hematoma frequently seen as a result of athletic injuries, and the more subacute lesion seen in the older population.

in the morning noncontact workout. Motion pictures of the afternoon live scrimmage did not demonstrate a significant blow to his head. Following the eighth play of that scrimmage, he returned to the huddle confused and disoriented and was helped to the side of the field where he collapsed and lost consciousness. A computerized tomographic (CT) scan demonstrated a small, acute, subdural hematoma on the left with marked left cortical edema that caused displacement of the ventricles to the right (Fig. 9-8). Treatment consisted of large intravenous doses of mannitol, dexamethasone (Decadron), and pentobarbital. Following initiation of treatment, his left pupil became reactive, and intracranial pressure, which was monitored by an intracranial pressure (ICP) bolt, could then be maintained within the normal range. During an induced coma that was maintained for 10 days, respirations were controlled and supported by a respirator. The patient's hospital course during this time was satisfactory, demonstrated on CT scans by resolution of the left hemispheric edema and subdural hematoma, and by the maintenance of normal vital signs. Three weeks after admission he was transferred to a rehabilitation center. Five weeks after his injury he was discharged from the center without apparent residual neurologic impairment, and has subsequently graduated from the university (Fig. 9-9).

The term "acute subdural hematoma" raises the image in most physicians' minds of a large collection of clotted blood in the intracranial cavity, compressing the brain substance and causing compromise due to the hematoma occupying space (Fig. 9-7). While this is not an infrequent consequence of closed head trauma, this type of subdural hematoma is more common in adults who have a degree of cortical atrophy.

Young athletes, and especially children, frequently develop only minimal subdural hematomas with underlying cerebral hemispheric swelling (Fig. 9-8). This type of brain injury is not the result of a space occupying mass from clotted blood caus-ing brain compression, but rather swollen brain tissue causing consequent rises in intracranial pressure. The advent of CT scanning permits accurate differential diagnosis between these two conditions, which frequently cause similar clinical pictures. The modalities of treatment for these two distinct types of acute subdural hematomas are quite different.

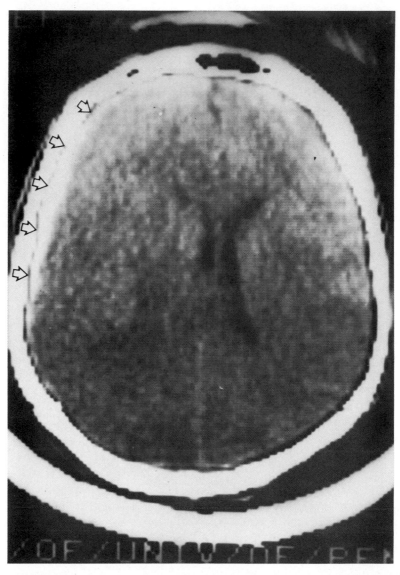

Fig. 9-8. *Case 5:* CT scan demonstrating a small, acute, subdural hematoma in the left temporoparietal area (arrows). There is associated marked left cortical edema that has caused displacement of the ventricles to the right.

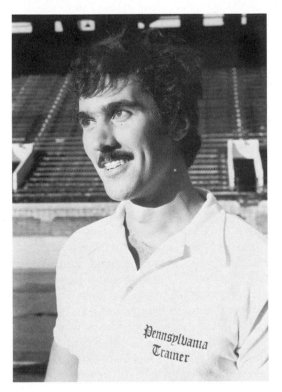

Fig. 9-9. Intercollegiate football player (Case 5) following nonoperative treatment for a subdural hemorrhage. He has made a complete recovery. Although not permitted to participate in contact sports following his injury, his interest in football has been sustained by his participation as a member of the University training staff.

PRINCIPLES OF MANAGEMENT

As our knowledge of physiology and pathophysiology increased, we have progressed through stages of development and gained the ability to successfully resuscitate seriously ill or severely injured people. We began in the 1950s to successfully treat acute respiratory and postoperative problems, followed by satisfactory cardiac resuscitation and emergency cardiac care in the 1960s. We have extended innovations in critical-care medicine in the form of brain resuscitation in the 1970s. Such care is based on the concept that the degree of permanent neurologic, intellectual, and psychologic deficits after brain trauma with coma is only partly the result of the initial injury, and is certainly in part due to secondary postinsult changes, which can be worsened or improved by the quality of the supportive care. Head injuries by their very nature require resuscitation, i.e., therapy initiated after the insult. The proper care of head-injured patients, athletic or otherwise, depends on a full appreciation and use of brain resuscitation measures in an intensive care setting.

Present management of focal intracranial hematoma resulting from athletic injury includes not only treatment for and removal of hematoma, but also recognition of and treatment for the underlying brain injury that results from severe head trauma. Included in this concept of treatment for the underlying brain injury is that of resuscitation of the brain. This is therapy designed to have specific neuron-saving potential once general resuscitation methods and supportive care have begun. Our concern in management of the athletic-injured patient is the same as those for any severely head-injured patient. Our current management and treatment protocol is outlined in Table 9-1.

First aid should consist of getting the patient safely into a supine position and determining vital signs and the significance of any associated injuries. Initial

TABLE 9-1. Head Injury

| First Aid—Hyperventilation | |
| Diagnosis—CT Scan | |
Surgery	*No Surgery*
Epidural hematoma	Small subdural
Large subdural	Contusion
Large intracerebral	Diffuse injury
	Most intracerebrals

ICP Monitoring and Treatment
Goal: Keep ICP less than 15 mmHg
Modalities: Hyperventilation (P_{CO_2} 22 to 30 mmHg)
Corticosteroids (1 mg/kg)
Mannitol (1 g/kg, serum osmolality 330-320)
Barbiturates (30 mg/kg loading and 0.5-3 mg/kg/hr maintenance)

treatment should consist of establishing an adequate and useful airway (Appendices I and II) and beginning hyperventilation maneuvers. This can be accomplished by using a manual resuscitation bag with supplemental oxygen, if it is available. The patient should then be transferred as quickly as possible to a medical facility where diagnosis and treatment of brain injury can begin. While these measures are important for all patients who have suffered concussion, they are of extreme importance for the patient who remains comatose following trauma. The use of an initial dose of corticosteroids given parenterally is specifically indicated, and 100 mg dexamethasone or 1 mg methylprednisolone sodium succinate can be administered to the average adult. Once the patient arrives in the emergency room and it is determined that he or she is stable from a cardiorespiratory point of view, endotracheal intubation is immediately performed on comatose patients and a CT scan is obtained as soon as possible. The CT scan provides an immediate diagnosis of the intracranial situation, and as can be seen from the management schema, patients are then divided into either a surgical or nonsurgical category, depending on the size of intracranial hematoma present.

Initial evaluation of all head trauma patients includes determination of their coma state by numerical ranking on the Glasgow Coma Scale (Table 9-2). This coma scale is based on the patient's response to stimulation by eye-opening, best motor response, and best verbal response. Scores of 15 to 3, from normal neurologic status to deeply comatose, are possible.

Patients with a Glasgow Coma Scale of 7 or lower should have immediate intracranial pressure (ICP) monitoring as part of their treatment. Intracranial hypertension, defined as a pressure over 15 mmHg, is seen in 50% or more of severely head-

TABLE 9-2.   Glasgow Coma Scale

	Open	Spontaneously	4
Eyes		To verbal command	3
		To pain	2
		No response	1
	To verbal command	Obeys	6
	To painful stimulus*	Localizes pain	5
		Flexion-withdrawal	4
Best motor response		Flexion-abnormal (decorticate rigidity)	3
		Extension (decerebrate rigidity)	2
		No response	1
		Oriented and converses	5
		Disoriented and converses	4
Best verbal response†		Inappropriate words	3
		Incomprehensible sounds	2
		No response	1
Total			3-15

* Apply knuckles to sternum; observe arms.
† Arouse patient with painful stimulus if necessary.

The Glasgow Coma Scale, based upon eye opening, verbal, and motor responses, is a practical means of monitoring changes in level of consciousness. If response on the scale is given a number, the responsiveness of the patient can be expressed by summation of the figures. Lowest score is 3; highest is 15.

injured patients. The poor correlation between alterations in ICP and the patient's neurologic status has been well described in the past. Therapy to treat intracranial hypertension can only be given correctly when the pressure is known. We are firmly convinced of the usefulness of continuous ICP monitoring in the intensive care of the severely head-injured patient. Because intermittent waves of increased pressure, which commonly occur without other signs or symptoms, can be diagnosed and treated before significant neurologic deterioration occurs, ICP monitoring facilitates titration of therapy.

When muscle paralysis or barbiturates are used to control elevated ICP, it is impossible to follow the patient's neurologic state. Other than brain-stem evoked potentials, ICP is the only parameter that can be followed. It would be inappropriate to use muscle paralysis or barbiturates without continuously recording ICP. Ideally, the ICP should be monitored from the earliest possible time after the patient's arrival in the hospital. In our unit, it is usually possible to obtain a CT scan within one hour of admission in all severe head injuries. The ICP monitor is usually inserted after the CT scan and within two hours of admission.

However, if any delay in diagnosis is foreseen or if the patient is rapidly deteriorating, an ICP bolt is inserted immediately following emergency resuscitation. This early insertion is especially important in patients with signs of shock from other injuries who require rapid fluid replacement. In these cases, we begin to monitor pressure in the emergency room with a portable recording system.

The ICP monitoring system must be simple, easily inserted, and reliable. The subarachnoid bolt, which can be easily inserted and maintained and does not require an operating room procedure, can be accomplished at bedside with local anesthesia.

We monitor ICP in comatose head-injured patients whether they are operated on initially for decompression or not. We rarely intervene surgically to remove contused brain, believing that if ICP can be controlled, the removal of potentially functional brain tissue is unacceptable as it may limit the patient's recovery. After surgical intervention in patients with hematoma, we routinely insert subarachnoid bolts and monitor ICP for possible further therapy.

The following principles of management of head-injured patients apply to those who do not have indications for surgical intervention, and to those postoperative. This management is guided by the monitored variables, and its goals are to prevent three major complications which cause most deaths if the patient is alive on arrival at the hospital: (1) intracranial hypertension, (2) inadequate cerebral oxygenation, and (3) systemic medical complications. These must be attacked vigorously for optimum results. Treatment for intracranial hypertension is also designed to maximize cerebral oxygenation, and the modalities are those previously listed.

Of all therapies for high ICP, hyperventilation is the first one that we use, and is extremely effective. With the patient intubated, we keep the P_{CO_2} at 22 to 30 mmHg and note that a fall in ICP is rapid after hyperventilation, and in some instances is all that is necessary for control.

Corticosteroids in large doses (1 mg/kg dexamethasone every 6 hr) are given routinely. Hyperosmotic agents decrease ICP by removing brain water due to an induced osmotic gradient from the brain to the intravascular component. Although slightly less rapid in its action, 20 to 25% mannitol has largely replaced 30% urea in this country because of less rebound after administration. Two forms of hyperosmotic therapy are available: intermittent bolus use and continuous infusion therapy. High-dose bolus therapy, 1 to 2 g/kg mannitol, is reserved for initial emergency control of ICP, usually in patients who have a rapid decrease in level of consciousness, dilating pupils, or decerebration. Maintenance therapy can then be carried out with smaller boluses of 0.15 to 0.3 g/kg mannitol every one to two hours or whenever the ICP exceeds 15 mmHg. Close attention must be given to the serum osmolality so that it does not rise above 320 mOsm/l. Significant cardiopulmonary and renal complications are frequent and often irreversible with serum osmolality above these levels. Clinicians utilizing this therapy should have a thorough understanding of the hyperosmolar state.

The most recent contribution to ICP control is the use of barbiturates. When initially used to protect the brain by lowering metabolism, it became apparent that reductions of ICP occurred regularly. Although the mechanism of barbiturate action on elevated ICP is not known, its successful use when other forms of therapy have failed to lower ICP is encouraging. The doses of barbiturates required have varied. Pentobarbital has been the most widely used agent, usually with loading doses of 10 to 30 mg/kg. Thereafter, infusions of 0.5 to 3 mg/kg/hr are maintained. We have been impressed with the wide variation of serum levels obtained by similar doses in different patients and no longer rely solely on serum levels as criteria. We prefer to titrate the dose until a burst-suppression pattern is present on the EEG monitor. Therapy is then closely regulated to keep the burst-suppressions of equal length. At this physiologic endpoint, the serum pentobarbital level may vary from 2.5 to 5.0 mg/dl. Care must be taken to prevent barbiturate cardiac toxicity and subsequent hypotension. This has not been a problem except in older patients, and the cerebral perfusion pressure can be adequately maintained without the use of pressor agents.

For the duration of barbiturate therapy, monitoring must be intensive because neurologic signs are abolished. Spontane-

ous respiratory activity is not present, and all other neurologic signs are generally absent. Although we have continued barbiturate therapy for as long as 21 days, the usual course is less than 5 days. By this time, the ICP rarely rises when an attempt is made to discontinue the barbiturate infusion. Once a patient's ICP is less than 15 mmHg for longer than 48 hours, we discontinue therapy in a sequential manner, stopping barbiturates first, then decreasing hyperosmolar therapy, and finally, ceasing hyperventilation.

The accepted treatment of a patient with acute subdural hematoma remains controversial. Some neurosurgeons believe that the majority of patients with acute subdural hematoma are not helped by an operation, and that the major problems are the control of brain swelling and elevated intracranial pressure. Others believe that because of obvious deterioration of the patient, evacuation of the hematoma, no matter how large, improves intracranial compliance and the neurologic state.

In those patients whose CT scans show a large localized subdural clot with an equal or larger shift of the midline structures, we surgically evacuate the hematoma. In patients with a "smear subdural," a few millimeters thick over the entire lateral aspect of one hemisphere, with the midline shift greater than the thickness of the subdural, we probably would not operate but would aggressively control ICP. Disagreements arise when a state between these two is seen. The argument against surgical intervention is that the major cerebral problem is brain injury, which cannot be helped by an operation. If there is a disruption of the blood-brain barrier with vasogenic edema, craniotomy decreases tissue pressure, increases hydrostatic pressure gradients between capillaries and tissue, and may therefore cause a marked increase in edema in the decompressed hemisphere. Thus, even if the clot is removed, the increased edema may cause swelling of the hemisphere, which rapidly returns the intracranial volume-pressure relationships to where they were prior to the operation.

If an operation is performed, we recommend a large temporofrontoparietal craniotomy flap with evacuation of the clot and control of the hemorrhage from bridging veins and cortical laceration. The patient with a sizable subdural hematoma as seen in Figure 9-7 should have an operation for evacuation of the clot followed by management of ICP. A patient with a subdural hematoma along the outside of the left hemisphere such as that seen in Figure 9-8 is best managed by aggressive treatment of brain swelling and therapy for increased ICP.

The mortality rates for the surgical treatment of acute subdural hematoma reported in the last 10 years vary from 42 to 63%. One important variable seems to be the level of consciousness of the patient at the time of the operation. We do not believe that an operation is necessary in all patients with acute subdural hematoma, but we do feel it is vital that all patients, including those who have had surgical intervention, have postoperative ICP monitoring and control. Of patients who died after surgical intervention, 25% died from uncontrollable elevated ICP. Thus, postoperative ICP monitoring plays a major role in the care of patients with acute subdural hematomas. We feel strongly that this will not only improve mortality rates, but also the quality of life.

In conclusion, we have come to recognize that in all patients with serious head injuries, including athletic head injuries, pathologic damage is usually diffusely distributed throughout the cerebral hemispheres and brain stem. Ideally, therapy should prevent secondary damage rather than modify any secondary injury once it occurs. With this approach, it should be possible to limit patient disability to the results of the primary biomechanical injury alone. Theoretically, no patient who is conscious after injury should die or suffer major disability.

Comatose patients require immediate and intensive therapy following their injury. The triage must include transport to a medical facility where rapid diagnosis and intensive care are available and routine.

Early effective diagnosis of surgically correctable lesions by CT scanning has decreased mortality from epidural and surgically treatable subdural hematoma. With no mass lesion, aggressive management can be started without undue concern that a mass lesion has been missed and negative exploratory surgery can be avoided. The use of ICP monitoring and monitoring of the systemic arterial pressure and blood gases, serum osmolality, and electrolytes allow any trend away from normal to be detected and corrected at the earliest possible time. The use of barbiturates is an effective way to control intracranial hypertension when other more common modes of treatment have failed.

Any athlete who has suffered loss of consciousness from head injury for more than one minute, or who has persistent headache with confusion or any disorientation which persists longer than one hour following trauma, or an athlete who has more than one episode of unconsciousness, however momentary, during any one playing season, should be referred for neurologic examination and CT scan evaluation. With the proper diagnosis and management of head-injury patients, we are convinced that the present distressingly high mortality and morbidity from severe head injury can be lowered without a decrease in the quality of life.

REFERENCES

1. Bruce, D.A., Gennarelli, T.A., and Langfitt, T.W.: Resuscitation from coma due to head injury. Crit. Care Med., 6:254, 1978.
2. Ommaya, A.K., and Gennarelli, T.A.: Cerebral concussion and traumatic unconsciousness: correlation of experimental and clinical observations on blunt head injuries. Brain, 97:633, 1974.

Section III

Neck Injuries

Chapter 10

Anatomy of the Cervical Spine and Its Related Structures

Robert J. Johnson

Eric I. Mitchell

THE CERVICAL SPINE

The seven cervical vertebrae stand as a slender articulated column between the head and the thorax. Thus, the cervical spine connects an approximately 15 lb object (the head) to a relatively immobile mass (the thorax). For its motions of flexion, extension, rotation, and lateral bending, the cervical spine must supply both flexibility and stability. To deliver these two requirements there are 17 diarthroses and 6 synarthroses between the skull and the thoracic spine. In addition, there are many more unions created by ligaments binding various elements of the cervical vertebrae together. In this enumeration the uncovertebral joints (of Luschka) are not considered to be distinct from the intervertebral discs. Thus, a large number of individual joints and ligaments contribute to the flexibility and stability of the cervical spine. The musculature of the neck is an additional important system that also aids in flexibility and stability.

There are many different anatomic aspects of the cervical spine, which give it special functions beyond those of the remaining spine. The cervical spine has the smallest bodies, and although these increase in size as we move caudally, the vertebral canal is larger at the cervical level of the spine than at all lower levels. The vertebral or neural foramen is triangular with rounded corners in each of the cervical vertebrae except the atlas, in which it is more circular. The series of vertebral foramina produces the vertebral or spinal canal. The transverse diameter at individual levels varies, decreasing as one progresses caudally. The sagittal diameter of the canal, which is somewhat smaller than the transverse diameter, decreases slightly down to the third cervical vertebra, then remains nearly constant.

Of the cervical vertebrae, four may be considered typical (the third to the sixth inclusive), and three are referred to as atypical or special (the first, second, and seventh).

Typical Cervical Vertebrae

As previously mentioned, the typical cervical vertebrae have small, rather ovoid bodies, with the long axis transversely oriented. The right and left lateral margins of the superior surface of each body are raised upward as uncinate processes, which relate to equivalent beveled surfaces at the right and left lateral margins of the inferior surface of the next vertebral body above (Fig. 10-1). Thus, the superior aspects of the vertebral bodies of typical vertebrae are curved and resemble some-

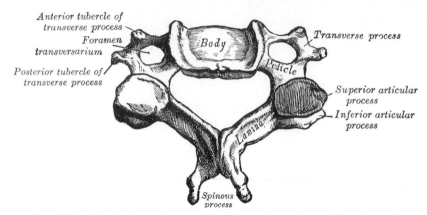

Anterior tubercle of transverse process
Foramen transversarium
Posterior tubercle of transverse process
Body
Pedicle
Transverse process
Superior articular process
Inferior articular process
Lamina
Spinous process

Fig. 10-1. A typical cervical vertebra viewed from above. (From Goss.[6])

what the contour of a bucket seat in a sports car. Stability is gained by this partial interlocking of vertebral bodies. The right and left tilted portions of the intervertebral disc space have long been called the uncovertebral joints, as if they were truly distinct from the intervertebral disc. However, these ten uncovertebral joints are developmentally lateral parts of the intervertebral joints and discs in which early degenerative change becomes evident after the first decade. These so-called joints acquire particular importance, because the posterior part of each forms a part of the margin of the intervertebral foramen, and thus relate to the emergent spinal nerve. Furthermore, they lie immediately medial to the vertebral artery, which ascends through the foramina transversaria. Thus, osteophytes may impinge upon the artery as well as the nerve.

The right and left transverse processes have a groove on their superior aspect to support the emerging spinal nerve. The transverse foramina, which transmit the vertebral artery, are far enough anterior in the roots of the transverse processes as to place the ascending vertebral artery in front of each of the emergent spinal nerves.

The right and left superior and inferior articular processes are situated at the junction of the pedicle (root) with the lamina of the neural (vertebral) arch. Projecting cranially and caudally, these two processes together create a short bony column for each vertebra, and from this column the lamina extends posteromedially to unite with its partner from the opposite side. The several superior and inferior articular processes thus create a posterior column of bones and joints on the right and left. These, together with the anterior column of intervertebral discs and vertebral bodies, create three parallel columns of bones and joints in the cervical spine. The articular facets of the two posterior columns of bones and joints are in a plane that has been tilted from the coronal to an oblique position in such a way that the superior facets face upward and dorsally and the inferior facets face downward and ventrally. Each is nearly flat and is surrounded by an articular capsule.

The spinous processes of the typical vertebrae are usually bifid at their tips and extend dorsally with a slight caudal slant. The long axis of the spinous process is directed so that if a line were extended dorsally from each, these lines would tend to converge at a central point posterior to the cervical spine. Therefore, an abnormality must be suspected at any level where the axes of these processes diverge.

Atypical Cervical Vertebrae

These vertebrae are the atlas (first), the axis (second), and the vertebra prominens (seventh).

The Atlas. The atlas, which has two superior articular facets that support the condyles of the occipital bone of the skull, is particularly unusual in that it lacks a body. Weight is borne through right and left lateral masses with articular facets above and below on each. The superior articular facets that surmount the lateral masses are ovoid and elongated, with their long axes convergent anteriorly (Fig. 10-2). Each of these facets is concave and conforms in size and orientation to the equivalent occipital condyle so that these condyles may glide and roll upon the atlas in nodding (flexion and extension) motions of the head.

The inferior articular facets that face downward on the underside of the lateral masses are rounded in outline to match the equally rounded outline of the superior articular facets of the axis (second cervical vertebra). The plane of the joint formed by these two facets is nearly horizontal and is thus designed for rotatory movements. However, the face of the inferior facet of the atlas is almost flat, while the surface of the superior facet of the axis is slightly convex upward, having a central summit. Accordingly, when the inferior facet of the atlas moves anteroposteriorly upon the superior facet of the axis, as in rotation, the lateral mass of the atlas rises slightly as its inferior facet centers over the superior facet of the axis, and the atlas descends

slightly as its facet moves anteriorly or posteriorly off the higher central area on the facet of the axis. This telescoping effect can be seen on rotational roentgenograms as a relative narrowing or widening of the joint space. The joint capsules of the atlanto-axial joints are loose, giving these joints the greatest mobility of any between the vertebrae in the spine.

The atlas has anterior and posterior arches, each with a slight median tubercle. The posterior arch is provided with a groove just behind each lateral mass. In this groove, the first cervical (suboccipital) nerve exits from the neural (vertebral) canal and the vertebral artery enters into the neural canal. Here these two structures pierce the atlanto-occipital membrane as they cross the posterior arch. Occasionally the lower border of the membrane is ossified where it bridges over the artery and nerve (the posterior ponticulus), and is therefore discernible on roentgenograms.

The Axis. The axis, or second cervical vertebra, has a body that supports the upright odontoid process. This process represents the phylogenetically displaced body of the atlas, and serves as a pivot about which the atlas rotates. The superior articular facets of the axis are nearly horizontal to coincide with the inferior articular facets of the atlas (Fig. 10-3). However, the inferior articular processes of the atlas have facets that face forward and down-

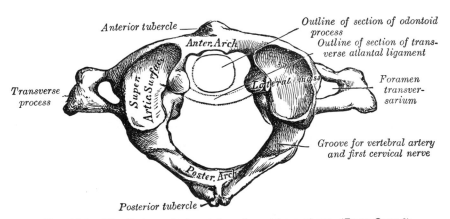

Fig. 10-2. The first cervical vertebra viewed from above. (From Goss.[6])

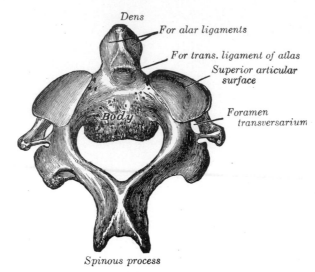

Dens

For alar ligaments

For trans. ligament of atlas

Superior articular surface

Foramen transversarium

Body

Spinous process

Fig. 10-3. The second cervical vertebra viewed from above. (From Goss.[6])

ward to fit the superior articular facets of the third cervical vertebra. The neural arch of the axis is formed of right and left flattened laminae with a median spinous process projecting dorsally.

The Vertebra Prominens. The seventh cervical vertebra is a transitional vertebra that has several distinctive features. The spinous process is longer than that of the other cervical vertebrae and is easily palpated clinically. Hence, this bone is called the vertebra prominens. Its body is proportionally broader than the bodies of the vertebrae above, and its transverse process is larger and more posteriorly placed. However, the costal element of the transverse process is less well developed, and the anterior tubercle is small or absent. Occasionally the costal element develops excessively and becomes a cervical rib with its potential for producing neurovascular symptoms.

Articulations and Relations Between Cervical Vertebrae

The atlas is held in proper relationship to the axis, not only by the articulation of its right and left lateral masses with the axis, but by the transverse ligament of the atlas. This ligament forms a sturdy band bridging across the interval between the lateral masses, to each of which it is securely attached. Thus, it subdivides the central foramen (or space ringed by the anterior and posterior arches and the lateral masses) of the atlas into a smaller anterior compartment for the odontoid process, and a larger posterior compartment for the upper end of the spinal cord. The space relationships here have been schematized by Steel's "rule of thirds," in which the anterior third of the anteroposterior diameter of the central foramen of the atlas is occupied by the odontoid process, leaving one third for the spinal cord, and a remaining third, which contains only the arachnoid and cerebrospinal fluid.[4] This latter third, however, is distributed both anteriorly and posteriorly to the spinal cord.

Anterior dislocation of the atlas upon the axis, especially when the transverse ligament ruptures but the odontoid process does not fracture, dangerously reduces the available space for the spinal cord and may result in its anteroposterior compression. Since the odontoid process is located anteriorly within the bony ring of the atlas, it is apparent that this process functions as an eccentrically placed pivot, and that rotatory motions of the atlas upon the axis significantly diminish the transverse diameter of the vertebral canal.

When the atlas rotates far to the left upon the axis, the right transverse foramen of the atlas moves forward relative to the transverse foramen of the axis, thereby increasing the distance between the two foramina, thus stretching the vertebral artery and increasing its angulation at the transverse foramen of the atlas. In extremes of rotation, as might occur with rotational dislocations and subluxations of the atlas on the axis, the vertebral artery may be so stretched and angulated as to impair circulation to the brain stem and upper spinal cord.

The major motions that occur in the cervical spine are flexion, extension, lateral bending, and rotation, while minor motions are distraction, anteroposterior translation, and lateral translation in the frontal plane. Although an occasional individual has an essentially straight cervical spine, there is generally a variable degree of lordosis in the cervical spine when it is in the neutral position. About 10° of flexion occurs at the atlanto-occipital joint, with further increments being added at the lower joints. In extension, the normal lordosis of the neutral position increases, with about 25° of extension occurring at the atlanto-occipital joint. A slight and variable amount of flexion and extension (up to 15°) also occurs at the atlantoaxial joint. Further increments of extension occur in the lower joints. The full range of extension plus flexion is about 100° in the young adult. Age must be considered, because the range of all cervical spine motions is greater in the child and lesser in the older adult.

The rotational range is approximately 80° to the right and 80° to the left, for a total of 160°. Approximately 50% of this rotational motion occurs at the atlantoaxial articulation, with decreasing increments occurring at joints below this level. The

atlanto-occipital joint does not contribute to rotation, but is involved only in flexion and extension.

Because of the oblique plane of the superior and inferior articular facets, lateral bending of the cervical spine is always associated with a certain degree of rotation at all levels of the cervical spine. In lateral bending to the right, the upper articular facet of an individual right-sided joint glides downward and posteriorly on the inclined plane of the facet below it, while on the left side the upper facet is gliding upward and forward. This small posterior motion by the right articular process and anterior motion by the left articular process add a rotatory component to lateral bending. A small amount of lateral bending (up to 5°) occurs at the atlantoaxial joint.

Below the axis, intervertebral discs fill each interval between the vertebral bodies. Naturally, the disc follows the same curved contour as does the upper surface of each vertebral body. The disc is thinner at the upcurving right and left margins (the so-called uncovertebral joints of Luschka). It is here that the disc degenerates early, leaving the hyaline cartilage plates intact above and below a fissure, which therefore simulates a diarthrodial joint cavity. As discs are elsewhere, the central, flatter portion of the disc is composed of a peripheral annulus fibrosus and a central nuclear pulposus. In flexion of the cervical spine, the anterior part of the disc is compressed and the posterior part is extended. Since in flexion the articular facets of the upper vertebra not only slide upward but somewhat forward, the vertebral body also shifts forward to the same degree (anterior translation). In extension there is a comparable posterior translation of the vertebral body.

Ligaments of the Cervical Spine

Ligamentous structures add to the stability of the cervical spine. Space does not permit a complete analysis of all of the ligaments related to the cervical spine. Certain ligaments, however, are so unique and important to an understanding of the upper cervical spine that they require discussion.

The right and left alar ligaments extend upward and obliquely laterally from the sides of the apex of the odontoid process (Fig. 10-4). Each attaches laterally to the medial aspect of the anterior part of the occipital condyle, thus anchoring the skull to the second cervical vertebra. Each ligament is sturdy and cylindric in form and creates a strong occipitoaxial connection. These two ligaments help check lateral and rotational movement, but play no significant role in restraining flexion and extension movements. After rupture of the transverse ligament of the atlas in dislocations, the alar ligaments become the next structures to resist further forward translation of the atlas upon the axis. When they fail (usually by avulsion from the apex of the odontoid), there is no other significant defense against compression of the cord. There are right and left accessory bands, which extend from the axis to the margin of the foramen magnum, passing behind the transverse ligament of the atlas and functioning somewhat like the alar ligaments. These accessory ligaments blend with the fibers of both the atlantoaxial and atlanto-occipital joints as they pass beside these capsules.

The transverse ligament of the atlas is a horizontal ligament extending from the medial side of one lateral mass of the atlas to the equivalent site on the opposite lateral mass. As it crosses the central area of the space surrounded by the ring of the atlas, it passes behind the odontoid process, coming into contact with the posterior surface of the process. Here the ligament is flattened and has a fibrocartilaginous surface for apposition against the reciprocal groove on the posterior side of the odontoid process (Fig. 10-5). Laterally the ligament is thicker and more rounded. It is a

structure of considerable strength, serving to capture the odontoid process and hold it against the posterior surface of the anterior arch of the atlas, where reciprocal articular facets are found on the apposed surfaces. A joint cavity occurs here as it does between the odontoid and the transverse ligament.

A slender, weak, apical dental ligament ascends from the odontoid tip to the anterior margin of the foramen magnum (Fig. 10-4). Posterior to the apical dental ligament and paralleling it is another vertical bundle of fibers, extending from the odontoid tip to the intracranial aspect of the occipital bone at the anterior margin of the foramen magnum. This bundle has a caudally placed counterpart extending from the odontoid apex downward to attach to the posterior surface of the body of the axis. The cranial and caudal parts of this vertical bundle are in the same plane as, and in part extensions from, the fibers of the transverse ligament. These vertical bands form a cross with the transverse ligament, and all four limbs are collectively called the cruciate ligament of the atlas (Fig. 10-4). The transverse ligament is by far the most important component.

Each of the ligaments on the anterior wall of the vertebral canal is overlaid by the posterior longitudinal ligament, which in the cervical region is broad and obscures the posterior surfaces of all the vertebrae and intervertebral discs (Fig. 10-5). As this ligament ascends behind the axis and atlas, it broadens still more and becomes laminated into a deeper stratum and a superficial stratum. The deeper stratum, called the tectorial membrane, is a strong, flat sheet that lies upon the cruciate ligament and extends above through the foramen magnum to attach intracranially to the clivus and adjacent areas of the basilar part of the occipital bone. The superficial stratum is thinner but is not fundamentally distinct, for it also extends upward to attach to the clivus. The tectorial membrane gives additional support to the

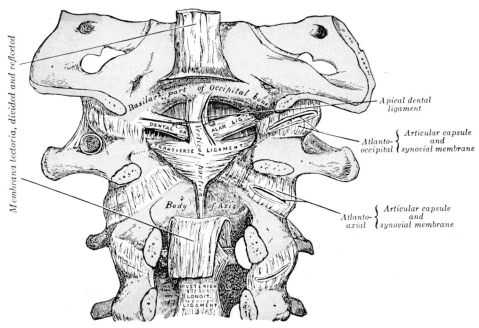

Fig. 10-4. Ligaments of the upper cervical spine viewed from behind. The neural arches have been removed. (From Goss.[6])

atlanto-occipital and atlantoaxial joints, and aids in the prevention of vertical translation or distraction.

Posteriorly, the ligamenta flava bridge the gap between the laminae of the neural arches from the axis downward. These are thick membranes of yellow elastic tissue that restrain flexion of the spine. Interspinous ligaments are poorly developed only in the cervical region. The supraspinous ligament does not exist in the cervical region, for its place has been taken by the ligamentum nuchae.

The ligamentum nuchae is a thin septum of collagenous and elastic fibers. When the neck is flexed, its posterior border may be felt to tense under the skin. Its anterior border attaches to the tips of the spinous processes of all the cervical vertebrae and extends in the midline onto the skull to reach the external occipital protuberance. The surfaces of this ligamentous sheet serve as the attachment for a number of muscles.

THE SPINAL CORD

The junction of the medulla and the spinal cord lies at approximately the level of the foramen magnum of the skull. Structures on the neuraxis that mark this junction are the lower limit of the decussation of the pyramids and the upper rootlets of the right and left first cervical nerves. The spinal cord ends below, at or near the level of the first lumbar intervertebral disc. Below this level the spinal nerve roots, from the second lumbar downward, pass to their respective intervertebral foramina to exit from the vertebral canal. The relatively greater length of the spinal column compared to the spinal cord accounts for the difference in length and the descending obliquity of the ventral and dorsal nerve roots. Only in the cervical region do the spinal nerve roots maintain the nearly horizontal course that they all followed until the third fetal month, when disproportionate growth begins. Even here a

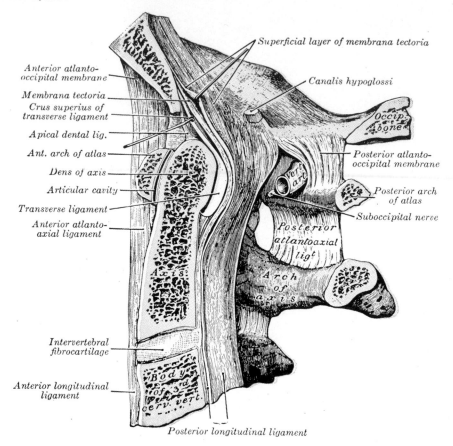

Superficial layer of membrana tectoria

Anterior atlanto-occipital membrane

Membrana tectoria

Crus superius of transverse ligament

Apical dental lig.

Ant. arch of atlas

Dens of axis

Articular cavity

Transverse ligament

Anterior atlanto-axial ligament

Canalis hypoglossi

Occip. bone

Posterior atlanto-occipital membrane

Posterior arch of atlas

Suboccipital nerve

Intervertebral fibrocartilage

Anterior longitudinal ligament

Posterior longitudinal ligament

Fig. 10-5. Ligaments of the upper cervical spine as seen in midsagittal section. (From Goss.[6])

slight degree of obliquity develops below the second cervical nerve.

There are eight pairs of cervical nerves. The first is exceptional in that it emerges not through an intervertebral foramen, but through the atlanto-occipital membrane just above the posterior arch of the atlas. The eighth nerve emerges through the foramen between the seventh cervical vertebra and the first thoracic vertebra. Each of the remaining six emerges through an intervertebral foramen formed between cervical vertebrae.

The three white columns of the spinal cord carry the long ascending and descending tracts. In both the ascending sensory pathways and the descending motor tracts there is a laminar pattern of the fibers

such that the cervical segment representation is nearest the gray substance, and then moving progressively toward the periphery of the cord, come the thoracic, the lumbar, and the sacral fibers. The latter, therefore, are closest to the surface of the cord (Fig. 10-6). This somatotopical laminar pattern of the fibers is seen in the lateral corticospinal tract (motor), the lateral spinothalamic tract (pain and temperature sense), the ventral spinothalamic tract (light touch), and the fibers of the posterior white column (tactile and deep pressure sense, position and motion sense, two-point discrimination, and vibratory sense).

The fibers of the lateral and ventral spinothalamic tracts carry impulses

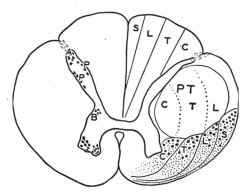

Fig. 10-6. Laminar pattern of the somatotopical arrangement of fiber tracts in the white columns. (From Goss.[6])

originating in the opposite side of the body (are crossed), while the fibers of the posterior white column are uncrossed. There are two ascending tactile pathways representing any given portion of the trunk or limbs. One of these is uncrossed and in the ipsilateral posterior white column, while the other is crossed and in the contralateral ventral spinothalamic tract. For this reason, unilateral spinal cord lesions do not produce a recognizable tactile sensory loss.

The lateral corticospinal tract is also laminated in the same somatotopical fashion as are the sensory pathways. Its fibers terminate ipsilaterally in relation to anterior horn cells. The ventral corticospinal tract, which represents some 10 to 20% of the descending voluntary motor fibers, is uncrossed. Its fibers cross to the opposite side before terminating about anterior horn cells of the cervical and upper thoracic levels only. This ventral motor tract is occasionally absent, and since it represents only a modest percentage of the descending motor fibers is not clinically important in diagnosis of spinal cord injury; whereas the somatotopical laminar patterns of representation of fibers in the long tracts are important clinically, because of their localizing value. An encroachment upon the spinal cord or other lesion that proceeds from the exterior in-

ward destroys representation of the lower parts of the body first, and as the damage progresses centrally into the cord, ever higher parts of the body are successively affected. The reverse is also true. A lesion that begins centrally in the cord and expands peripherally produces a sensory or motor loss in higher parts of the body first, with progression caudally, as the lesion expands toward the periphery of the cord.

Throughout the H-shaped gray substance of the cord there is a segmental representation of the muscles supplied by the ventral root of any spinal nerve and an equivalent segmental representation of the sensory fibers that enter over the dorsal root. Thus, specific muscle paralysis and dermatomal losses have great localizing value diagnostically. For example, the posture of the upper limbs may be of value in localizing the level of a total transverse injury of the cervical cord. With fracture-dislocations of C6 and C7, the upper limbs are likely to be in a posture with elbows at the sides of the chest, the forearms flexed to 90°, and the hands together in front of the chest. This posture is due to the persisting and unopposed function of the forearm flexors and the arm adductors and medial rotators. With fracture-dislocations of C5 and C6, the upper limbs may assume a posture in which the arms are abducted and the forearms flexed so that the hands lie upon the bed alongside the patient's head. This posture is due to the persisting and unopposed function of such muscles as the deltoid and supraspinatus, the biceps, and the trapezius. With still higher fracture-dislocations, as at the C4 and C5, the upper limbs tend to lie flail and at the sides, for now all the roots to the brachial plexus are at or below the cord lesion. If the fracture-dislocation is at the level of C3 and C4, there is also likely to be respiratory paralysis, because the phrenic nerve comes from the third and fourth cervical cord segments, which are probably included in the crushing lesion.

Blood Supply of the Cervical Cord

The entire length of the spinal cord is supplied by longitudinal arteries arranged as a single median anterior spinal artery and right and left posterolateral arteries. The latter vary greatly and each is frequently duplicated so that two posterolateral arteries lie on either side of the posterior rootlets of the spinal nerves as these enter the cord. The anterior spinal artery is the largest of the three sets of arteries and forms sulcal branches at fairly regular and close intervals (Fig. 10-7). These branches pass alternately to the left and to the right sides. Each sulcal artery supplies the anterior gray horn, the intermediate gray matter, and all but the peripheral or superficial portions of the anterior and lateral white funiculi. At irregular intervals the anterior spinal artery is connected to the posterolateral spinal arteries on either side by slender surface vessels known as the vasa coronaria. It is these anastomosing vessels traversing the surface of the anterior and lateral funiculi that supply the superficial zone of the two white columns. The posterior white column on each side and the associated posterior gray column are supplied by branches of the posterolateral artery.

Occlusion of one sulcal artery is followed by ipsilateral loss of function of the anterior horn cells through approximately one segment of the cord, plus loss of the function of the ventral and lateral spinothalamic tracts and at least the medial (upper-limb) portion of the lateral corticospinal tract. Because tactile sensory fibers ascend in both the ipsilateral posterior white column and the contralateral ventral spinothalamic tract, it is evident that tactile sense will not be lost. Thus, the major signs of such sulcal artery occlusion in the cervical cord are contralateral loss of pain and temperature sensation below the segment in question, plus ipsilateral upper limb motor loss. Depending on the extent of the damage in the lateral white column, there may be various other deficits such as bladder dysfunction. It must be em-

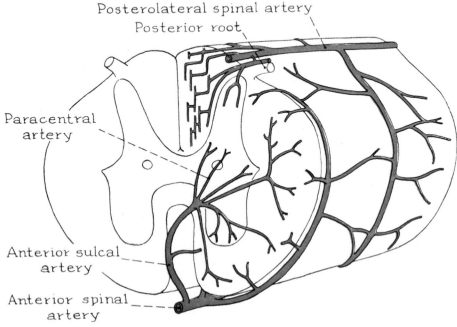

Fig. 10-7. Diagram of the arterial supply of the human spinal cord (after Herren and Alexander, 1939). (From Everett.[7])

phasized that the motor loss is due both to the segmental damage to anterior horn cells and to destruction of the more medial fibers of the lateral corticospinal tract.

Occlusion of the anterior spinal artery for some of its length is equivalent to obstructing several sulcal arteries, and therefore causes effects such as those described for a single sulcal artery. However, the lesion and signs are bilateral. The three-dimensional pattern of capillaries and smaller arterioles in the gray substance of the cord is a dense plexus with vessels arranged both in the horizontal plane and along the vertical axis. Small vessels in the white substance are arranged more along the longitudinal axis to supply the long ascending and descending tracts. Longitudinal or vertical strain more readily disrupts the plexus of capillaries in the gray substance with consequent hemorrhage, than it does in the white substance. With compressive forces on the cord, there is not only a horizontal strain at the level of the compression, but a longitudinal strain above and below this level.[1,3] This explains why hematomyelia spreads upward and downward beyond the local level of compression.

CERVICAL NERVE ROOTS

Each dorsal root ganglion is found just inside the intervertebral foramen. Immediately beyond and frequently at the level of the ganglion, the ventral and dorsal roots unite to form the spinal nerve, which emerges through the foramen with a sheath of dura mater. This sheath merges imperceptibly into the epineurium, which is the connective tissue sheath that surrounds the entire spinal nerve. The epineurium sends prolongations into the interior of the nerve to invest the various bundles of which the total nerve is composed. These connective tissue investments of the bundles are referred to as the perineurium. Proceeding to a finer level of organization, we find the individual

nerve fibers surrounded by a thin reticular connective tissue called the endoneurium. These three levels of connective tissue investments hold the nerve trunk together and give it integrity as a single structure. The ventral and dorsal nerve roots within the dural sheath and spinal canal have no such investments of connective tissue corresponding to the perineurium and epineurium. They possess only the connective tissue prolongations from the pia mater.

At the cervical levels, the ventral and dorsal nerve roots each pierce the dura separately, and thus create two small tubes of dura that fuse into one as the ventral and dorsal roots fuse together. Each root is surrounded by a sleeve of arachnoid, which is inside the dural sleeve as the roots approach the intervertebral foramen. Thus, a short extension of the subarachnoid space briefly follows the ventral and dorsal roots as they penetrate the dural sac (Fig. 10-8).

A thin lateral expansion of the pia mater extends like a flange from the midlateral line of the cord and is prolonged by 21 toothlike processes to points of anchorage on the internal aspect of the dural sac. These are the denticulate ligaments, and they serve to tether the spinal cord within the dural tube, resisting lateral and anteroposterior displacements of the cord.

Each spinal nerve promptly divides into anterior and posterior rami. The latter pass backward at once to supply the intrinsic spinal musculature and the overlying skin. The anterior primary rami continue their lateral course, and those from the fifth to the eighth cervical nerves (plus the first thoracic) enter into the formation of the brachial plexus. The epineurium of the anterior primary rami of the cervical spinal nerves is anchored to the periosteum of the transverse processes. This is especially so at the levels of the fourth, fifth, and sixth cervical nerves.[5] Lateral traction on the nerves is thereby resisted rather than being transmitted along the nerve and its ventral and dorsal roots to the spinal cord.

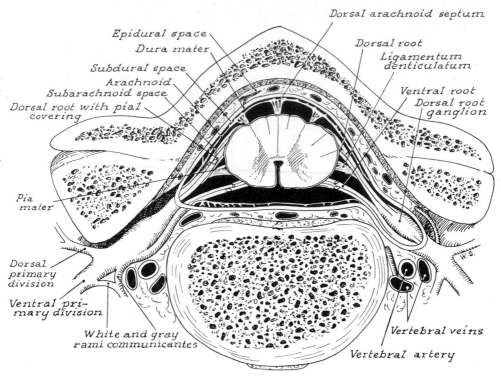

Fig. 10-8. Cross section of spine and cord showing relations of meninges to cord, nerve roots, and intervertebral foramina. (From Everett.[7])

A further resistance to lateral traction on the nerves is created by the funnel-shaped outpouchings of the dura at each level of exit of a nerve root. Under lateral traction, these funnels of dura impact into the inner aspect of the intervertebral foramen, and like a cork in a bottle offer resistance to further lateral displacement of the nerve.[5] By the two mechanisms cited, the individual nerve fibers of the roots are prevented from having to bear the stress of moderate traction on the brachial plexus. But for these two protective systems, the weakest point in the sequence of spinal cord, nerve roots, and spinal nerve would be torn asunder by traction. This weakest point is at the junction of the ventral and dorsal roots with the spinal cord. Avulsions do occur here when the protective arrangements fail due to excessive traction or to injuries of the cervical spine. In this circumstance, the sensory fibers are disrupted on the central side of the dorsal root ganglion cell. Avulsion of the rootlets from the cord, at the level of the first thoracic nerve, interrupts the preganglionic sympathetic fibers destined for the supply of the eye, and the ocular portion of a Horner's syndrome results.

Due to the direction of the nerves in the brachial plexus, downward traction on the arm or shoulder plus excessive lateral bending of the neck to the opposite side or severe hyperextension are likely to stretch the fibers of the fifth and sixth cervical nerves. Disruption of these nerve roots of the brachial plexus would manifest itself primarily by paresis of the muscles supplied by the suprascapular, deltoid, musculocutaneous, and long thoracic nerves. Fiber damage may occur in the roots as an upper radiculopathy or in the superior trunk as a plexopathy. Minimal damage or strain in fibers of the fifth and sixth nerves may give transitory episodes of burning paresthesia and paresis in the upper limb.[2]

REFERENCES

1. Gosch, H.H., Gooding, E., and Schneider, R.C.: Cervical spinal cord hemorrhages in experimental head injuries. J. Neurosurg., *33*:640, 1970.
2. Robertson, W.C., Eichman, P.L., and Clancy, W.G.: Upper trunk brachial plexopathy in football players. J.A.M.A., *241*:1480, 1979.
3. Schneider, R.C., Cherry, G., and Pantek, H.: The syndrome of acute central cervical spinal cord injury. J. Neurosurg., *11*:546, 1954.
4. Steel, H.H.: Anatomical and mechanical considerations of the atlanto-axial articulations. J. Bone Joint Surg., *50A*:1481, 1968.
5. Sunderland, S.: Meningeal-neural relations in the intervertebral foramen. J. Neurosurg., *40*:756, 1974.
6. Goss, C.M. (ed.): Gray's Anatomy of the Human Body. 29th American ed. Philadelphia, Lea & Febiger, 1973.
7. Everett, N.B.: Functional Neuroanatomy. 6th ed. Philadelphia, Lea & Febiger, 1971.

Chapter 11

Mechanisms and Pathomechanics of Athletic Injuries to the Cervical Spine

Albert H. Burstein

James C. Otis

Joseph S. Torg

The purpose of this chapter is to describe and clarify the mechanisms and pathomechanics of the most frequently occurring athletic injuries to the cervical spine on the basis of existing clinical, epidemiologic, and laboratory evidence. White and Panjabi have published a definitive text describing, in detail, three-dimensional vector analyses of a variety of cervical spine injuries.[8] It is not intended that their work be summarized here, and the reader is referred to their publication for further details.

Schneider has observed "there is probably no better experimental or research laboratory for human trauma in the world than the football fields of our nation."[4] An analysis of available information pertaining to cervical spine injuries resulting in quadriplegia substantiates this thesis.

Accurately describing the mechanism or mechanisms responsible for a particular injury transcends simple academic interests. In order that appropriate measures be implemented to effect prevention, the manner in which injury occurs must be accurately defined. Similarly, erroneous concepts regarding injury causation only act to impede the implementation of proper preventive measures. Consequently, anecdotal examples and unusual case reports must be examined critically, lest inaccuracies become established as "fact."

A variety of mechanisms have been proposed as being responsible for cervical spine injuries occurring in athletics, and more specifically, tackle football. Two concepts, one which has implicated the facemask as acting as a lever, forcing the head and neck into hyperflexion; and the other, which has implicated the posterior rim of the football helmet acting as a "guillotine," have not survived close scrutiny. This discussion of the mechanisms of cervical spine injuries must necessarily dismiss these two concepts as erroneous when evaluated in the light of existing scientific evidence.

Regarding the role of the facemask acting as a lever, causing cervical spine fracture or dislocation with or without quadriplegia, in no instance has this been a factor in 209 severe injuries that occurred between 1971 and 1975 (Table 11-1).

The proposal that the upward sweep of a long-lever arm, the faceguard, can cause a marked mechanical advantage as the posterior rim of the rigid helmet guillotines the cervical cord has been effectively refuted on the basis of radiographic, biomechanical, and epidemiologic data.

Virgin performed a cineradiographic study to evaluate the possible role of the

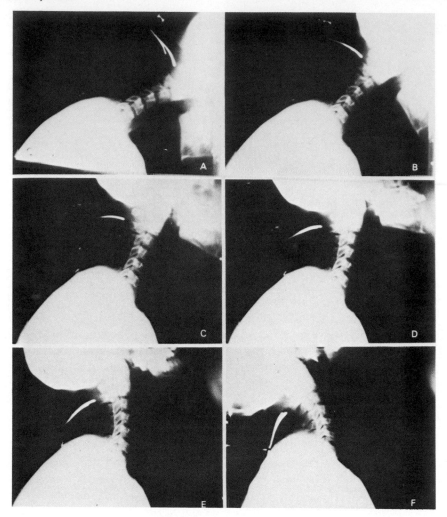

Fig. 11-1. *A-F,* A series of cineradiograms demonstrating the failure of the posterior rim of one of five different brand football helmets to impinge on the soft tissue overlying the spinous processes of C1 through C6. (From Virgin, H.: Cineradiographic study of football helmets and the cervical spine. Am. J. Sports Med., *8*:310, 1980.)

posterior rim of the football helmet in causing neck injuries.[7] Motion pictures were produced in a series of lateral view cineradiograms taken to document the path and position of the posterior rim of the football helmet relative to the spinal column of 16 subjects as they moved their heads from the fully-flexed to fully-extended position under several loading conditions. Five different football helmets were used in the study. No contact occurred at any time between the posterior rim of any of the five helmets on the spinous processes of the cervical vertebrae (Fig. 11-1*A-F*). Virgin's conclusion was that the notion of the posterior rim and the helmet striking the cervical spine above the C7 level is without foundation (Fig. 11-2*A-E*).

Carter and Frankel studied the biomechanics of cervical spine hyperextension injuries in football players using quasi-static-free body analysis.[2] The study examined the guillotine mechanism of in-

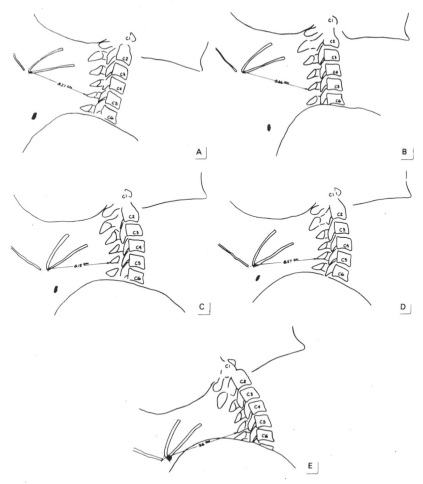

Fig. 11-2. *A-E,* Measurements of the distance from the posterior rim of the helmet to the spinous processes C5 from the neutral position to point of impingement: A = 8.27 cm; B = 8.06 cm; C = 8.12 cm; D = 8.27 cm; and E = 9.6 cm. Determined from cineradiographic studies, these measurements refute the contention that the posterior rim of the football helmet can act as a guillotine in the extremes of forced cervical extension. (From Virgin, H.: Cineradiographic study of football helmets and the cervical spine. Am. J. Sports Med., *8*:310, 1980.)

jury. The static-free body analysis was undertaken to determine the forces imposed on the cervical spine, when the faceguard was struck in such a manner as to create hyperextension of the cervical spine. Three situations that corresponded to the loading conditions created by three different helmet designs were examined. In the first condition it was assumed that the helmet rim was cut high enough posteriorly so that it did not impinge on the posterior cervical spine (Fig. 11-3*A*-*C*). In the second condition it was assumed that

the helmet rim impacted at the level of the fourth cervical vertebra (Fig. 11-4*A*-*C*). In the third case it was assumed that the posterior rim of the helmet struck the shoulder pads (Fig. 11-5*A*-*C*). The results of the analysis (Fig. 11-6) suggest that the most dangerous hyperextension situation occurs with the first condition, which leads to high forces and possible serious injuries to the upper cervical spine. The impact of the posterior rim of the helmet at the fourth cervical vertebra significantly reduced these forces. This finding directly conflicts

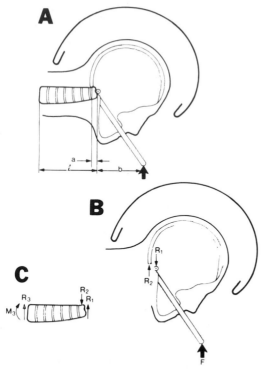

Fig. 11-3. *A,* A loading condition of hyperextension limited by bony contact of occiput on the atlas. *B,* Free body diagram of the head and helmet. *C,* Free body diagram of the cervical spine. (From Carter, D., and Frankel, V.H.: Biomechanics of hyperextension injuries to the cervical spine in football. Am. J. Sports Med., *8*:302, 1980.)

with the so-called "guillotine" mechanism of injury. The impact of the posterior rim of the helmet on the shoulder pads is the least hazardous of loading conditions.

Data dealing with the mechanisms of cervical spine injuries resulting from tackle football both with and without neurologic involvement further tend to refute the hyperextension-guillotine concept. Torg et al.[5] identified only 3% of injuries that resulted in quadriplegia as being due to hyperextension, while 8% of those resulting in fracture or dislocation without quadriplegia were due to this mechanism.

To reiterate, the concept of the posterior rim of the football helmet acting as a guillotine and incurring injury to the cervical spinal cord in extreme forced hyperextension is without foundation.

The commonly acknowledged mechanism responsible for fracture-dislocation of the cervical spine has been that of accidental forced hyperflexion. The subject is an unsuspecting victim of some untoward circumstance, such as an accidental fall, a dive into shallow water, an unexpected blow to the head or, in the case of the athlete, a poorly executed physical act in which the cervical spine is unwittingly forced into hyperflexion with resulting injury (Fig. 11-7). In the majority of fracture-dislocations of the cervical spine that occur to football players, two major factors differentiate them from the classic injury: (1) the circumstances surrounding the event are not accidental, and (2) the mechanism of injury is not cervical spine hyperflexion.

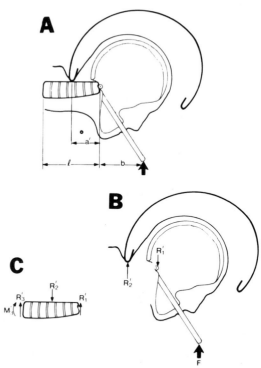

Fig. 11-4. *A,* Loading condition with hyperextension limited by the impingement of the helmet rim at the fourth cervical vertebra. *B,* Free body diagram of the head and helmet. *C,* Free body diagram of the cervical spine. (From Carter, D., and Frankel, V.H.: Biomechanics of hyperextension injuries to the cervical spine in football. Am. J. Sports Med., *8*:302, 1980.)

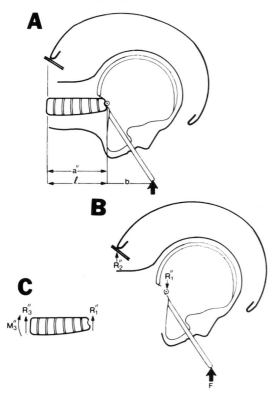

Fig. 11-5. *A,* Loading condition for hyperextension limited by impingement of the helmet rim on the shoulder pad. *B,* Free body diagram of the head and helmet. *C,* Free body diagram of the cervical spine. (From Carter, D., and Frankel, V.H.: Biomechanics of hyperextension injuries to the cervical spine in football. Am. J. Sports Med., *8*:302, 1980.)

the high school level, 52% of the injured players were defensive backs, 13% were on specialty teams, and 10% were linebackers. At the college level, 73% of those players rendered quadriplegic were defensive backs (Table 11-2).[6]

The data indicate that 52% of all cervical spine quadriplegias that occurred from 1971 to 1975 resulted from "spearing," or direct compression head-on type collisions, in which initial contact is made with the top or crown of the helmet. These figures clearly identify the individuals at greatest risk of sustaining a cervical spine injury resulting in quadriplegia as the defensive backs, linebackers, or specialty team members who tackle by using their heads as the initial point of contact (Fig. 11-8 and Table 11-3).

In the majority of injuries that resulted in quadriplegia, the subject was, of his own volition, executing a maneuver in which the head was used as a battering ram, the initial point of contact being made with the top or crown of the helmet in a high-impact situation. Thus, rather than an accidental, untoward event, a technique was deliberately implemented that placed the cervical spine at the risk of catastrophic injury (Fig. 11-9*A-D*).

When a force applied to the cervical spine exceeds the elastic capabilities of the involved structures, injury results. In the course of a contact activity such as tackle football, the cervical spine is repeatedly exposed to potentially injurious energy

Of those cervical spine injuries resulting in quadriplegia, between 1971 and 1975 at the high school level, 72% resulted from tackling. At the college level, 78% of the quadriplegias resulted from tackling. At

TABLE 11-1. Mechanism of Injury Resulting in Permanent Cervical Quadriplegia 1971-75

	Injuries Resulting in Quadriplegia, % (n = 73)	Injuries Not Resulting in Quadriplegia, % (n = 136)
Hyperflexion	10	11
Hyperextension	3	8
Vertical compression (spearing)	52	39
Knee or thigh to head	15	17
Collision, pileup, or ground contact	11	19
Tackled	7	7
Machine-related	3	0
Facemask acting as lever	0	0

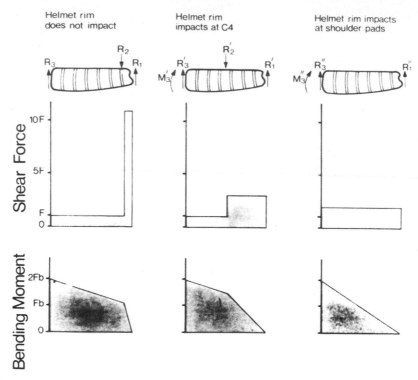

Fig. 11-6. Diagram showing the distribution of cervical spine shear forces and bending movements created in each of the three loading conditions examined. (From Carter, D., and Frankel, V.H.: Biomechanics of hyperextension injuries to the cervical spine in football. Am. J. Sports Med., *8*:302, 1980.)

levels. Fortunately, however, most energy inputs on the cervical spine are effectively dissipated in lateral bending, flexion, or extension by the energy-absorbing capabilities of the cervical paravertebral musculature, the intervertebral discs, or to a lesser extent, the ligaments. However, the bones, discs, and ligamentous structures can be injured when contact occurs on the top or crown of the helmet with the head, neck, and trunk positioned in such a way that forces are transmitted along the axis of the cervical spine, obviating the energy-absorbing capacities of these structures.

Considering the alignment of the cervical spine from the lateral perspective, with the neck in the neutral position, the normal alignment of the spine is one of extension because of the normal cervical lordosis (Fig. 11-10*A*, *B*). It is with forward flexion of the neck that the cervical spine is straightened (Fig. 11-11*A*, *B*). With impact exerted along the vertical axis of a straight spine, loading of a segmented column occurs (Fig. 11-12). When the energy input

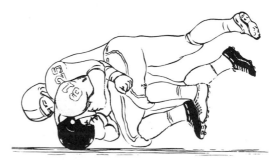

Fig. 11-7. Hyperflexion injury to the cervical spine occurs when it is forced beyond the limits of motion and the applied force exceeds the elastic capabilities of the involved structures. Recent evidence indicates that contrary to past thinking, this mechanism is an infrequent cause of cervical spine injury in athletes. (From Melvin W.J.S.: The role of the face guard in the production of flexion injuries to the cervical spine in football. Can. Med. Assoc. J., *93*:1110, 1965.)

TABLE 11-2. Injury by Activity

	Permanent Cervical Quadriplegia, 1971-75		Cervical Fracture-Dislocations Without Quadriplegia, 1971-75	
	High School % (n = 77)	College % (n = 18)	High School % (n = 105)	College % (n = 46)
Tackling	72	78	59	49
Tackled	14	22	15	24
Blocking	6	0	7	16
Drill	3	0	5	7
Collision pileup	3	0	12	4
Machine-related	2	0	2	0

exceeds the energy-absorbing capacities of the involved structure, intervertebral disc space injury, vertebral body fracture, ligamentous disruption, or posterior element fracture can ensue. When maximum vertical compressive deformation is reached, cervical spine flexion or rotation occurs with fracture, subluxation, or unilateral or bilateral facet dislocation. The majority of cervical spine injuries that result in quadriplegia occur in tackle football and are due to purposeful vertical loading of the vertebral elements.

In order to understand the biomechanics of this injury mechanism, first consider a seemingly unrelated injury, the jammed finger. This is an injury common to basketball players that occurs when the tip of a fully outstretched finger is struck by an oncoming basketball. The resulting injury is a dislocation of the proximal interphalangeal (PIP) joint. This dislocation occurs because the phalanges behave as a segmented, elastic column. The kinetic energy of the ball is transferred to strain energy in the column, and when sufficient strain energy has been stored to make the column unstable, buckling occurs. Buckling is a mechanism of energy release that can be produced in slender structures by subjecting them to excessive axial compressive loads.

Axial loading fractures, dislocations, and fracture-dislocations of the cervical spine result from the same compressive loading mechanism. Since the typical burst fracture of the cervical vertebral body can be produced by direct compressive loads, it is reasonable that axial compression of the cervical spine can produce compressive loads on the vertebral bodies. What then is the mechanism for producing dislocations, which must apparently derive from excessive angulation, i.e., flexion of the proximal vertebral body over the contiguous distal vertebral body? As seen in the example of the jammed finger, the buckling phenomenon is really a large local angulation that develops somewhere

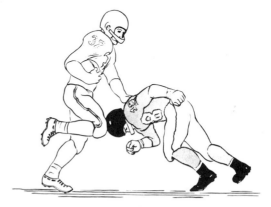

Fig. 11-8. Axial loading of the cervical spine due to impact on the crown of the head or helmet is responsible for the majority of serious injuries that occur in football. The same mechanism is responsible for diving injuries. (From Melvin, W.J.S.: The role of the face guard in the production of flexion injuries to the cervical spine in football. *93*:1110, 1965.)

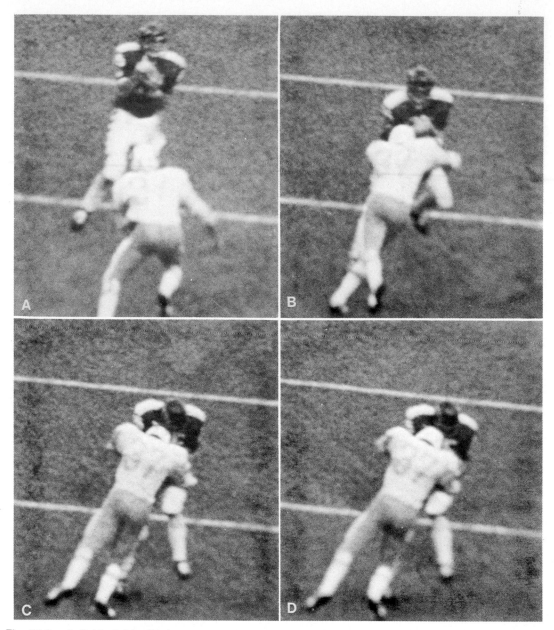

Fig. 11-9. *A*, Subject (No. 37, foreground) lines up in front of ball carrier in preparation for tackling. *B*, Preimpact position shows tackler about to ram ball carrier with crown of his helmet. *C*, At impact, contact is made with the top of the helmet. Although the neck is slightly flexed, it is clearly not hyperflexed. The major force vector is transmitted along the axial alignment of the cervical spine. *D*, The tackler recoils following impact.

along the length of the compressed column. This angulation, or buckling, occurs whenever there is more energy due to compression stored in the column than can

be stored in that same column in a bending mode.

Several factors affect the stability of the system. These factors, which control the

TABLE 11-3. Injuries by Position, 1971 to 1975

	Permanent Cervical Quadriplegia		Cervical Fracture-Dislocations Without Quadriplegia	
	High School % (n = 52)	College % (n = 15)	High School % (n = 89)	College % (n = 47)
Defensive back	52	73	23	33
Linebacker	10	0	18	17
Specialty team	13	7	2	0
Offensive back	12	7	20	21
Defensive line	10	0	28	12
Offensive line	4	13	8	15

point at which buckling occurs, include the size and shape of the vertebral bodies and discs, the elastic characteristics of surrounding ligamentous tissue, and the preload imposed by muscles crossing the cervical spine. The local changes or damage that may occur in any part of the cervical spine also control the buckling phenomenon. If, while under compressive load, one vertebral body collapses (compression fracture), then the whole system becomes unstable at that point and reverts

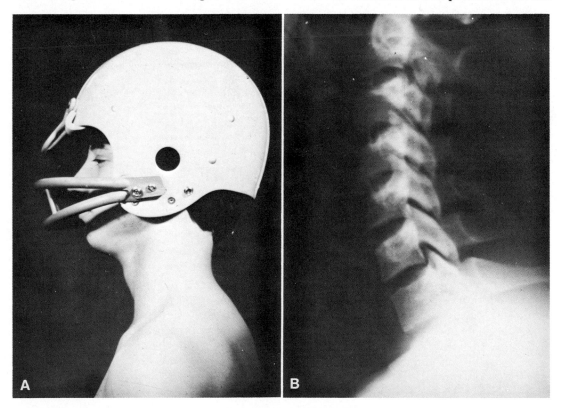

Fig. 11-10. *A, B,* With the head and neck held in the neutral position, because of normal cervical lordosis, the posture of the cervical spine is one of extension. (From Torg, J.: National Football Head and Neck Injuries Registry: report on the cervical quadriplegia from 1971 to 1975. Am J. Sports Med., 7:127, 1979.)

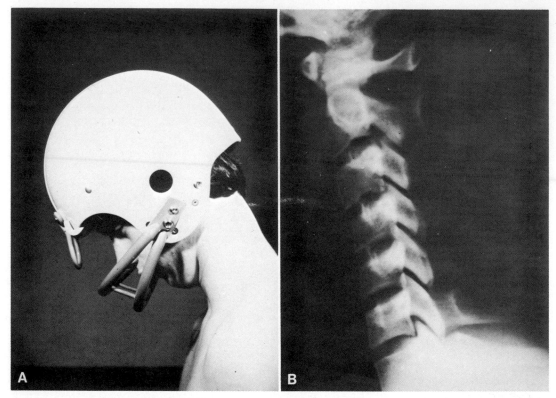

Fig. 11-11. *A, B,* When the neck is flexed approximately 30°, the cervical spine becomes straight; from the standpoint of force, energy absorption, and the effect on tissue deformation and failure, the straightened cervical spine, when axially loaded, acts as a segmented column. (From Torg, J.: National Football Head and Neck Injuries Registry; report on the cervical quadriplegia from 1971 to 1975. Am. J. Sports Med., 7:127, 1979.)

into a buckling mode failure. It is likely that the first damage mode to occur in many instances is a compression fracture of the vertebral body. Following this fracture, local buckling is triggered and excessive flexion occurs in that same region.

Buckling may also be triggered by failure of the intervertebral disc. The local flexion that follows produces a dislocation, and this is the major damage mode observed. The ability to predict whether a crush fracture or a collapsing disc is the initiating mechanism has to date eluded exact analytic definition.

The experimental literature contains sufficient information to put critical limits on the magnitude of a compressive load that can be supported by vertebral bodies. While most of these data have been ac-

cumulated for lumbar and thoracic vertebral bodies, extrapolation of the data gives compressive load limits for cervical vertebral bodies somewhere between 750 and 1000 lbs.

In order for the cervical spine to carry load under direct compression, it is necessary that the spine be in a straight or anatomically slightly flexed position. In this position, the spine is capable of sustaining compression load directly without assistance from the muscles or supporting ligamentous structures. If the spine is not in a straightened position, then axial loads simply cause bending moments and bending deformation that result in further asymmetries of loading.

Therefore, if a load of 750 to 1000 lbs is reached while the spine is loaded in an

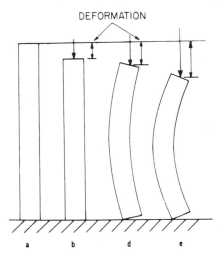

Fig. 11-12. Axial loading of a segmented column first results in compressive deformation (a and b). At a point (d), angular deformation occurs, and if a significant amount of force has been applied, marked deformation occurs (e). When the cervical spine is loaded in such a manner, absorption of excessive amounts of energy can result in buckling with resulting fracture or dislocation of the segmented column. (From Frankel, V.H., and Burstein, A.: Orthopaedic Biomechanics. Philadelphia, Lea & Febiger, 1970.)

axial compressive mode, a compression failure of the vertebral body occurs, and this is the initiating factor in a compression, buckling, local flexion failure mode.

Experimental substantiation of the field observations and subsequent analyses identifying axial loading as the mechanism responsible for the majority of football-related cervical spine injuries has been demonstrated previously by Roaf[3] and Bauze.[1] In addition, an analytic model has been constructed allowing a numerical solution on a digital computer.

Roaf has published results of studies in which spinal units were subjected to forces differing in magnitude and direction, i.e., compression, flexion, extension, lateral flexion, rotation, and horizontal shear. He stated unequivocally that he had never succeeded in producing pure hyperflexion injuries in a normal intact spinal unit, and concluded that hyperflexion of the cervical spine is an anatomic impossibility. Of

equal significance is the fact that Roaf was able to produce almost every variety of spinal injury by a combination of compression and rotation.[3]

Bauze has reported experimental production of forward dislocation of the cervical spine by subjecting it to pure vertical loads. The spine in human cadavers was subjected to loads in a compression apparatus to simulate the clinical situation for dislocation. The movements were recorded by lateral cineradiography. The lower part of the spine was flexed and fixed, and the upper part extended and free to move forward. Vertical compression then produced bilateral dislocation of the facet joints without fracture. If lateral tilt or axial rotation occurred as well, a unilateral dislocation was produced. The maximum vertical loading required was 145 kg (319 lbs), and coincided with rupture of the posterior ligament and capsule, and severing of the anterior longitudinal ligament prior to dislocation. The low vertical load indicates the peculiar vulnerability of the cer-

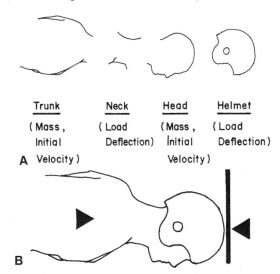

Trunk	Neck	Head	Helmet
(Mass,	(Load	(Mass,	(Load
Initial	Deflection)	Initial	Deflection)
A Velocity)		Velocity)	

Fig. 11-13. *A,* The composite model consists of a trunk mass, a nonlinear spring cervical spine, a head mass, and a nonlinear spring-damped helmet load-deflection function. The basic law of dynamics (F = MA) characterizes system. *B,* The model, representing the axial loading injury condition, illustrates how the cervical spine is compressed between an abruptly deaccelerated head mass and the continued momentum of the body.

vical spine in this position. Bauze concluded that this low load correlated well with the minor trauma often seen in association with forward dislocation.[1]

ANALYTIC MODEL

What type of impact situation gives rise to the particular mode of failure described as a compression, buckling, local flexion failure? An analytic model has been constructed that allows a numerical solution on a digital computer to answer this question. The model uses measured load vs deformation parameters for a helmet, and ap-

proximate load vs deformation parameters for the neck of a football player, in order to examine those situations that might give rise to the aforementioned cervical spine failures.

The model assumes that the cervical spine is in an anatomically straight position and that a football player encounters a relatively immovable object with his helmet while proceeding at some forward velocity. To duplicate actual observed configurations, the model allows the helmet, head, cervical spine, and a portion of the trunk to move along a straight line coincident with the axis of the neck. It is assumed that contact is made at the top of the helmet in the same area that the central axis of the neck crosses the top of the helmet. This is illustrated in Figure 11-13*A, B*. The mathematical model uses a two degree of freedom, nonlinear analysis for the dynamic nonsteady state solution. Computation is on the basis of a small time interval approximation with an iterative solution.

The mechanical characteristics of several helmets have been determined experimentally by placing the helmets on a rigid head form. An MTS hydraulic servocontrolled test machine was used to apply step displacement to the crown of the helmet (Fig. 11-14). The load vs displacement tests were conducted so that the test cycle was completed in 60 msec. While the final solutions indicate that the actual sequence of events occurs in less than 60 msec, it was nevertheless felt that a 60 msec-duration test would portray the characteristics of the helmet with reasonable accuracy. The resulting load vs deformation curves were recorded on an oscilloscope and then digitized for use in the computer simulation. For each test the helmet was preconditioned by several loading cycles and adjusted on the head form in accordance with the fitting instructions. Therefore, all data represent reproducible load-deformation cycle curves.

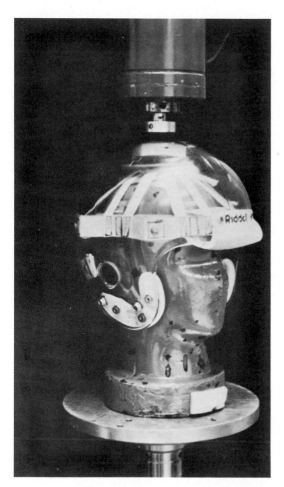

Fig. 11-14. The MTS hydraulic servocontrolled test machine used to apply step displacement to the crown of the helmet in load vs displacement test.

The amplitude of the deformation was chosen as that amplitude at which the helmet system starts to display an almost vertical asymptote on the load vs deformation curves. For modeling purposes the curve was assumed to be infinitely stiff at that point.

Three parametric studies were carried out to determine whether conditions existed that would allow development of between 750 and 1000 lbs of compressive force on the neck. The first examined the influence of varying the helmet performance characteristics, the second examined variations in impact velocity, and the third examined the influence of the effect of the trunk mass.

The parameters that the designer can vary within the helmet are the stiffness and thickness of the lining. These two parameters are responsible for the shape and extent of the load-deformation curve. If a helmet is to be used in football, it must possess reversible deformation characteristics. This limits the material choice to those that either display straight-line load deflection characteristics (the so-called "linear materials"), or in a more realistic representation, those that display curves that may be described as exponential.

The impact velocities examined were 7.5, 15, and 20 ft/sec, which range from fast walking speed to about two thirds of the top speed of a well-conditioned athlete.

In football impact situations, since the trunk, legs, and arms are not always traveling in exactly the same direction as the head and neck, the third study was conducted to see what the effect of the mass of the trunk would have been in providing kinetic energy in the impact, in order to cause catastrophic cervical spine failure. Therefore, the weight of three effective trunk masses was considered: 20 lbs, 50 lbs, and 80 lbs. A conservative estimate of the weight of the trunk mass (less limbs) was 80 lbs, while the 20-lb figure was used to represent that portion of the trunk as-sociated only with the shoulders and upper thoracic region. This last estimate is probably a minimum, since that portion of the trunk is virtually always traveling in almost the same direction as that of the neck at the time of impact.

TEST RESULTS

The suspension type helmet (Riddell Tk-2) tested showed a displacement capability of slightly over one inch when it developed a resisting force of approximately 1500 lbs. When this load-deflection curve was put into the computer model, it was determined that all impact conditions, with a single exception, from the lowest velocity upward and from the least body mass up to the fully effective trunk mass produced force readings in the neck that exceeded the 1000-lb threshold level. All cases exceeded the 750-lb level.

A similar result was obtained for all other helmets examined. Results are also shown for a padded-suspension type helmet (MacGregor 100 MH). The results for each of the cases tested are shown graphically (Figs. 11-15 to 11-20). Each pair of graphs depicts the force-displacement characteristics of the neck and the helmet. In each case, the time, in milliseconds, required to achieve a particular displacement, and the corresponding force are shown by the horizontal lines on the curve.

In Case 1 an initial velocity of 7.5 ft/sec was utilized with an effective torso weight of only 20 lbs. As can be seen in Figure 11-15, the helmet performance (interrupted line) demonstrated that the head ceased penetration into the helmet suspension and thereafter started rebounding away from the helmet at 12.0 msec. The corresponding displacement pattern of the neck (solid line) showed that at 12.0 msec the neck had only compressed approximately 1/3 of the total 0.7-in. displacement that it would undergo. During the remainder of the impact period, between 12.0 and 20.0 msec, the head moved backward into

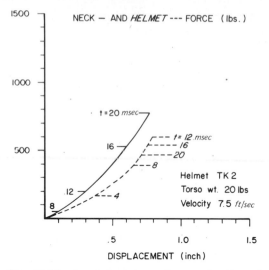

Fig. 11-15. Load-displacement curve for Case 1. The helmet performance is represented by the interrupted line and the neck displacement pattern by the solid line. At t = 20.0 msec, the resulting neck load is over 800 lbs.

the trunk. The trunk then stopped, with a resulting neck load of over 800 lbs. Even in this situation, in which a low impact velocity is coupled with a low effective torso weight, the neck probably developed sufficient force to cause fracture.

In Case 2 (Fig. 11-16), we see the results

of the same impact velocity, but with a higher equivalent torso mass of 80 lbs. In this case the time sequence of events hardly changes. It takes the head slightly more than 12.0 msec to come to a complete stop and rebound toward the body. At the end of 19.0 msec the neck has developed a compressive load of 1000 lbs. At this time the remaining velocity of the body is 6.4 ft/sec, with a remaining kinetic energy of 50 ft-lbs. This remaining kinetic energy is sufficient to continue to cause neck deformation, dislocation, and soft-tissue injury after the 1000-lb point at which the compression fracture would occur.

When the impacting velocity is raised to 15 ft/sec with a 40-lb weight for the trunk mass, as in Case 3 (Fig. 11-17), the head comes to rest after slightly more than 8.0 msec, and it takes the trunk only 10.8 msec to impart sufficient energy to the neck to exceed the 1000-lb compressive failure load. Notice that at the end of 8.0 msec the neck has barely started its compression, while the head has come to a complete stop and is starting to rebound. The velocity of the trunk at the 10.8 msec mark, at which the neck has theoretically fractured, is still

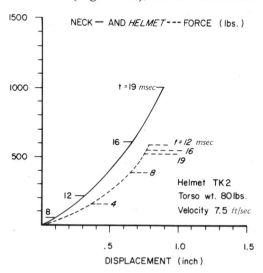

Fig. 11-16. Load-displacement curve for Case 2. The helmet performance is indicated by the interrupted line and the neck displacement by the solid line. The graph indicates that at 19.0 msec after impact, the neck has developed a compressive load of 1000 lbs.

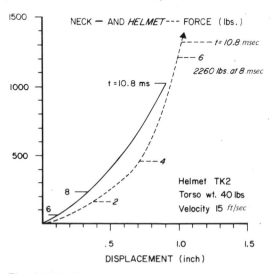

Fig. 11-17. Load-deflexion curve for Case 3. The helmet performance is indicated by the interrupted line and the neck displacement by the solid line. The velocity of the trunk at 10.8 msec, at which the neck has theoretically fractured, is still 14.1 ft/sec, i.e., 88% of its initial kinetic energy.

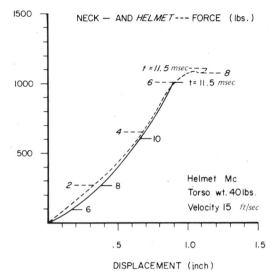

Fig. 11-18. Load-deflexion curve for Case 4. The helmet performance is represented by the interrupted line, and the neck displacement by the solid line. Time sequence is slightly different, but the consequences are identical to that of Case 3. The neck would fracture at 11.5 msec at contact, at which time the body still has a velocity of 13.4 ft/sec, and 80% of its initial kinetic energy.

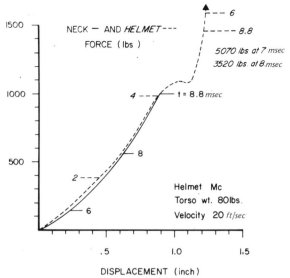

Fig. 11-20. Load-deflexion curve for Case 6. The neck reaches a fracture load in 8.8 msec with the trunk retaining 475 ft-lbs of energy at a velocity of 19.6 ft/sec.

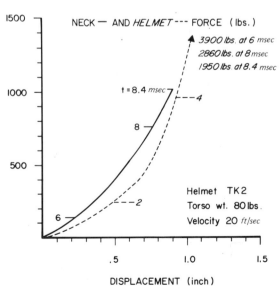

Fig. 11-19. Load-deflexion curve for Case 5. The head (interrupted line) comes to a complete stop in 6.0 msec and the neck (solid line) develops 1000 lbs of compressive force at 8.4 msec, at which time only 2% of the initial 497 ft-lbs of kinetic energy is dissipated.

14.1 ft/sec, i.e., 88% of its initial kinetic energy. This same impact situation is illustrated for the MacGregor MH helmet (Fig. 11-18). Note that the time sequence is slightly different, but that the consequences are identical. In this case, the neck would fracture at 11.5 msec after contact, at which time the body still has a velocity of 13.4 ft/sec and 80% of its initial kinetic energy.

When the impacting velocity is 20 ft/sec and the trunk weight is 80 lbs, as in Case 5 (Fig. 11-19), the head comes to a complete stop in approximately 6.0 msec, and the neck requires 8.4 msec to develop the 1000 lbs of compressive force. In this case, only 2% of the initial 497 ft-lbs of kinetic energy is dissipated at 8.4 msec.

The model behavior is similar with the MacGregor MH helmet (Fig. 11-20). The neck reaches the fracture load in 8.8 msec with the trunk retaining 475 ft-lbs of energy at a velocity of 19.6 ft/sec.

In all of these studies, the head came to rest within 6 to 12.0 msec because of the energy absorption of the helmet. After that the head rebounded away from the helmet. Although the head, in most cases, comes to a complete stop some time before fracture, the trunk mass does not. The trunk mass loses only a small fraction of its velocity by the time it has imparted enough energy to the neck to create an excessive axial compressive load. Thus in Case 2 (Fig. 11-16), although the velocity of the trunk mass is only 7.5 ft/sec, the decrease in velocity is only 1 ft/sec when the critical load is reached.

From these results, it appears that the typical helmet is able to bring the head to rest in anywhere between 6 and 12.0 msec, depending on the initial velocity of the head. It does this while keeping the head accelerations well within intended limits. Since the kinetic energy of the head is under 50 ft-lbs, while the kinetic energy of the torso can easily exceed 600 ft-lbs, it is obvious that a structure such as the helmet cannot be relied upon to absorb the kinetic energy from the torso. Moreover, if the primary function of the helmet is to provide protection for the skull, a redesigned helmet, which would also be capable of absorbing all the kinetic energy of the body, would be a disproportionate and totally useless structure.

The mechanism that is displayed in the computation is one of the helmet stopping the head while the trunk continues its motion and applies kinetic energy to the neck. Under the alignment conditions previously described, the neck, a relatively fragile structure in compression, cannot absorb the kinetic energy without exceeding its dynamic load limits. Therefore, fractures or dislocations occur.

The model that has been examined describes the conditions under which cervical spinal fractures or dislocations can occur. Based on observed geometry during actual cervical spine injury in football, it has a coincident anatomic axis for the head, neck, and trunk. In addition, the velocity of these segments is parallel to this anatomic axis, and the impact is allowed to occur between the helmet and a relatively immovable object. This study shows that the helmet successfully stops the head. However, in all dynamic conditions examined, the trunk continues to input kinetic energy into the neck in the form of strain energy until a sufficient amount of energy is stored to damage the cervical spine. The damage mode may be compression, which produces crush fractures of the cervical vertebrae; buckling, which produces a flexion dislocation acutely at one junction, or a combination of these two modes. Because of disparity between the kinetic energy of the body and the kinetic energy of the head, the helmet is not a suitable structure for absorbing all kinetic energies, and therefore is not useful in preventing neck injury.

The one meaningful conclusion to be drawn from the available data is that axial loading of the cervical spine must be avoided if injuries are to be prevented. Cervical spine injuries are a function of technique, i.e., head tackling or diving into shallow water, and cannot be prevented by equipment, i.e., helmets. The implications of this fact for coaches, game officials, and athletic administrators are obvious.

REFERENCES

1. Bauze, R.J.: Experimental production of forward dislocations in the human cervical spine. J. Bone Joint Surg., *60-B*:239, 1978.
2. Carter, D.R., and Frankel, V.H.: Biomechanics of hyperextension injuries to the cervical spine in football. Am. J. Sports Med., 8:302, 1980.
3. Roaf, R.: A study of the mechanics of spinal injuries. J. Bone Joint Surg., *42-B*:810, 1960.
4. Schneider, R.C.: Head and Neck Injuries in Football. Baltimore, Williams & Wilkins, 1973.
5. Torg, J.S., et al.: Spinal injury at the level of the third and fourth cervical vertebrae from football. J. Bone Joint Surg., *59-A*:1015, 1977.
6. Torg, J.S., et al.: The National Football Head and Neck Injury Registry: report and conclusions 1978. J.A.M.A., 241:1477, 1979.
7. Virgin, H.: Cineradiographic study of football helmets and the cervical spine. Am. J. Sports Med., 8:310, 1980.
8. White, A.A., and Panjabi, M.M.: Clinical Biomechanics of the Spine. Philadelphia, J.B. Lippincott, 1978.

Chapter 12

Radiographic Evaluation of the Cervical Spine

Helene Pavlov

The purpose of the radiographic examination of a patient with possible head and neck injuries is to rapidly obtain diagnostic radiographs without further injuring the patient. Following a brief preliminary clinical examination to determine the vital signs, neurologic status, and the possible sites of injury, the radiologic examination is started. Whenever there is a possible cervical spine injury, initial radiographs are obtained without moving the patient from the litter. Radiographs taken on the litter are never as good as those done on the radiographic table, but they are usually sufficient to diagnose an unstable cervical spine fracture. An anteroposterior and a horizontal crosstable lateral view of the cervical spine, using grid cassettes, can demonstrate a fracture or fracture-dislocation. The examination is best performed in the x-ray department with a machine that minimizes the radiographic distortion produced by involuntary patient movement instead of in an emergency room with a low-powered portable machine. The technologist must be alerted not to turn the patient's head during the initial examination, because any manipulation of the head and neck in the presence of an unstable cervical spine fracture could damage the spinal cord and result in paralysis or death. Not until an unstable

fracture is excluded, or if present properly braced, should the patient be transferred from the litter to the radiographic or computed tomographic table for additional studies. The vital signs and neurologic status must be monitored continuously, and no patient, especially an unconscious one, should ever be left unattended during the radiologic examination.

RADIOGRAPHIC TECHNIQUES AND ANATOMY

The radiographic examination and interpretation of the cervical spine can be challenging because each of the seven individual segments has complex and varying anatomy.

As with any body part, the routine radiologic examination requires at least two projections taken at right angles to each other, the anteroposterior (AP) and lateral views. For the cervical spine, the complete AP study requires two films. The complete lateral study requires one film and is the most important view. Additional plain film examination of the cervical spine includes oblique and pillar views and mobility studies that can be performed after an unstable fracture is excluded. Tomography, fluoroscopy, and computed tomography (CT) provide further detail and information about the vertebrae and spinal canal. The spinal cord and nerve roots are protected by the cervical spine, and are examined by myelography.

Plain Films

The normal anatomic relationship of the cervical vertebrae must be recognized in order to interpret the abnormal.

The *AP view* of the cervical spine requires two films; both can be obtained with the patient sitting, or with a critically injured patient supine on the litter. The lower cervical spine, C3 through C7 is demonstrated on the *routine view*. The atlas and axis are visualized on an *open-mouth view* (Fig. 12-1*A, B*). In the AP view of the lower cervical spine (Fig. 12-1*C*) the joints of Luschka, the superior and inferior cortices of the vertebrae, and the spinous processes are examined for integrity and anatomic alignment. There is a symmetric undulation of the lateral cortical margins of the articular masses. The tracheal air shadow should be midline. On the open-mouth view (Fig. 12-1*D*), the odontoid is equidistant from the lateral masses of C1, and the lateral masses of C1 and C2 are aligned. The spinous processes are midline. Occasionally, the margin of the posterior arch of C1 projects over the odontoid, simulating a fracture at the base of the dens. This is known as a Mach effect.[15]

The *lateral view* of the spine is the most important film in the cervical spine examination. In the critically injured patient with possible cervical spine and spinal cord damage, the lateral view should be obtained without moving the patient from the litter. A cassette is placed vertically alongside the patient's neck and the roentgenographic beam or central ray is horizontal, perpendicular to the cassette. This view is called a crosstable lateral (Fig. 12-2*A*). The entire spine, from C1 to C7, should be included on the lateral view. Sometimes the odontoid is obscured by the

mastoids and mandible; C7 and occasionally even C6 may not be demonstrated because of the shoulder girdle. The odontoid can be visualized by slightly tilting the head, provided an unstable fracture has been excluded, or by tomography. The lower cervical spine can be demonstrated by having the shoulders pulled out of the way. If the patient is supine and not fully conscious, someone can gently pull on the patient's arms. If the lower cervical vertebrae are still not demonstrated, a *swimmer's view* should be obtained. This is a horizontal crosstable view obtained with the patient prone or supine. The arm closest to the cassette is raised over the patient's head, simulating a swimming position. The central ray is directed through the shoulder girdle (Fig. 12-2*B*). If all these attempts fail, routine tomography or CT may be used.

On the lateral view, the prevertebral soft tissues should be examined (Fig. 12-2*C*). If the lateral cervical spine film is overexposed and only the bones are detailed, the film should be repeated with proper

---

Fig. 12-1. *A,* An AP view of the cervical spine is obtained with the roentgenographic tube (central ray) angled 5 to 10° cephalad. The cassette is placed behind the patient's neck. The patient may be sitting or supine. *B,* An open-mouth view is obtained with the patient supine and the cassette behind the head and neck. The central ray is perpendicular to the cassette and directed through the open mouth. This view may be facilitated in a conscious patient by having the patient chew during the exposure so the mandible is blurred and does not obscure the odontoid. *C,* An AP view of the cervical spine delineating C3 through C7. The lateral margins of the lateral masses form a gentle undulating line, bilaterally. The joints of Luschka (arrowheads), the spinous processes (S), the vertebral body end-plates (arrows), the intervertebral disc spaces, and the pedicles (P) are identified at each level. The tracheal air shadow is midline. *D,* The atlas and axis are identified on the open-mouth view. The lateral margins of the articular masses of C1 and C2 should be in alignment (arrows). The odontoid is equidistant from the lateral masses of C1. Occasionally, the posterior arch of C1 overlaps the odontoid simulating a horizontal fracture. This is known as a Mach effect (arrowheads).

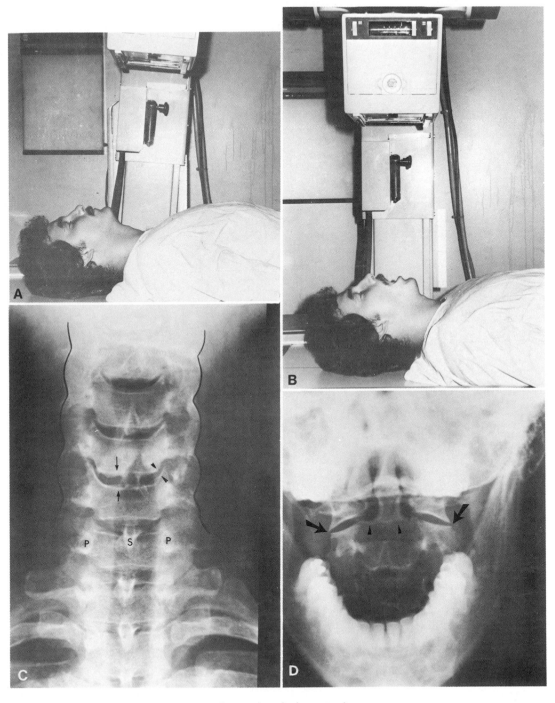

(Legend on facing page.)

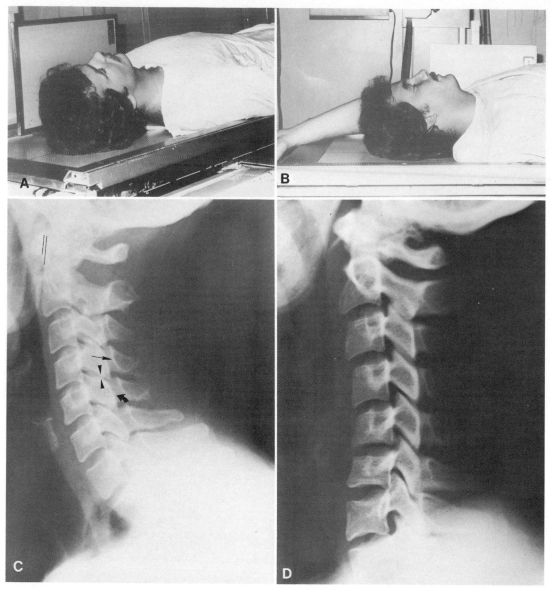

Fig. 12-2. *A,* A horizontal crosstable lateral view of the cervical spine is the most important film in the examination of an acutely injured patient. The central ray is perpendicular to a vertical cassette, which is placed alongside the patient's neck. *B,* The swimmer's view is obtained with the patient prone, or if critically injured, supine. It is a crosstable lateral view using a horizontal beam and a vertical cassette. The arm closest to the cassette is raised above the head. This view demonstrates the lower cervical vertebrae through the shoulder girdle. *C,* On the lateral view of the cervical spine, C1 through C7 should be visualized. Gentle lordotic curved lines are formed by the anterior cortical margins of the vertebral bodies, the posterior cortical margins of the vertebral bodies, the posterior cortical margins of the articular processes (short arrow), and also the spinolaminar lines (arrow). The intervertebral disc spaces should be the same height anteriorly to posteriorly and equal in height at each level. The superior and inferior articular facets of the interfacetal joints should be parallel to each other (arrowheads). The vertebral body heights are equal. The spinous processes should be almost parallel to each other, and the interspinous distances equal. The ADI distance between lines must be less than 3 mm, even in flexion. The prevertebral soft tissues are normal. *D,* The cervical lordosis may be straightened or reversed by spasm or voluntary guarding, and it is a normal variant in 20% of the population. When intact, the reversal should be gradual, and the alignment of the intervertebral spaces, interfacetal joints, and the spinous processes are normal. (Fig. 12-2*D*: Courtesy of Jay W. MacMoran, M.D., Director, Department of Radiology, Germantown Hospital, Philadelphia, PA.)

technique factors that delineate the soft tissues. The normal prevertebral soft tissues have specific measurement.[17] The most important soft tissue determination is at the level of C3. In adults this should be an absolute maximum of 4.8 mm or approximately one half the AP width of the C3 vertebral body.[34] At the C6 level the average width of the soft tissues is 14 mm with a maximum of 22 mm in adults, approximately equal to the AP width of the C6 vertebral body. At the C1-C2 level any soft tissue visualization is abnormal and anterior to C2, 3.5 to 7 mm is acceptable.

On the lateral view, there is a gentle lordosis to the normal cervical spine. The anterior and posterior borders of the vertebral bodies, the posterior cortices of the lateral masses, and the spinolaminar lines of C2 through C7 align to form four uninterrupted lordotic curved lines. The posterior arch of C1 is normally smaller than the rest. The spinous processes each converge slightly toward a hypothetical posterior point and the interspinous distances are equidistant at each level, except between C2-C3, which is larger. The intervertebral disc spaces should be uniform in height from anterior to posterior and the disc spaces should be of equal height at each level, except at C2-C3, which is larger. The interfacetal joints are angled 35° caudally from the vertical plane, and the superior and inferior facets of each joint are parallel to each other. Each vertebral body is equal in vertical height, with the exception of C4, C5, or C6, which on occasion may be slightly smaller. Finally, the atlantodens interval (ADI), the distance between the anterior arch of C1 and the anterior aspect of the odontoid, must be measured. A measurement over 3 mm in adults is abnormal, regardless of flexion or extension.[11,18]

The roentgen pattern of a cervical spine in the lateral view can be affected by numerous factors. The cervical lordosis can be reversed or straightened by muscular spasm, voluntary guarding, ligamentous disruption, a fracture, or dislocation.

Approximately 20% of the population normally have a straight or kyphotic spine, and a one inch depression of the chin straightens the cervical spine in 70% of the population (Fig. 12-2D).[34] Also, lateral views of the cervical spine occasionally are inadvertently obtained with the head or body slightly rotated. Rotation produces a lack of superimposition of the posterior margins of the vertebral bodies and lateral masses. Rotation of the head mainly affects the upper cervical spine, and rotation of the body produces a gradual increasing lack of superimposition from C1 to C7. This rotation is normal when the lack of superimposition at each level throughout the spine is gradual.[16]

Mobility studies are lateral views performed in maximum voluntary flexion and extension to locate and document ligamentous stability and disruption.[10,16,24,33] In flexion, there is an increase in the intraspinous distances, widening of the posterior aspect of the interfacetal joints and intervertebral disc spaces, and narrowing of the anterior aspect of the intervertebral disc spaces (Fig. 12-3A). The vertebrae may normally slide anteriorly up to 3 mm on the subjacent vertebrae. These changes should be gradual and consistent throughout the cervical spine but are more extreme in the upper cervical spine. All these changes are reversed in extension (Fig. 12-3B).[16] Flexion and extension views must not be performed following trauma until the initial radiographs have been reviewed and an unstable fracture excluded.

Oblique views are important for a complete trauma series; both right and left obliques are obtained. This view demonstrates the interfacetal joints, the lamina, the intravertebral foramina, the pedicles, and the lateral masses (Fig. 12-4A, B). The lateral elements of the superior vertebrae should always be slightly lateral to that of the subjacent vertebrae. The radiographic appearance of these structures depends on the degree of obliquity. The oblique views are usually obtained with the patient sit-

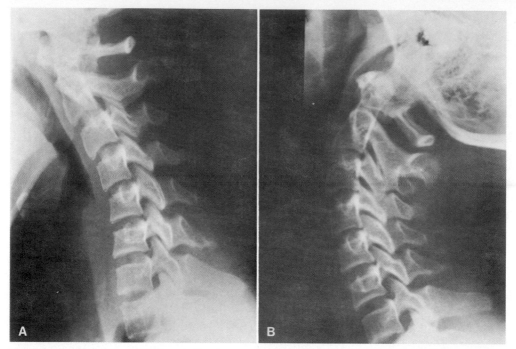

Fig. 12-3. Mobility studies of the cervical spine are lateral views obtained in maximum voluntary flexion and extension. They are useful to determine ligamentous disruption. *A,* In flexion, the cervical lordosis is reversed. Each vertebral body moves slightly anteriorly to the vertebra below, and the anterior aspect of the intervertebral disc spaces are narrowed. The interspinous distance and the posterior aspect of the interfacetal joints are increased. These changes are present at all levels, but are greatest in the upper segments. *B,* In extension, the cervical lordosis is increased and the changes that occur in flexion are reversed.

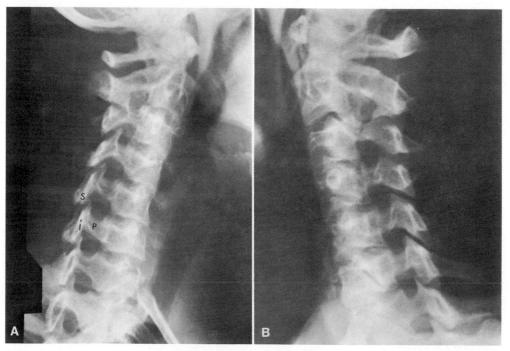

Fig. 12-4. Oblique views of the cervical spine demonstrating the interfacetal joints. *A,* Left posterior oblique view demonstrates the right side. The superior facet (S) should be lateral to the inferior facet (i). The pedicles (P) connect the vertebral body to the articular mass and form the border of the intervertebral foramen. The intervertebral foramen should be patent at each level. The laminae are seen en face as corticated oval structures. Each lamina, as each articular process, should be lateral to that of the subjacent vertebra. *B,* The configuration of the articular masses, laminae, pedicles, foramen, and interfacetal joints is slightly different due to a different degree of obliquity.

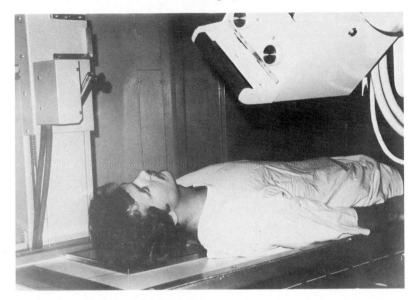

Fig. 12-5. An oblique view can be obtained with the patient supine on the litter, if necessary, by angling the tube 45° from one side of the patient toward a cassette placed flat on the litter either under or alongside the neck. Both right and left oblique views should be obtained.

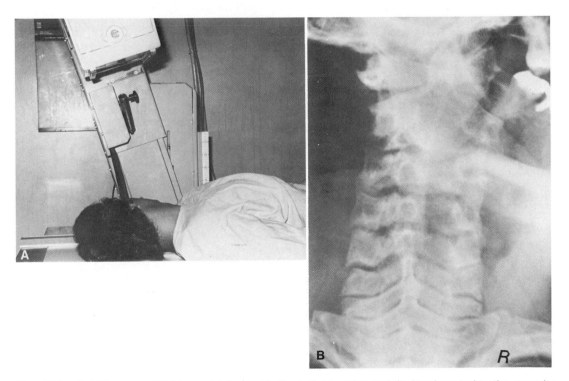

Fig. 12-6. *A,* Pillar views (Weir) are obtained with the patient supine and the head rotated to the opposite side of interest. The head rotation is necessary to eliminate superimposition of the mandible and face on the lateral masses. The central ray is moved 2 cm off midline toward the side of interest and angled 35° caudad. This is an important view but must not be obtained until it has been established that the head can be rotated safely. *B,* Pillar view demonstrating the articular masses in the coronal plane.

ting, but can be obtained while the patient is still on the litter by placing the film cassette posterior to the neck, and angling the central ray 45° toward the cassette from the opposite side of the patient (Fig. 12-5).[15]

Pillar views are designed to examine the lateral masses and are obtained with the patient supine, and with the tube angled caudally and centered 2 cm from midline toward the side of interest.[34] The chin is rotated to the opposite direction; this position is not recommended for a patient who might have an unstable fracture (Fig. 12-6A, B).

Fluoroscopy and Tomography

The use of fluoroscopy, tomography, or CT is occasionally required in the examination of the cervical spine. Fluoroscopy is an excellent method of obtaining coned-down views under direct visual control and at different degrees of obliquity.

Tomography is useful to demonstrate a part of a vertebra that is otherwise superimposed by adjacent vertebrae. Tomography can be performed in the AP, lateral, oblique, or pillar views.

The CT examination displays the vertebrae in cross section and is especially helpful in determining the integrity of the lamina, pedicles, and the spinal canal (Fig. 12-7A-C).

Myelography and Computed Tomography

The central nervous system in the region of the cervical spine is the spinal cord and nerve roots. A cervical myelogram demonstrates the subarachnoid space, spinal cord, and the roots of the spinal nerves. A myelogram involves the subarachnoid injection of a radiopaque contrast agent. The

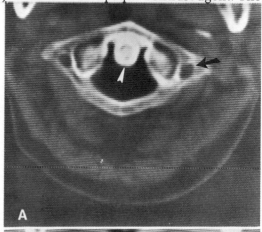

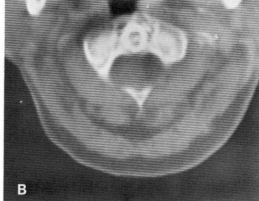

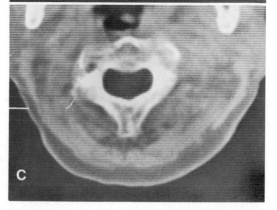

Fig. 12-7. CT sections of the atlas and axis. *A,* Cross-sectional tomogram of the atlas demonstrating the anterior and posterior arches, lateral masses, and vertebral artery foramina (arrow). The odontoid (arrowhead) is seen in anatomic relation to the anterior arch of C1, and the shape and integrity of the spinal canal can be determined. The window setting is for bone and the marrow cavity and cortex can be distinguished in the lateral masses and the odontoid. *B,* A slightly caudad section demonstrating the top of the lateral masses of C2 and the still corticated odontoid. *C,* A still further cauded section through the anterior and posterior arches of C2. (Courtesy of James C. Hirschy, M.D., New York, NY.)

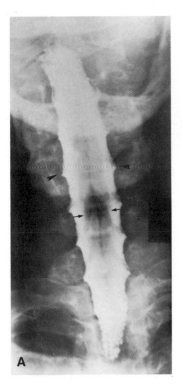

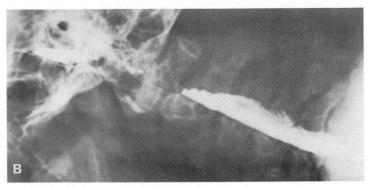

Fig. 12-8. *A,* An AP view of a normal cervical myelogram. The spinal cord (arrows) and nerve roots (arrowheads) are lucent and surrounded by the white contrast material. *B,* A crosstable lateral view of a normal cervical myelogram, obtained with the patient prone. The radiopaque contrast is adjacent to the posterior aspect of the cervical vertebrae, the cord is dorsal.

contrast is heavier than cerebrospinal fluid, and can be maneuvered to surround the cord and the nerve roots by adjusting the patient's position (Fig. 12-8*A, B*).[27] With the contrast agent in place, posteroanterior, both obliques, and a crosstable lateral view of the cervical spine are obtained with the patient in a prone position.

The CT has been used for analysis of the bony architecture of the spinal canal for several years. The newer CT models have increased resolution capabilities and can also demonstrate the spinal cord, and may provide more information about the cord in the future (Fig. 12-9).[8, 21, 30]

Fractures and Injuries to the Cervical Spine

In examining roentgenograms of the cervical spine for fractures and dislocations, it is important to remember to examine the soft tissues in addition to the bones. On the lateral view, a localized or generalized increase in the prevertebral soft tissues following injury indicates a hematoma or edema. On the AP view, a soft-tissue swelling may be evident by deviation of the tracheal air shadow from the midline (Fig. 12-10*A, B*). In addition to confirming a serious injury and localizing the area of abnormality, soft-tissue swelling, in and of itself, can be life threatening. Soft-tissue swelling can obstruct the airway and must not be ignored. If the soft tissues cannot be evaluated on a lateral view of the cervical spine, the radiograph should be repeated.

Cervical spine injuries can be stable or unstable. Stable injuries are those in which additional spinal cord or nerve root damage is not anticipated with gentle spine

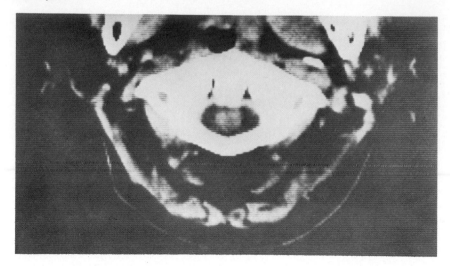

Fig. 12-9.   This cross section of C1 is identical to Figure 12-7A; however the window setting is for soft tissue in order to demonstrate the spinal cord within the spinal canal. (Courtesy of James C. Hirschy, M.D., New York, NY.)

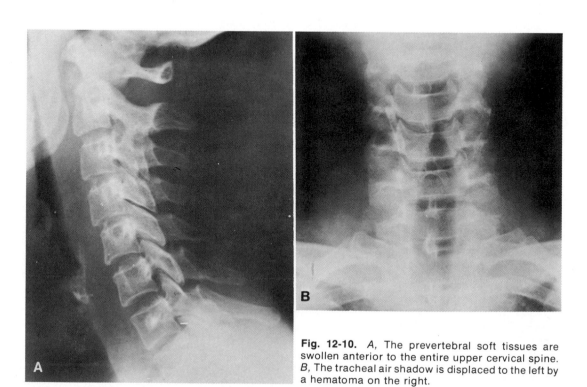

Fig. 12-10.   *A,* The prevertebral soft tissues are swollen anterior to the entire upper cervical spine. *B,* The tracheal air shadow is displaced to the left by a hematoma on the right.

movement. Unstable fractures are those in which there is significant ligamentous damage, and any movement of the spine may further compromise the neurologic status by injuring the nerve roots or the spinal cord.[2, 12, 16] Roentgenograms must be evaluated to specifically determine signs of ligamentous injury in addition to bony pathologic change.

Radiographically, ligamentous injury as well as bony fractures and dislocations are evident by a change in the anatomic configuration and alignment. The cervical spine can be divided into anterior and posterior elements (Fig. 13-14). The anterior elements include the vertebral body, intervertebral discs, and the anterior and posterior longitudinal ligaments. The posterior elements include the vertebral arch, spinous process, the capsule of the interfacetal joints, the ligamentum flavum, and the intraspinous and supraspinous ligaments. Injury to either the anterior or posterior elements is evidenced by impaction or narrowing due to compressive forces, and by separation or widening due to distracting forces. Ligamentous injuries, avulsions, fractures, and dislocations vary according to the position of the cervical spine and the strength and direction of the forces as they are transmitted through the cervical spine segments. The lower cervical spine (C3 through C7) is subject to different forces than the atlas and axis (C1-C2). The injuries of the lower and upper cervical spine will be discussed separately.

Lower Cervical Spine

Lower cervical spine injuries are divided into three categories: (1) ligamentous injuries, (2) fractures, and (3) dislocations.

Ligamentous Injuries. Ligamentous injuries are diagnosed indirectly by malalignment of the osseous structures. An *anterior subluxation*[7, 16, 19, 33] is the mildest injury that has radiographic manifestations; it is diagnosed on the lateral

view. The radiographic findings include a localized reversal of the normal cervical lordosis, increase in the intraspinous distance or fanning, widening of the intervertebral disc space posteriorly, and loss of parallelism at the interfacetal joints (Fig. 12-11A). All of these findings are more obvious when the cervical spine is flexed; flexion views are recommended whenever this injury is clinically suspected and the initial films are normal or inconclusive. The posterior ligaments, interfacetal joint capsule, and occasionally even the posterior aspect of the disc are disrupted; however the majority of the disc and the anterior spinous ligament remain intact. When there is disruption of the intervertebral disc and posterior longitudinal ligament, anterior angulation and translation of the superior vertebrae can occur (Fig. 12-11B).

Fractures. Fractures of the lower cervical spine are divided into fractures of the vertebral body, isolated or in combination with posterior element injuries, and fractures of the posterior neural arch and spinous process.

The mildest vertebral body fracture is the *wedge fracture*.[16, 33] This fracture is diagnosed on the lateral view by a decrease in the anterior height of the vertebral body (Fig. 12-12). The anterior superior or inferior corner is compressed and the area is flattened and dense. Occasionally, when the inferior corner is fractured, a beak forms. A wedge fracture is usually a stable fracture because the anterior longitudinal ligament and intervertebral disc are intact. The posterior longitudinal ligament and ligamentous complex may be lax or disrupted; flexion views should always be obtained if a wedge fracture is present or suspected on the routine films. Disruption of the posterior ligamentous complex results in fanning, and there may be an anterior subluxation above the fractured vertebrae.

More severe vertebral body fractures are *burst fractures*. These fractures are diagnosed on the lateral and AP views by col-

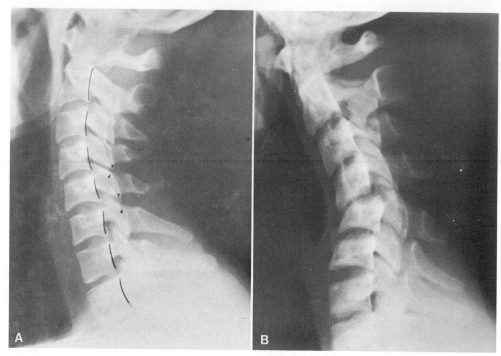

Fig. 12-11. *A,* An anterior subluxation may be roentgenographically subtle. There is interruption of the cervical lordosis at C5-C6, widening of the interspinous distance (fanning), and loss of parallelism of the posterior aspect of the interfacetal joint (lower set of arrowheads). *B,* A more severe anterior subluxation is demonstrated in this patient in which, in addition to fanning, there is anterior translation of C4 on C5 and acute angulation of the spine. All of these findings are accentuated in flexion.

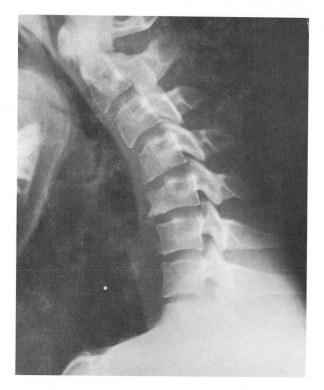

Fig. 12-12. A wedge fracture of C5 with decreased anterior vertebral body height involving both the superior and inferior borders. There is localized increased density anteriorly and inferiorly and a small chip fracture. The interspinous distances are normal in flexion, indicating an intact posterior ligamentous complex.

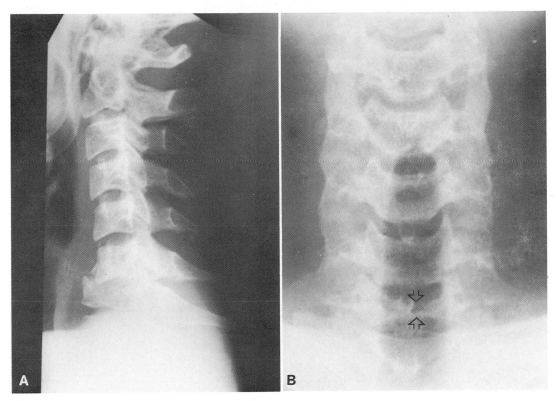

Fig. 12-13. *A,* A burst fracture of C7 in which only the vertebral body is involved. The superior end-plate is fractured (cupping), and the intervertebral disc space is narrowed. The posterior ligamentous complex is intact so there is no fanning. *B,* On the AP view, this compression fracture is demonstrated by loss of height of the involved vertebrae (arrows). The margins of the lateral masses are normal. This patient was injured during a football game and continued to play. One month later the patient escorted his brother who had a broken arm to the emergency room. While there, the patient mentioned to the doctor that his neck had ached for the past month, and these films were obtained.

lapse of the superior and/or inferior end-plate and reduction in the anterior and posterior height of the vertebral body (Fig. 12-13*A*, *B*). These changes of compression of the vertebral body result when the intervertebral disc "explodes" into the vertebral body[23]; the disc itself remains intact. This fracture is stable if the posterior elements are intact.[12]

A burst fracture of the vertebral body combined with fractures of the posterior neural arch is unstable. This injury is diagnosed on the AP view by the interruption of the normal symmetric undulating curves of the lateral masses and a vertical fracture through the vertebral body (Fig. 12-14*A*). A tomogram in the AP view delineates the fracture and the lateral dis-

placement of the lateral masses more clearly (Fig. 12-14*B*). On the lateral view, the comminuted vertebral body fracture and posterior displacement of the posterior fracture fragment can be identified. If the posterior ligamentous complex is intact, the interspinous distances are normal (Fig. 12-14*C*). Neurologic involvement is secondary to the degree of motion of the involved fracture segments.

A burst fracture of the vertebral body, combined with disruption of the posterior ligamentous complex, is unstable and is also diagnosed on the lateral view. This injury has been called a "teardrop fracture," named for the triangular fracture fragment at the anterior inferior corner of the vertebral body, which resembles a

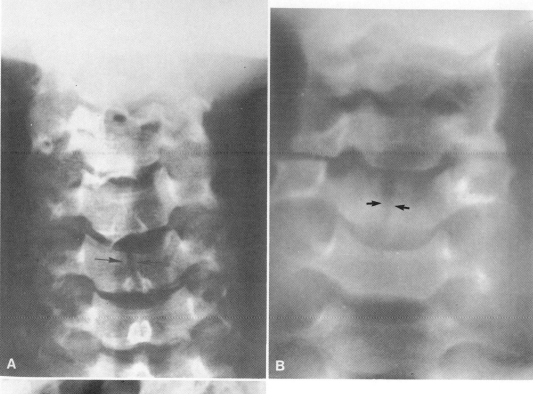

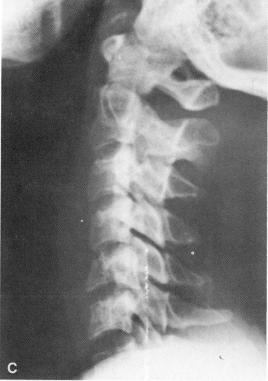

Fig. 12-14. *A,* A burst fracture of C5 involving the vertebral body and posterior neural arch. On the AP view, a vertical fracture (arrows) through the vertebral body is demonstrated. The symmetric lateral mass margins are interrupted, indicating a posterior neural arch fracture. *B,* On an AP tomogram, the lateral displacement of the lateral masses and disruption of the undulating curves of the lateral margins, as well as the vertical fracture of the vertebral body are better demonstrated. *C,* On the lateral view, there is a comminuted fracture through the vertebral body involving both the inferior and superior end plates. The posterior fracture fragment is posteriorly displaced without tilting. There is no fanning, because the posterior ligamentous complex is intact. (Courtesy of Jay W. MacMoran, M.D., Director, Department of Radiology, Germantown Hospital, Philadelphia, Pa.)

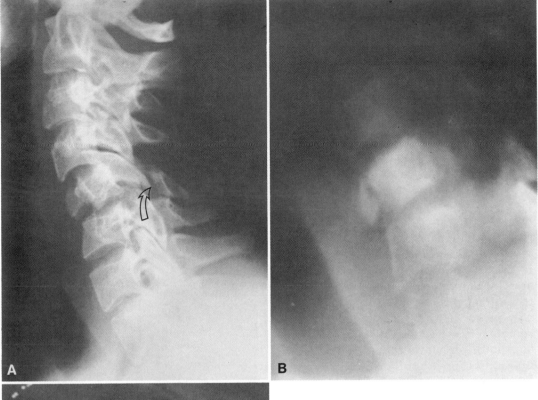

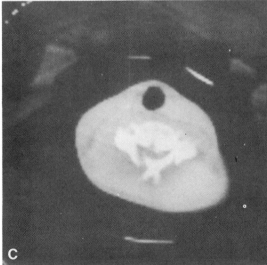

Fig. 12-15. *A,* Teardrop fracture of C5 involving the vertebral body, the posterior neural arch, and the posterior ligamentous complex. There is acute angulation of the spine at the level of injury. The posterior vertebral fracture fragment is posteriorly displaced and tilted. There is fanning of the C4-C5 spinous processes due to disruption of the posterior ligamentous complex. This patient also has associated fractures of the lamina of C5 (curved arrow). *B,* A tomogram of C5 demonstrating the tear-shaped fracture fragment for which this fracture is named. Widening of the posterior aspect of the disc space indicates disruption of the disc in this area and the posterior longitudinal ligament. *C,* CT section demonstrates the fracture in cross section. The severe encroachment of the spinal canal from both anterior and posterior fracture fragments is displayed.

teardrop (Fig. 12-15*A, B*). The fracture of the vertebral body is comminuted and there is acute kyphotic angulation of the spine at this level. The posterior fracture fragment of the vertebral body is posteriorly displaced and posteriorly tilted, which narrows the spinal canal and con-tributes to spinal cord compromise.[16, 25] Disruption of the posterior ligamentous complex is indicated by fanning. Widening of the posterior aspect of the intervertebral disc space at the involved level indicates a tear of the posterior longitudinal ligament and posterior aspect of the disc.

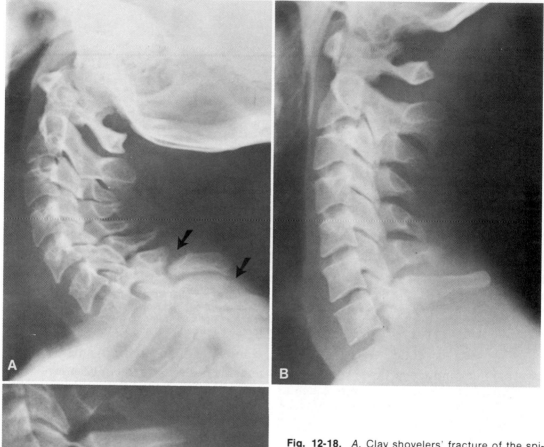

Fig. 12-18. *A,* Clay shovelers' fracture of the spinous process of C7 and T1 (arrows). Whenever one spinous process fracture is identified, attention to the spines of the vertebrae above and below is mandatory. *B,* Normal lateral view that includes C1 through C7. The broad shoulders obliterate T1, where the patient specifically located his pain. *C,* A coned-down view of the spinous processes of C7 and T1 demonstrating the fracture (arrow).

Fig. 12-20. *A,* Demonstration of a locked right facet on the oblique view. The superior facet of C6 is displaced medially to the inferior facet (arrow). *B,* Oblique view, demonstrating a subluxed left facet joint (arrow). The superior facet of C5 is medially displaced but has not fallen over the inferior facet into the intervertebral foramen.

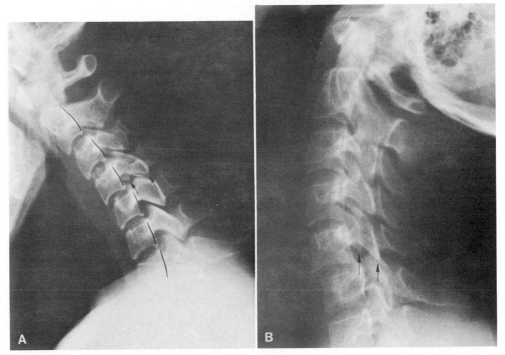

Fig. 12-19. *A,* Lateral view of a unilateral facet dislocation of C4. The C4 vertebra is slightly anteriorly displaced. Both inferior articular processes (arrows) of C4 and the higher vertebrae are seen, i.e., the vertebrae are oblique; the articular processes of C5 and the lower vertebrae are superimposed on each other, i.e., the vertebrae are lateral. *B,* Unilateral facet dislocation of C5 demonstrating both articular processes (arrows) at this level and above are demonstrated and there is slight anterior displacement of C5 on C6, and fanning of C5-C6 spinous processes. The articular masses are superimposed normally at C6.

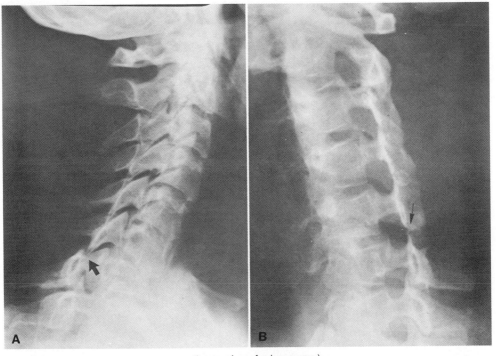

(Legend on facing page.)

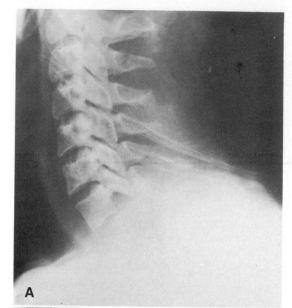

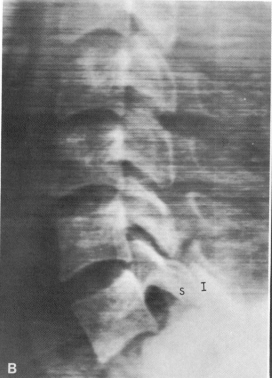

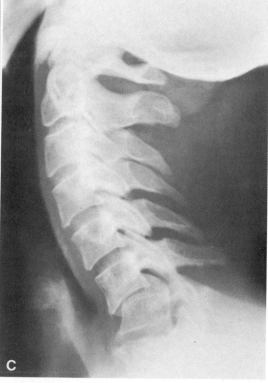

Fig. 12-21. *A,* Crosstable lateral view demonstrating anterior displacement of C7 on T1. *B,* A coned-down view, using a grid cassette, delineates more clearly the anterior displacement of C7 on T1. This displacement is over 75% of its AP width and is a bilateral facet dislocation. The superior facets of the interfacetal joints (S) (the inferior articular processes of C7) are completely anterior and locked in front of the inferior facets of the interfacetal joint (I) (the superior articular processes of T1). *C,* A bilateral facet subluxation of C6-C7. C6 is anteriorly displaced less than 50% of its AP width. The interfacetal joints are subluxed but not locked. The superior facets of C6 are displaced upward and forward but are not anterior to the inferior facets of C7. There is fanning of the spinous processes at this level.

AP width (Fig. 12-21C). Oblique views are necessary to evaluate the facet status. Flexion and extension views are contraindicated in these injuries as there is a high incidence of cord damage. These are un-stable injuries in which there is complete disruption of the posterior ligamentous complex, the intervertebral disc, and the anterior longitudinal ligament.[2,5]

A *posterior dislocation* should be sus-

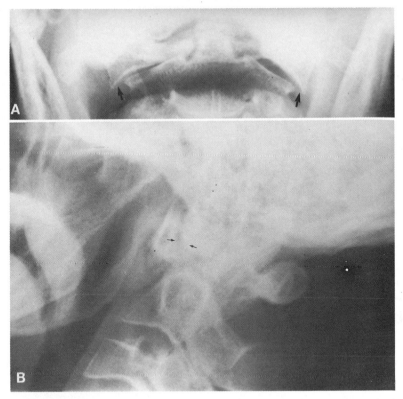

Fig. 12-22. *A,* A Jefferson fracture is best demonstrated on an open mouth view by the lateral displacement of the masses of C1 (arrows) compared with those of C2. *B,* Lateral view of a Jefferson fracture demonstrates an increased ADI (distance between arrows).

pected when a patient is quadriplegic and the radiographs seem normal.[3, 13, 16, 22, 31, 32] The radiographic changes, although subtle, are best observed in the lateral view as prevertebral soft-tissue swelling, a small posterior displacement of the vertebrae above the level of injury, a vacuum in the anterior aspect of the intervertebral disc at the level of injury, and occasionally an avulsion fracture of the inferior border of the vertebral body or superior corner of the subjacent vertebra. Any one of these signs is a strong indication that this injury has occurred and the cervical spine should be immediately immobilized.

Upper Cervical Spine

Radiographic evidence of upper cervical spine injuries are divided into fractures of the atlas and fractures of the axis.

Atlas. A Jefferson fracture is a bursting fracture of C1 and is diagnosed on the AP open-mouth view. On this view there is lateral displacement of the lateral masses of the atlas with respect to the lateral masses of the axis. The odontoid is usually intact (Fig. 12-22*A*, *B*). On the lateral view there is usually an increased ADI (distance between the anterior arch of C1 and the odontoid is over 3 mm) and prevertebral soft-tissue swelling. This is an unstable fracture produced by a compressive force of the occipital condyles into the lateral masses of the atlas, in which both the anterior and posterior elements of the atlas are fractured.[16, 20]

A fracture of the *posterior arch* of C1 is a stable injury without neurologic symptoms and it is diagnosed on the lateral view. The fracture may be isolated or in combination with more serious injuries (Fig. 12-23).[29]

Axis. Fractures of the odontoid have been classified by Anderson and D'Alonzo according to where the dens is fractured.[1] A *Type I* fracture occurs at the tip of the dens, and is a rare and stable injury. A *Type II* fracture occurs at the base of the dens where it joins the body of the axis, and is best diagnosed on a lateral view tomogram (Fig. 12-24A). This is usually initially unstable. A *Type III* fracture extends into the body of the axis and is best seen on an AP open-mouth view tomogram (Fig. 12-24B). This is usually a stable injury.

Odontoid fractures can be associated with dislocations of C1. *A C1-C2 dislocation* is best diagnosed on the lateral view, while the state of the odontoid is best identified on the AP open-mouth view (Fig. 12-25A, B). On the lateral view, the ADI should be measured. The ADI is usually increased in anterior dislocations and

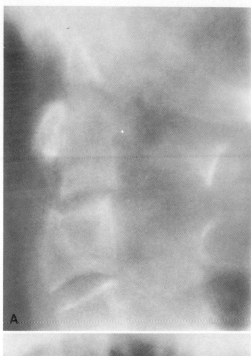

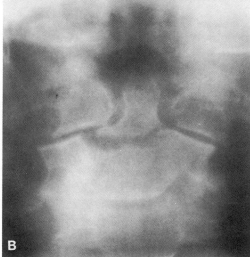

Fig. 12-24. *A*, Type II fracture of the odontoid. Tomogram demonstrates the fracture at the base of the dens where it joins the body of C2. There is slight posterior displacement of the odontoid. The ADI is intact. *B*, Type III fracture of the odontoid in which the fracture extends into the body of C2.

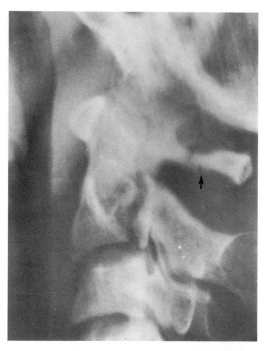

Fig. 12-23. A fracture through the posterior arch of C1 (arrow) associated with a hangman's fracture. There is also a teardrop avulsion fracture of C2.

normal in posterior dislocations.[1, 14] In the open-mouth view, the odontoid fracture and the degree of odontoid fragmentation can be appreciated. Because the spinal canal is largest in this area, the cord is

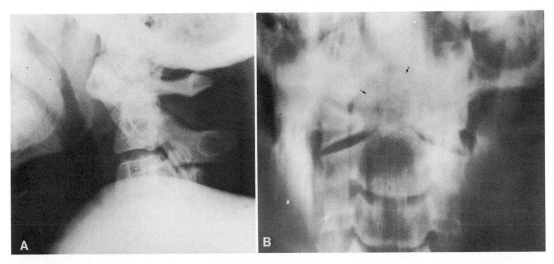

Fig. 12-25. *A,* Lateral view of the upper cervical spine demonstrating an anterior fracture-dislocation of C1 on C2. The top of the odontoid is not seen, but the ADI measured from a projected line continued cephalad along the anterior cortex of the visualized odontoid to the anterior arch of C1 is increased. *B,* A tomogram in the AP open-mouth view documents the fragmentation of the odontoid as seen by several cortical surfaces (arrows).

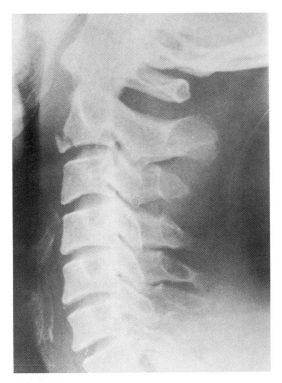

Fig. 12-26. A teardrop avulsion fracture of the anterior inferior corner of C2. There is soft-tissue swelling. The vertebrae are in normal alignment.

usually not compressed and the patient may be without neurologic damage.

An *avulsion teardrop fracture* of C2 results at the insertion site of the anterior longitudinal ligament. The "teardrop" refers to the triangular shape of the fracture fragment (Fig. 12-26).[4, 16] The posterior ligaments and interfacetal joint capsules are intact and there is normal vertebral alignment. This injury is usually stable in flexion and unstable in extension.

A *hangman's fracture* is a traumatic spondylolysis or pedicle fracture of C2 with a spondylolisthesis of C2 on C3. It is best diagnosed on the lateral view.[3, 9, 16, 26, 28] There is prevertebral soft-tissue swelling, narrowing of the C2-C3 disc, and anterior dislocation of C2 on C3. Occasionally a wedge fracture of C3 is also present (Fig. 12-27A).[3, 12, 26, 28] The ADI remains normal, less than 3 mm, because the transverse ligament remains intact. A unilateral pedicle fracture should be suspected when there is slight C2-C3 spondylolisthesis, and a tomogram should be obtained (Fig. 12-27B, C). A hangman's fracture is unstable, with

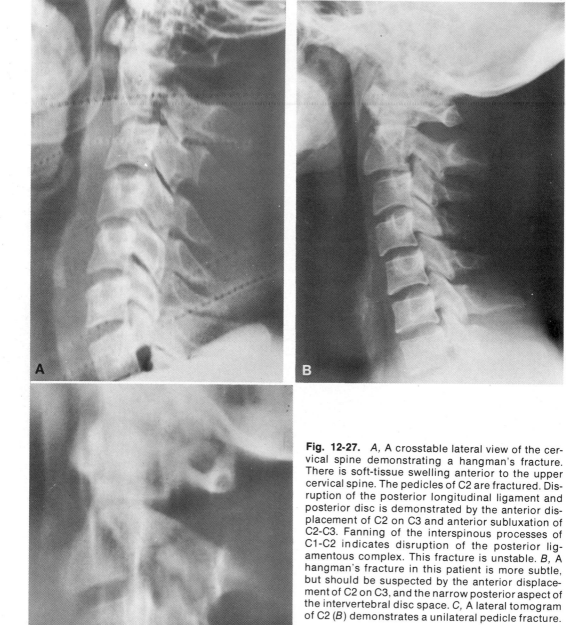

Fig. 12-27. *A,* A crosstable lateral view of the cervical spine demonstrating a hangman's fracture. There is soft-tissue swelling anterior to the upper cervical spine. The pedicles of C2 are fractured. Disruption of the posterior longitudinal ligament and posterior disc is demonstrated by the anterior displacement of C2 on C3 and anterior subluxation of C2-C3. Fanning of the interspinous processes of C1-C2 indicates disruption of the posterior ligamentous complex. This fracture is unstable. *B,* A hangman's fracture in this patient is more subtle, but should be suspected by the anterior displacement of C2 on C3, and the narrow posterior aspect of the intervertebral disc space. *C,* A lateral tomogram of C2 (*B*) demonstrates a unilateral pedicle fracture.

the only protection to the cord being the autodecompression secondary to the bilateral pedicle fractures, and the increased diameter of the canal in this region.

Central Nervous System

Trauma to the cervical spine can damage the spinal cord, the surrounding ligamentous, dural and vascular structures, the intervertebral disc, and the nerve roots. Myelography is the best method to demonstrate these lesions and is especially useful prior to surgery.[27]

Injury to the vessels surrounding the cord most commonly results in an *extradural hematoma*. On the myelogram a complete or partial block to the contrast agent may be demonstrated. When this defect is dorsal, it is best seen on the horizontal lateral view performed with the patient prone. A unilateral extradural defect displaces the cord to the opposite side and is best seen on the AP view. The hematoma normally extends over several vertebral segments (Fig. 12-28*A*).

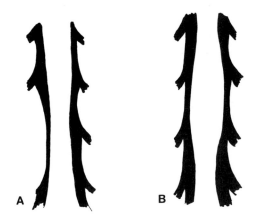

Fig. 12-28. A diagram of a myelogram in AP view. The cord is white and the contrast-filled subarachnoid space is black. *A,* An epidural hematoma narrows the subarachnoid space and displaces the cord to one side. The hematoma is localized but extends over several segments and does not correspond to an intervertebral disc space. *B,* Cord swelling, due to hematoma or edema, is seen as a localized widening of the cord. The cord can appear widened when compressed dorsally or ventrally, so true cord swelling must be confirmed by two right-angle films.

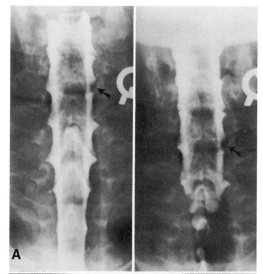

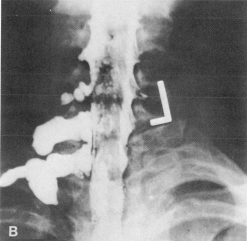

Fig. 12-29. *A,* An AP cervical myelogram demonstrating a herniated nucleus pulposus (disc). There is a horizontal lucency at the level of the intervertebral disc space and unilateral compression of the nerve root, demonstrated by widening of the nerve root and truncation of the contrast. *B,* An AP myelogram demonstrating an avulsion injury to the right brachial plexus. The contrast material extends along the enlarged and saccular nerve root sheaths.

Injury to the spinal cord secondary to a fracture or dislocation can result in *hemorrhage or localized edema*. This can occur immediately or several days following the injury. The injured cord swells, and as indicated on the myelogram, symmetrically narrows the surrounding contrast column or produces a complete block (Fig. 12-

28B). AP and lateral views are required to confirm that the cord is actually widened and not compressed from either front or back.

An *intervertebral disc herniation* can occur at the time of trauma. A disc herniation is diagnosed on the myelogram as a local defect in the anterior aspect of the contrast column localized at the intervertebral disc space. Occasionally, the associated nerve root may be blunted (Fig. 12-29A).

The arachnoid and dura accompany the nerve root through the intervertebral foramina. These structures may tear or the nerve root may be avulsed and retract. These injuries result in the formation of a *traumatic meningocele*, which is an irregular outpouching of the subarachnoid space along the path of the injured nerve root, and can be demonstrated when filled with a contrast agent (Fig. 12-29B).

REFERENCES

1. Anderson, L.D., and D'Alonzo, R.T.: Fractures of the odontoid process of the axis. J. Bone Joint Surg., 56A:1663, 1974.
2. Apley, A.L.: Fractures of the spine. Ann. R. Coll. Surg. Engl., 46:210, 1970.
3. Babcock, J.L.: Cervical spine injuries. Arch. Surg., 111:646, 1976.
4. Beabrook, G.M.: Stability of spinal fractures and dislocations. Int. J. Paraplegia, 9:23, 1971.
5. Beatson, T.R.: Fractures and dislocations of the cervical spine. J. Bone Joint Surg., 45B:21, 1963.
6. Braakman, R., and Vinken, P.J.: Unilateral facet interlocking in the lower cervical spine. J. Bone Joint Surg., 49B:249, 1967.
7. Cheshire, D.J.E.: The stability of the cervical spine following conservative treatment of fractures and dislocations. Int. J. Paraplegia, 7:193, 1970.
8. Coin, C.G., et al.: Diving type injuries of the cervical spine. Contribution of computed tomography to managment. J. Comput. Assist. Tomog., 3:362, 1979.
9. Cornish, B.L.: Traumatic spondylolisthesis of the axis. J. Bone Joint Surg., 50B:31, 1968.
10. Evans, K.D.: Anterior cervical subluxation. J. Bone Joint Surg., 58B:318, 1976.
11. Fielding, J.N., et al.: Tears of transverse ligament of the atlas. J. Bone Joint Surg., 56A:1683, 1974.
12. Fielding, J.N., and Hawkins, R.J.: Roentgenographic diagnosis of the injured neck. In AAOS Instructional Course Lectures. Vol. 25. St. Louis, C.V. Mosby, 1976.
13. Forsyth, H.F.: Extension injuries of the cervical spine. J. Bone Joint Surg., 46A:1792, 1964.
14. Gehweiler, J.A., et al.: Cervical spine trauma— the common combined conditions. Radiology, 103:77, 1979.
15. Harris, J.H., Jr.: Acute injuries of the spine. Semin. Roentgenol., 13:53, 1978.
16. Harris, J.H., Jr.: The Radiology of Acute Cervical Spine Trauma. Baltimore, Williams & Wilkins, 1978.
17. Hay, P.D.: Measurement of the soft tissues of the neck. In Atlas of Roentgenographic Measurements. 3rd Ed. Edited by L.B. Lusted, and T.E. Keats. Chicago, Yearbook Medical Publishers, 1972.
18. Hinck, V.C., and Hopkins, C.E.: Measurement of the atlanto dental interval in the adult. Am. J. Roentgenol., 84:945, 1965.
19. Holdsworth, F.: Fractures, dislocations and fracture/dislocations of the spine. J. Bone Joint Surg., 52A:1534, 1970.
20. Jefferson, G.: Fracture of the atlas vertebrae. Report of 4 cases, and a review of those previously recorded. Br. J. Surg., 7:407, 1920.
21. Kershner, M.S., et al.: Computed tomography in the diagnosis of an atlas fracture. Am. J. Roentgenol., 128:688, 1977.
22. Marar, B.C.: Hyperextension injuries of the cervical spine. The pathogenesis of damage to the spinal cord. J. Bone Joint Surg., 56A:1655, 1974.
23. Roaf, R.: A study of the mechanics of spinal injuries. J. Bone Joint Surg., 42B:810, 1960.
24. Scher, A.T.: Anterior cervical subluxation; an unstable position. Am. J. Roentgenol., 133:275, 1979.
25. Schneider, R.C., and Kahn, E.A.: Chronic neurologic sequelae of acute trauma to the spine and spinal cord. Part I: The significance of the acute-flexion or "teardrop" fracture dislocations of the cervical spine. J. Bone Joint Surg., 38A:985, 1956.
26. Schneider, R.C., et al.: "Hangman's fracture" of the cervical spine. J. Neurosurg., 22:141, 1965.
27. Shapiro, R.: Myelography. 2nd Ed. Chicago, Yearbook Medical Publishers, 1968.
28. Sherk, H.H.: Lesions of the atlas and axis. Clin. Orthop., 109:33, 1975.
29. Sinbert, S.E., and Berman, M.S.: Fracture of the posterior arch of the atlas. J.A.M.A., 114:1996, 1940.
30. Tadmor, R., et al.: Computed tomographic evaluation of traumatic spinal injuries. Radiology, 127:825, 1978.
31. Taylor, A.R., and Blackwood, W.: Paraplegia in hyperextension cervical injuries with normal radiographic appearances. J. Bone Joint Surg., 30B:245, 1948.
32. Taylor, A.R.: The mechanism of injury to the spinal cord in the neck without damage to the vertebral column. J. Bone Joint Surg., 33B:543, 1951.
33. Webb, J.K., et al.: Hidden flexion injury of the cervical spine. J. Bone Joint Surg., 58B:322, 1976.
34. Weir, D.C.: Roentgenographic signs of cervical injury. Clin. Orthop., 109:9, 1975.

Chapter 13

Diagnosis and Management of Cervical Spine Injuries

Joseph S. Torg

Sam W. Wiesel

Richard H. Rothman

Athletic injuries to the cervical spine may involve the bony vertebrae, intervertebral discs, annulus fibrosus, ligamentous supporting structures, the spinal cord, roots, and peripheral nerves, or any combination of these structures. The panorama of injuries seen run the spectrum from the "cervical sprain syndrome" to fracture-dislocations with permanent quadriplegia. Fortunately, severe injuries with neural involvement occur infrequently. However, those responsible for the emergency and subsequent care of the athlete with a cervical spine injury should possess a basic understanding of the variety of problems that can occur.

Roaf has proposed an international classification for spinal injuries.[8] The reader is encouraged to acquire an understanding of his system. He also delineated criteria for the ideal classification to include: (a) etiologic factors; (b) mechanism of injury; (c) anatomic and pathologic features of the lesion; and (d) means for restoring normal alignment and stability.

For purposes of obtaining a descriptive understanding of those cervical spine injuries observed to occur in athletics, we propose the following schemata:

I. Activity
    (a) Water sports—diving, surfing, waterskiing, others
    (b) Gymnastics—tumbling, trampoline, others
    (c) Wrestling
    (d) Football—position, activity, (e.g., blocking, tackling)
    (e) Skiing
    (f) Other

II. Mechanism of Injury
    (a) Axial compression—flexion
    (b) Axial compression—flexion-rotation
    (c) Flexion-rotation
    (d) Lateral flexion
    (e) Extension

III. Level of the Lesion
    (a) Upper cervical—C1-C3
    (b) Midcervical—C3-C4
    (c) Lower cervical—C4-C7

IV. Extent of the Lesion
    (a) Single vertebra
    (b) Single disc space
    (c) Vertebra and disc space
    (d) Disc space and adjacent vertebrae
    (e) Multiple levels
    (f) Other

V. Signs and Symptoms
    (a) Pain
    (b) Paresthesia
    (c) Paralysis
        (1) One extremity
        (2) Two extremities
        (3) Four extremities

VI. Roentgenographic Findings
  (a) Normal
  (b) Subluxation
  (c) Unilateral facet dislocation without fracture
  (d) Bilateral facet dislocation without fracture
  (e) Fractured vertebrae—anterior elements
    (1) Wedge compression fracture of vertebral body
    (2) Comminuted burst fracture of vertebral body
    (3) Comminuted burst fracture of vertebral body with displacement into vertebral canal
    (4) Comminuted burst fracture of vertebral body with associated fracture of vertebral body with associated posterior instability
    (5) Combined fractures of anterior and posterior bony elements
  (f) Fractured posterior elements
    (1) Pedicles
    (2) Lamina
    (3) Superior and inferior articular processes
    (4) Spinous processes
  (g) Special fractures
    (1) Jefferson fracture
    (2) Odontoid fracture
    (3) Hangman's fracture
  (h) Cervical spine instability
    (1) Acute
      (a) Anterior
      (b) Posterior
      (c) Combined
    (2) Chronic
      (a) Anterior
      (b) Posterior
      (c) Combined
VII. Paralysis Pattern
  (a) Quadriplegia—permanent. Complete motor deficit below level of the lesion.
  (b) Quadriplegia—transient. Temporary motor deficit with complete recovery.
  (c) Quadriparesis—permanent. Incomplete motor and sensory deficit with characteristic recovery pattern depending on area of cord involved.
    (1) Syndrome of acute anterior spinal cord injury—characterized as an immediate acute paralysis of all four extremities with a loss of pain and temperature sensation to the level of the lesion, but with preservation of posterior column sensation of motion, position, vibration, and part of touch.
    (2) Syndrome of acute central cervical spinal cord injury—characterized by disproportionately more motor impairment of the upper than lower extremities, bladder dysfunction, usually urinary retention, and varying degrees of sensory loss below the level of the lesion.
    (3) Other

ACUTE CERVICAL SPRAIN SYNDROME

An acute cervical sprain is an injury frequently seen in contact sports; the patient complains of having "jammed" his neck with subsequent pain localized to the cervical area. Characteristically, the patient presents with limitation of cervical spine motion (Fig. 13-1*A-G*), without radiation of pain or paresthesia. Neurologic examination is negative and roentgenograms are normal.

In the absence of findings other than pain and limitation of neck motion, identifying the exact nature of the injury may be difficult or impossible. However, it is assumed that either the intervertebral disc structures, ligamentous supporting structures, or the joints between the articular processes have been injured.

In general, treatment of athletes with "cervical sprains" should be tailored to the degree of severity. Immobilizing the neck in a soft collar and using analgesics and anti-inflammatory agents until there is a full, spasm-free range of neck motion is appropriate. If the patient has severe pain and muscle spasm of the cervical spine,

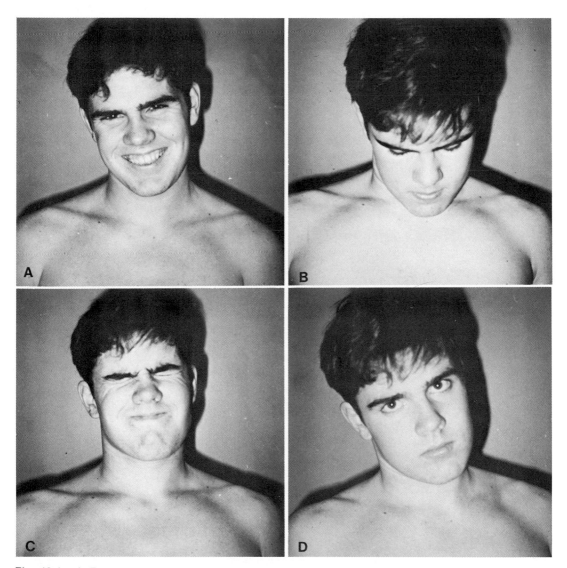

Fig. 13-1. *A,* Examining the athlete with complaints referrable to his neck, cervical spine, cervical nerve roots, or brachial plexus first involves observing the postural relationship between the head, neck, and torso. Although apparently comfortable and smiling, torticollis or wryneck posture indicates the possibility of a significant cervical injury. *B,* Active flexion of the neck and cervical spine accentuates the torticollis. As a general rule, the patient who presents with a wryneck following trauma should have a roentgenographic examination of the cervical spine. *C,* Active extension of the neck and cervical spine is markedly limited by pain and muscle spasm. Discomfort is vividly portrayed by his facial expression. *D,* Limitation of lateral bend to his right is evident by inability to actively touch right ear to right shoulder.

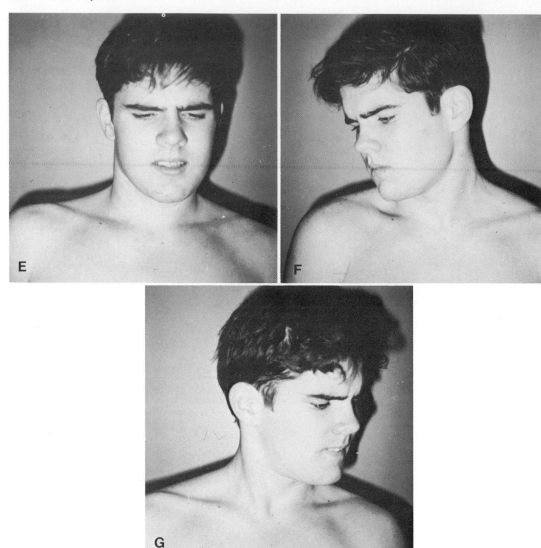

Fig. 13-1 (Cont'd). *E,* Marked limitation of lateral bend to the left is demonstrated when he attempts to touch his left ear to his left shoulder. The discomfort is vividly portrayed by his facial expression. *F,* Rotation of the cervical spine to the right is evaluated by having the patient actively touch his chin to his right shoulder. None of these maneuvers should involve manual assistance on the part of the examiner, nor should the patient be encouraged to attempt to move his neck at the point of pain. *G,* Rotation of the cervical spine to the left is evaluated by instructing the patient to actively touch his chin to his left shoulder.

hospitalization and the head-halter traction may be indicated. It should be emphasized that individuals with a history of collision injury, pain, and lack of normal range of cervical motion should have a routine cervical spine roentgenographic study. Also, lateral flexion and extension roentgenograms are indicated after the acute symptoms subside.

INTERVERTEBRAL DISC INJURIES

Roaf has provided insight to the sequence of events involved during compressive loading of the vertebrae in trauma.[7] The disc is less compressible than the vertebra and initial deformation occurs by vertebral end-plate bulging. He noted that the process continues to subsequent end-plate failure, which is the first structure to fracture. Cortical shell fracture and cancellous bone compression occur as deformation proceeds. Roaf further recognized that there was asymmetric compression, and that the pressure transmitted to the annulus resulted in tearing of the annulus or a general collapse of the vertebra due to buckling at its side. His study included determining the resistance of the annulus fibrosus with and without the presence of a fluid nucleus pulposus. After removing the nucleus pulposus, compressive loading produced the type of typical annulus prolapse seen in disc protrusion. Thus, Roaf suggested that compressive loading results in vertebral end-plate fracture with extrusion of nucleus pulposus into the vertebral body.

Albright has reported a study involving 75 University of Iowa freshmen football recruits who had roentgenograms of their

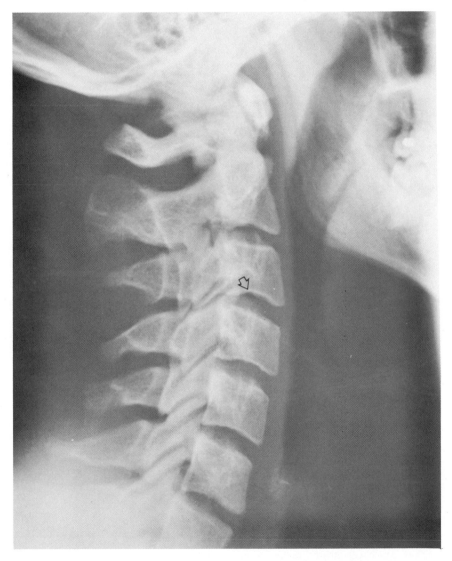

Fig. 13-2. Lateral roentgenogram of the cervical spine of a 20-year-old football player with neck pain demonstrates an abnormality involving the C3-C4 disc space. Specifically, there is a small area of radiolucency (arrow), the so-called vacuum phenomenon, that represents intervertebral disc injury.

cervical spines after having played in high school, but before playing in college.[1] Of the group, 32% had one or more of the following: "occult" fractures, vertebral body compression fractures, intervertebral disc-space narrowing, or other degenera- tive changes. Of this group, only 13% admitted to a positive history of neck symptoms. The development of early degenerative changes or intervertebral disc-space narrowing in this group was attributed to the effect of repetitive loading on

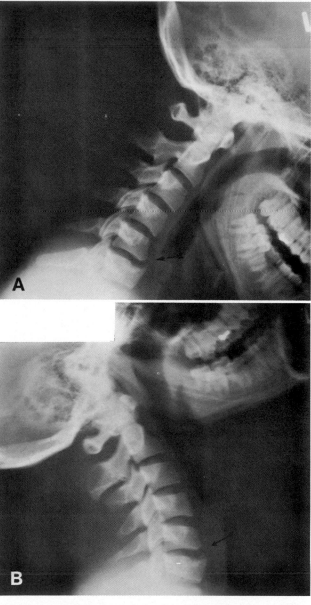

Fig. 13-3. *A, B,* Lateral flexion and extension roentgenograms demonstrate a lesion involving the superior end-plate of C6. The defect in the end-plate associated with an area of vertebral body sclerosis is in keeping with the history of the youngster having injured his neck 3 years prior while playing football. Following a head-impact injury, he had a "stiff neck" that caused him to miss 2 games. At that time he had not been seen by a doctor or examined radiographically. To be noted is the absence of evidence of instability on flexion and extension films.

the cervical spine as a result of head impact from blocking and tackling.

Although not completely documented, the findings of Roaf and Albright suggest the occurrence of intervertebral disc injury without herniation of the nucleus pulposus results from axial compression of the cervical spine. More careful clinical and roentgenographic examinations will determine whether "occult" injury to the intervertebral disc space occurs more frequently than is currently appreciated (Figs. 13-2 and 13-3*A, B*).

Acute herniation of the nucleus pulposus as an isolated entity resulting from athletic injuries is rare. However, there is documentation in the National Football Head and Neck Injury Registry of an injury involving a 19-year-old intercollegiate player who was 168-cm tall and weighed 84 kg, who sustained such an injury while spear blocking a dummy during Spring practice. Initially, there was complete motor and sensory deficit distal to the lesion. Complete return of neurologic function occurred over the next 72 hours. However, because of persistent pain a

myelogram was performed, which demonstrated posterior herniation of the C3-C4 disc (Fig. 13-4). Six weeks postinjury, anterior discectomy and interbody fusion was performed. The patient subsequently retained full neurologic function and had a stable spine with no residual disability.

Acute onset of quadriplegia occurring in an athlete who has sustained head impact with negative cervical spine roentgenograms suggests acute rupture of a cervical intervertebral disc. The syndrome of acute anterior spinal cord injury, as described by Schneider, may be observed.[9] The pressure of the disc is on the anterior and lateral columns, while the posterior columns are protected by the denticulate ligaments. Myelography should be performed to substantiate the diagnosis. Anterior discectomy and interbody fusion for a patient with neurologic involvement or persistent disability because of pain should be considered.

CERVICAL VERTEBRAL SUBLUXATION WITHOUT FRACTURE

Axial compression-flexion injuries incurred by spearing or tackling an opponent with the top of the helmet can result in disruption of the posterior soft-tissue supporting elements with angulation and anterior translation of the superior cervical vertebrae. Fractures of the bony elements are not demonstrated on roentgenograms and the patient has no neurologic deficit. Flexion-extension roentgenograms (Fig. 13-5*A, B*) demonstrate instability of the cervical spine at the involved level manifested by motion, anterior intervertebral disc-space narrowing, anterior angulation and displacement of the vertebral body, and fanning of the spinous processes. We believe that demonstrable instability on lateral flexion-extension roentgenograms in a young, vigorous individual requires aggressive treatment. When soft-tissue disruption occurs without an associated frac-

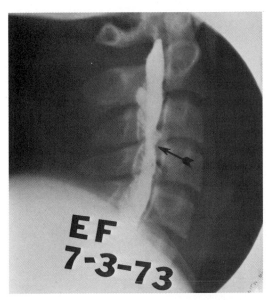

Fig. 13-4. Myelographic demonstration of C3-C4 intervertebral disc herniation that resulted from axial loading of the cervical spine.

ture, it is likely that instability will result despite conservative treatment (Fig. 13-5C). When anterior subluxation greater than 20% of the vertebral body is due to disruption of the posterior supporting structures, a posterior cervical fusion is recommended.

CERVICAL FRACTURES AND/OR DISLOCATIONS: GENERAL PRINCIPLES

Fractures and/or dislocations of the cervical spine may be stable or unstable, and may or may not be associated with neurologic deficit. When fracture or dis-

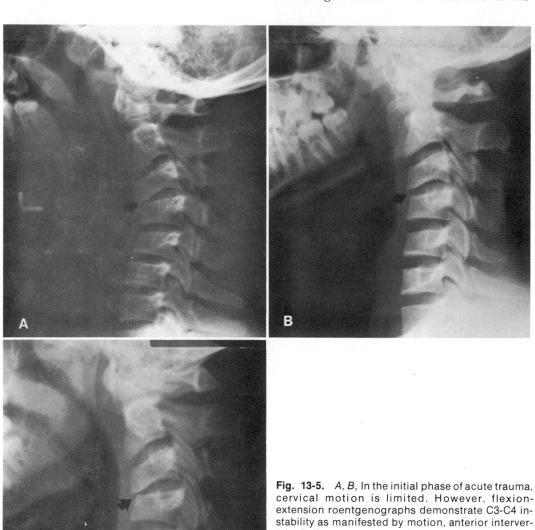

Fig. 13-5. *A, B,* In the initial phase of acute trauma, cervical motion is limited. However, flexion-extension roentgenographs demonstrate C3-C4 instability as manifested by motion, anterior intervertebral disc space narrowing, anterior angulation and displacement of the superior vertebral body, and fanning of the spinous processes. *C,* Four and one-half months postinjury, following treatment in a cervical brace, posterior instability at the C3-C4 level persists.

ruption of the soft-tissue supporting structure immediately violates or threatens to violate the integrity of the spinal cord, implementation of certain management and treatment principles is imperative.

The first goal is to protect the spinal cord and nerve roots from injury through mismanagement. It has been estimated that 50% of neurologic deficits occur after the initial injury. That is, if a patient with an unstable lesion is carelessly manipulated when being transported to a medical facility or subsequently inappropriately managed, further encroachment on the spinal cord can occur. The principles of emergency immobilization and transporting techniques have been delineated in Chapter 4.

Second, traumatic malalignment of the cervical spine should be reduced as quickly and gently as possible. This will effectively decompress the spinal cord. When dislocation or anterior angulation and translation are demonstrated roentgenographically, immediate reduction is attempted with skull traction utilizing Gardner-Wells tongs. These tongs can be easily and rapidly applied under local anesthesia, without shaving the head, in the emergency room or in the patient's bed. They are spring-loaded, thus precluding the necessity for drilling the outer table of the skull. The tongs are attached to a cervical-traction pulley and weight is added in 5 lb increments every 15 minutes, using the rule of thumb of 5 lbs per disc space level up to 25 to 40 lbs for lower cervical injury. Reduction, is substantiated by a lateral roentgenogram obtained 15 minutes after each addition of weight.

Experience indicates that unilateral facet dislocations, particularly at the C3-C4 level, are not always reducible using skeletal traction. In such instances, closed skeletal or manipulative reduction under nasotracheal anesthesia may be necessary. The expediency of early reduction of cervical dislocations is illustrated by the following two case reports.

Case 1: An 18-year-old collegiate football player sustained a C3-C4 unilateral facet dislocation while playing defensive back and making a tackle (Fig. 13-6*A*). Initial examination within one hour of the injury revealed complete motor and sensory deficit distal to the lesion. Gardner-Wells tongs with 40 lbs of traction were unsuccessful in reducing the dislocation (Fig. 13-6*B*). An immediate closed manipulative reduction under nasotracheal anesthesia was then performed (Fig. 13-6*C*). Within 24 hours there was return of posterior column function. Cervical myelogram demonstrated complete block at C3 (Fig. 13-6*D*). Five-days postinjury a C3-C4 discectomy and anterior interbody fusion was performed (Fig. 13-6*E, F*). Over the following six months there was gradual, incomplete return of neurologic function. At one-year postinjury he exhibited residua of the syndrome of acute central cervical spinal cord injury. Lower extremity function was excellent, upper extremity function was good, and hand function was fair. There was return of all sensation, as well as bowel and bladder function.

Case 2: A 30-year-old automobile driver sustained a bilateral C5-C6 facet dislocation in a vehicular crash. He was immediately transported to a hospital where initial evaluation revealed no sensation or motor function below the level of injury. Within three hours of the time of injury he was taken to the operating room, where a closed manipulative reduction was performed under general anesthesia. Over the next three months he regained both sensory and motor function in the involved arms and legs.

Traumatic malalignment of the cervical spine should be reduced as quickly as possible. In most instances, this is effected by skeletal traction; however, if necessary, manipulative or open reduction under general anesthesia should be effected.

It has been proposed that the presence of a bulbocavernous reflex indicates that spinal shock has worn off, and that except for recovery of an occasional root at the injury, the paralysis, both motor and sensory, does not recover regardless of treatment. The bulbocavernous reflex is produced by a pulling on the urethral catheter, which stimulates the trigone of the bladder, pro-

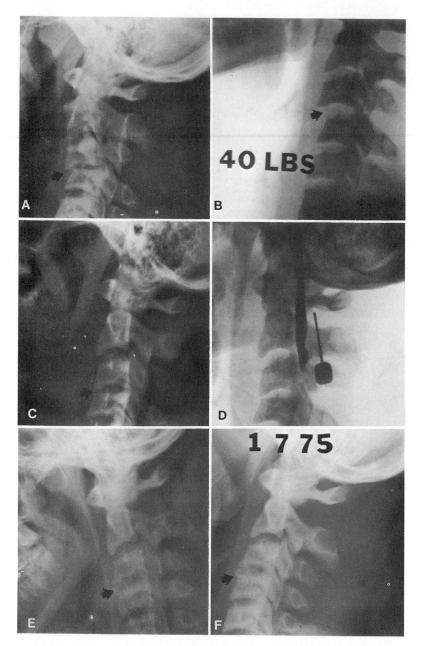

Fig. 13-6. *A,* Unilateral C3-C4 facet dislocation resulting in complete motor and sensory deficit distal to the lesion. *B,* Despite strong skeletal traction (40 lbs), the dislocation was irreducible. *C,* Manipulative reduction under nasotracheal anesthesia resulted in reduction of the dislocation. However, there is persistence of fanning of the C3-C4 spinous processes. *D,* Cervical myelogram demonstrates complete block at C3. *E, F,* Flexion and extension roentgenograms performed 2 months after anterior intervertebral disc excision and interbody fusion demonstrate a stable cervical spine with complete reduction of both anterior and posterior elements of the dislocation.

ducing a reflex contraction of the anal sphincter around the examiner's gloved finger. Although the presence of a bulbocavernous reflex is generally a sign that there will be no further neurologic recovery below the level of injury, this is not always completely accurate. The presence of this reflex should not give the clinician license to handle the situation in an elective fashion. Cervical spine subluxations and dislocations associated with quadriparesis should be reduced as quickly as possible, by whatever means necessary, if maximum recovery is to be expected.

Regarding the role of operative decompression for cervical fractures and/or dis-

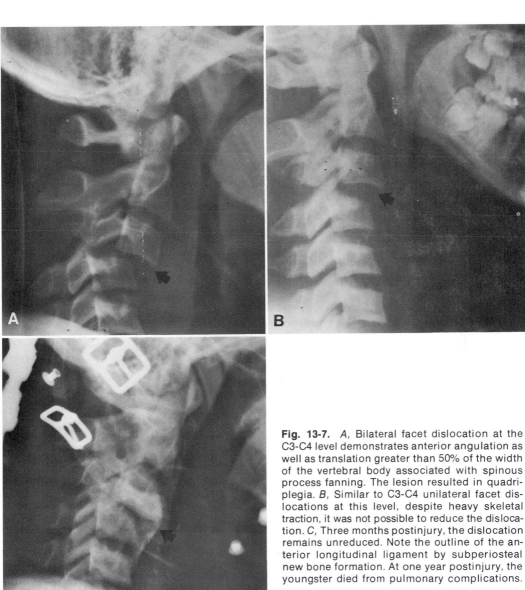

Fig. 13-7. *A,* Bilateral facet dislocation at the C3-C4 level demonstrates anterior angulation as well as translation greater than 50% of the width of the vertebral body associated with spinous process fanning. The lesion resulted in quadriplegia. *B,* Similar to C3-C4 unilateral facet dislocations at this level, despite heavy skeletal traction, it was not possible to reduce the dislocation. *C,* Three months postinjury, the dislocation remains unreduced. Note the outline of the anterior longitudinal ligament by subperiosteal new bone formation. At one year postinjury, the youngster died from pulmonary complications.

locations, we believe there is a limited role for cervical laminectomy in their treatment. Only rarely, when excision of foreign bodies or bony fragments in the spinal canal is necessary, is a posterior laminectomy indicated. Realignment of the spine is the most effective method for decompression of the cervical cord.

In most instances in which a vertebral body burst fracture is associated with anterior compression of the cord, decompression is logically effected through an anterior approach with an interbody fusion. Likewise, traumatic intervertebral disc herniation with cord involvement is best managed through an anterior discectomy and interbody fusion.

Indications for surgical decompression of the spinal cord have been delineated. A documented increase in neurologic signs is the clearest mandate for surgical decompression. Further observation, expectancy, and procrastination in this situation is contraindicated. Persistent partial cord or root signs, with objective evidence of mechanical compression, is also an indication for surgical intervention. However, in this instance, the procedure may be delayed 7 to 14 days. There is no evidence that a ten-day delay will impair the final return of neurologic function, and from the standpoint of patient homeostasis, mortality and morbidity is decreased by this period of re-equilibration.

Preceding and following reduction of cervical spine fractures and/or dislocations, the use of parenteral corticosteroids (dexamethasone) to decrease the inflammatory reactions of the injured cord and surrounding soft-tissue structures is very important. Drugs that inhibit norepinephrine synthesis or deplete catecholamines have been advocated to prevent autodigestion of the cord. However, there is no evidence as yet that this is of value in altering prognosis of cord recovery. Procedures such as durotomy, myelotomy, and rhizotomy require extensive laminectomy, adding further instability to the spine, and are contraindicated.

The third goal in managing fractures and/or dislocations of the cervical spine is to effect rapid and secure stability in order to prevent residual deformity and instability with associated pain, and the possibility of further trauma to the neural elements. The method of immobilization depends on the post-reduction status of the injury. Thompson et al. have concisely delineated indications for nonsurgical and surgical methods for achieving stability.[10] These concepts for managing cervical spine fractures and dislocations may be summarized as follows:

1. Patients with stable compression fractures of the vertebral body, undisplaced fractures of the lamina or lateral masses, or soft-tissue injuries without detectable neurologic deficit can be adequately treated with traction and subsequent protection by using a cervical brace until healing occurs.

2. Stable, reduced facet dislocation without neurologic deficit can also be treated conservatively in a Minerva jacket brace until healing has been demonstrated by negative lateral flexion-extension roentgenograms.

3. Unstable cervical spine fractures or fracture-dislocations without neurologic deficit may require either surgical or nonsurgical methods to insure stability.

4. Absolute indications for surgical stabilization of an unstable injury without neurologic deficit are late instability following closed treatment, and flexion-rotation injuries with unreduced locked facet.

5. Relative indications for surgical stabilization in unstable injuries without neurologic deficit are anterior subluxation greater than 20%, certain atlantoaxial fractures or dislocations, and unreduced vertical compression injuries with neck flexion.

6. Cervical spine fractures with complete cord lesions require reduction followed by stabilization by closed or open means as indicated.
7. Cervical spine fractures with incomplete cord lesions require reduction followed by careful evaluation for surgical intervention.

The fourth and final goal of treatment is rapid and effective rehabilitation started early in the treatment process.

A more specific categorization of athletic injuries to the cervical spine can be made. Specifically, these injuries can be divided into those that occur in the upper cervical spine, the midcervical spine, and the lower cervical spine.

Upper Cervical Spine Fractures and Dislocations

Upper cervical spine lesions involve C1 through C3. Although rarely occurring in sports, there are several specific injuries that can occur to the upper cervical vertebrae that deserve mention. The transverse and alar ligaments are responsible for atlantoaxial stability. With rupture of these structures resulting from a flexion injury, with translation of C1 anteriorly, the spinal cord can become impinged between a posterior aspect of the odontoid process and the posterior rim of C1. Such a lesion is potentially fatal. The patient gives a history of head trauma and complains of neck pain, particularly with nodding, and may or may not present with cord signs. Roentgenographically, lateral views of the C1-C2 articulation demonstrate increase of the atlanto-dens interval (ADI). This interval is normally 3 mm in the adult. With transverse ligament rupture it may increase up to 10 to 12 mm depending on the status of the alar and accessory ligaments. Note that increase in the ADI may only be seen with the neck flexed. Fielding states that atlantoaxial fusion may be the "conservative" treatment for this lesion.[5] He recommended posterior C1-C2 fusion

using wire fixation and iliac bone graft.

Fractures of the atlas were described by Jefferson in 1920.[6] These may be of two types: posterior arch fractures, and burst fractures. Posterior arch fractures are the more common of the two, and with a brace support go on to satisfactory fibrous or bony union.

The burst fractures result from an axial load transmitted to the occipital condyles, which then disrupt the integrity of both the anterior and posterior arches of the atlas. Roentgenograms demonstrate bilateral symmetric overhang of the lateral masses of the atlas, in relationship to the axis, with increase in the para-odontoid space on the open-mouth view (see Fig. 12-22*A*). Clinically, the patient characteristically demonstrates pain on, and limitation of the nodding motion.

Treatment, as recommended by Fielding, includes head-halter traction until muscle spasm resolves, followed by brace support. If flexion-extension roentgenograms subsequently demonstrate significant instability, fusion may be indicated.

Fractures of the odontoid have been classified into three types by Anderson and D'Alonzo.[2] Type I is an avulsion of the tip of the odontoid at the site of the attachment of the alar ligament, and is a rare and stable lesion. Type II is a fracture through the base at or just below the level of the superior articular processes (see Fig. 12-24*A*). Type III involves a fracture of the body of the axis (see Fig. 12-24*B*). When not displaced, planograms may be required to identify the lesion.

The mechanism of odontoid fractures has not been clearly delineated. However, they appear to be due to head impact. All routine cervical spine roentgenographic studies should include the open-mouth view to identify lesions involving the odontoid as well as the atlas. If these are negative, and if a lesion in this area is suspected, planograms or bending films may further delineate pathologic changes.

Managing Type II fractures is a problem.

It has been reported that 36 to 50% of these lesions treated initially with plaster casts or reinforced cervical braces fail to unite. Cloward[3] has reported that 85% of his patients heal within three months when treated with the halo brace.[3]

Fibrous or nonunion fractures of the odontoid, associated with roentgeno-graphic demonstration of instability on flexion and extension views, indicate the necessity for surgical stabilization. This may be effected either through posterior C1-C2 wire fixation and fusion, or anterior fusion of C1-C2 by dowel grafts through the articular facets, as described by Cloward.[3]

Fractures through the arch of the axis are also known as traumatic spondylolisthesis of C2 or hangman's fracture (see Fig. 12-27A). These are relatively rare lesions, and have not been recorded to have occurred as a result of tackle football. The mechanism of injury is generally recognized to be hyperextension. However, there are instances where a compression fracture of C3 is associated with traumatic spondylolisthesis of C2, indicating that the lesion was due to flexion. This injury is inherently unstable; however, it has been shown to heal with predictable regularity without surgical intervention. After reduction is effected with traction, a halo cast is applied and the fracture immobilized until healing occurs, which usually takes 12 to 16 weeks. At that point, flexion and extension lateral roentgenograms are obtained. If instability is demonstrated, or the patient has persistent pain because of disruption of the C2-C3 intervertebral disc, fusion may be necessary. The anterior C2-C3 approach is recommended. To obtain stability by posterior fusion requires stabilization of C1 to C3, thus blocking C1-C2 rotation.

Midcervical Spine Fractures and Dislocations

Acute traumatic lesions of the cervical spine at the C3-C4 level are rare. Torg et al.[11] recently reported eight such lesions that resulted from tackle football, all of which were without associated fracture. Of note was the fact that the mechanism of injury was the volitional use of the top or crown of the helmet as a primary point of contact in high-impact collisions while blocking, tackling, or head butting.

Classification of C3-C4 lesions are as follows: (1) acute rupture of the C3-C4 intervertebral disc; (2) anterior subluxation of the third cervical vertebra on the fourth; (3) unilateral dislocation of the joint between the articular process; and (4) bilateral dislocation of the articular process (facet).

Acute onset of quadriplegia with a sensorimotor level of the fourth cervical nerve root in an athlete who has sustained head impact with a negative cervical spine roentgenogram suggests acute rupture of the C3-C4 intervertebral disc. The syndrome of acute anterior spinal cord injury, as described by Schneider,[9] may be observed. A cervical myelogram substantiates the diagnosis. Anterior discectomy and interbody fusion may be the most effective treatment of this lesion.

Anterior subluxation of C3 on C4 is a result of a shearing force through the intervertebral disc space disrupting the interspinous ligament, as well as the posterior supporting structure. Roentgenograms demonstrate narrowing of the intervertebral disc space, anterior angulation and translation of C3 and C4, an increase in the distance between the spinous processes of the two vertebrae, and instability without fracture of the bony elements (Fig. 13-5A, B). A posterior C3-C4 spine fusion may be necessary for adequate stabilization in such cases, in contrast with instances of cervical spine instability caused by fracture in which adequate reduction and subsequent bony healing results in stability. When the patient has posterior instability, posterior fusion is preferable to an anterior interbody fusion.

Unilateral facet dislocation at C3-C4 may result in immediate quadriparesis. This injury involves the intervertebral disc space, the interspinous ligament, the posterior ligamentous supporting structures, and the one facet with resulting rotatory dislocation of the third cervical vertebra on the fourth without fracture (Fig. 13-6*A*). At this level, strong skeletal traction does not yield a successful reduction (Fig. 13-6*B*), and closed manipulation under general anesthesia is necessary to disengage the locked joint between the articular processes. Manipulation may be done with the patient supine on a Stryker frame, with the head and neck maintained in axial alignment, and a sandbag placed under the shoulders. Traction is applied through Gardner-Wells tongs with gentle lateral bend away from the dislocated joint associated with extension and rotation toward the site of the lesion. Reduction is associated with a subtle click (Fig. 13-6*C*). In two reported cases,[11] the initial neurologic findings resembled those of acute anterior spinal cord injury. However, the recovery pattern was that of an acute central cervical spinal cord injury. Presumably, the injury involved initial compromise of the anterior lateral cord function associated with central cervical cord edema and hemorrhage. Following immediate reduction and subsequent anterior decompression and interbody fusion, months elapsed before there was significant motor improvement.

Bilateral facet dislocation at the C3-C4 level is a grave lesion (Fig. 13-7*A*–*C*); skeletal traction may not reduce the lesion, and the prognosis for this injury is very poor.

Lower Cervical Spine Fractures and Dislocations

Lower cervical spine fractures or dislocations are those involving C4 through C7. In those injuries that result from various athletic endeavors, the majority of fractures and/or dislocations of the cervical spine, with or without neurologic involvement, involve this segment. Although unilateral and bilateral facet dislo-

cations occur, they are relatively rare. The vast majority of severe athletically incurred cervical spine injuries are fractures of the vertebral body with varying degrees of compression or comminution.

Unilateral Facet Dislocations. Unilateral facet dislocations are the result of axial loading, flexion-rotation type mechanisms. The lesion may be truly ligamentous without associated vertebral fracture. In such instances, the facet dislocation is stable and is usually associated with neurologic involvement. Roentgenograms demonstrate less than 50% anterior shift of the superior vertebra on the inferior vertebra (see Fig. 12-11*A*, *B*). Attempts should be made to reduce the facet dislocation by skeletal traction. However, as with similar lesions described at the C3-C4 level, it may not be possible to effect a closed reduction. In this instance, open reduction under direct vision through a posterior approach with supplemental posterior element bone grafting should be performed.

Bilateral Facet Dislocations. Bilateral facet dislocations are unstable and are almost always associated with neurologic involvement. These injuries are associated with a high incidence of quadriplegia. Lateral roentgenograms demonstrate greater than 50% anterior displacement of the superior vertebral body on the inferior vertebral body (Fig. 13-7*A*). Immediate treatment, as previously delineated, is closed reduction with skeletal traction. Such lesions are generally reducible by skeletal traction and then treated by halo-cast stabilization and posterior fusion. To be noted is the fact that instability is directly related to the ease with which the lesion is reduced, since the easier it is to reduce, the easier it is to redislocate. If skeletal traction is unsuccessful, either manipulative reduction under sedation or general anesthesia, or open reduction under direct vision is recommended. When the dislocation is reduced closed, and the reduction maintained, immobilization should be effected by use of the halo cast for 8 to 12 weeks.

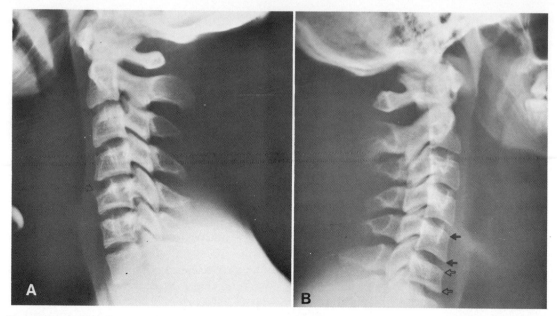

Fig. 13-8. *A,* Type I vertebral body wedge compression fracture involving the anterior aspect of C5. There is no evidence of subluxation at the joints between the articular processes. Also, there is absence of fanning of the spinous processes. The small fragment at the superior aspect of the vertebral body is of no significance. This is a stable lesion that can be effectively managed with a cervical collar or brace. *B,* A Type I simple wedge compression fracture of the sixth cervical vertebra with a uniform diminution of height of the vertebral body. Radiographic signs of instability are absent.

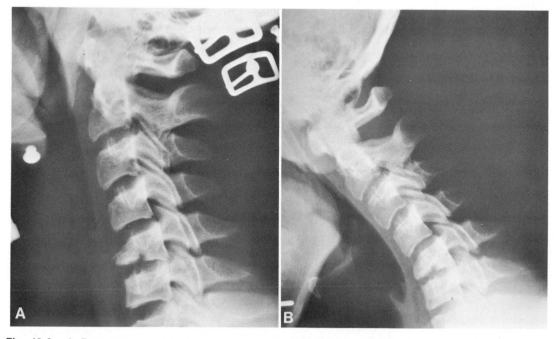

Fig. 13-9. *A,* Type II vertebral body compression fracture demonstrates the characteristic comminuted burst fracture of the vertebral body without displacement into the vertebral canal. *B,* Lateral flexion roentgenograms of the lesion demonstrate maintenance of adjacent disc space height, as well as a lack of subluxation or spinous process fanning. With no disruption of the posterior elements, this is a relatively stable lesion.

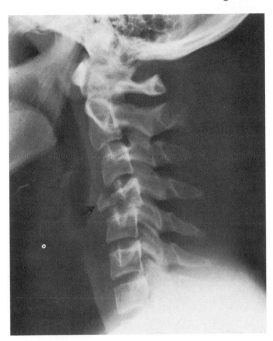

Fig. 13-10. Type III comminuted burst fracture of C4 with displacement of fragments into the vertebral canal.

Corrective bracing should continue for an additional four weeks.

Vertebral Body Compression Fractures. Compression fractures of the vertebral body are a result of axial loading. Vertebral body fractures of the cervical spine can be classified into five types:

Type I: Simple wedged compression fracture of vertebral body without associated ligamentous or bony disruption (Fig. 13-8*A*, *B*).

Type II: Comminuted burst fracture of the vertebral body without displacement into the vertebral canal (Fig. 13-9*A*, *B*).

Type III: Comminuted burst fracture of the vertebral body with displacement into the vertebral canal (Fig. 13-10). Usually, but not always, associated with neurologic involvement.

Type IV: Comminuted burst fracture of the vertebral body with associated posterior instability (Fig. 13-11). This is a severe injury that is almost always associated with quadriplegia.

Type V: Comminuted burst fracture of the vertebral body associated with fractures of the neural arch (Fig. 13-12*A*, *B*).

Type I wedged compression fractures of the cervical vertebrae are common injuries that respond to conservative management, and rarely, if ever, are associated with neurologic involvement. It is important that these lesions be differentiated from compression fractures that are associated with disruption of the posterior element soft-tissue supporting structures. The latter lesions are unstable and frequently associated with neurologic involvement, including quadriplegia.

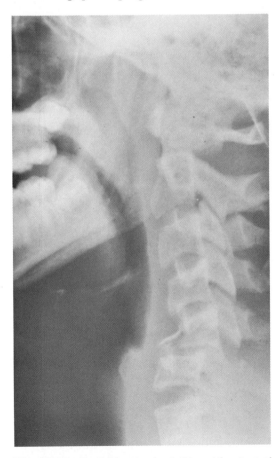

Fig. 13-11. Type IV comminuted burst fracture of the vertebral body of C5 with associated fanning or widening of the spinous processes between C5 and C6 indicating disruption of the posterior soft tissue structures. The combined anterior and posterior instability has resulted in settling and posterior displacement of the superior vertebral segment. This lesion is the result of a compression flexion injury.

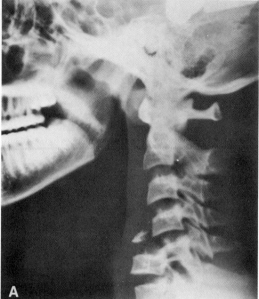

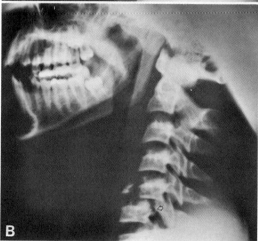

Fig. 13-12. *A,* Type V comminuted burst fracture of the vertebral body associated with fractures of the neural arch. There is settling and posterior displacement of the superior vertebral segment. *B,* Distraction of the superior vertebral segment with skeletal traction permits visualization of fractures through the pedicles (arrow) of C6 in addition to the burst fracture of the body of C5.

Type II comminuted burst vertebral body fractures without displacement are not usually associated with neurologic involvement. However, settling of the comminuted vertebral body fracture may result in late cervical instability. These patients should be considered for anterior exploration, decompression, and fusion.

Type III comminuted burst vertebral body fractures, with displacement of bony fragments into the vertebral canal, are serious injuries that place the spinal cord in jeopardy, and should be treated accordingly.

Type IV comminuted burst vertebral body fractures associated with disruption of the posterior elements are extremely unstable lesions with anterior subluxation or dislocation of the superior vertebral segments and associated quadriplegia. The prognosis is grave. Combined anterior and posterior procedures may be necessary to effect stabilization.

Type V comminuted burst vertebral body fractures are associated with fractures of the elements of the neural arch. Subsequently, there is both anterior and posterior instability. Because of the disruption of the posterior bony elements there is posterior displacement of the superior vertebral segment. As would be expected, quadriplegia is associated with this lesion. Note that posterior dislocation of the vertebral body cannot be realigned effectively without surgical intervention. Because of both anterior and posterior instability, combined anterior and posterior operative procedures may be necessary to effectively stabilize the spine.

Transient Quadriplegia. An infrequently occurring and not well-documented phenomenon is that of transient quadriplegia. This characteristically occurs to an athlete, most usually a football player, who sustains either forced hyperextension or hyperflexion to his neck and cervical spine. A painless paralysis ensues, which may manifest as weakness or complete absence of motor function in all four extremities. The episode is brief, lasting from five to ten minutes. The involvement of sensory function has not been established. Roentgenograms do not demonstrate findings indicating acute trauma to the cervical spine; however, examination of the lateral films reveals either a congenital fusion or a developmental decrease in the sagittal diameter of the spinal canal (Fig.

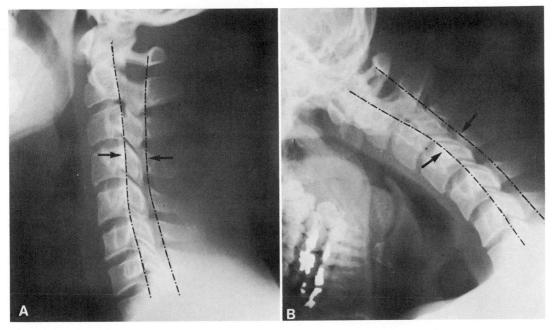

Fig. 13-13. *A,* Lateral roentgenogram of the cervical spine of an 18-year-old high school football player who had had two episodes of transient quadriplegia. There is narrowing of the spinal canal at C3-C4. *B,* Lateral flexion film demonstrating decrease in the width of the spinal canal at C3-C4. The mechanism of injury in both episodes of transient quadriplegia was reported to be hyperflexion.

13-13*A*). The degree of developmental cervical stenosis is increased on flexion and extension roentgenograms (Fig. 13-13*B*).

Until a clearer understanding of the mechanics and implications of this problem are established, an athlete who experiences weakness or paralysis associated with a flexion or extension injury of a narrowing cervical spine should be precluded from participation in contact sports.

CERVICAL SPINE INSTABILITY

The spectrum of late cervical spine instability following injury is a necessary consideration when an athlete is injured. Subsequent permanent or transient narrowing of the spinal canal with compression of the neural elements is well avoided if possible. For each particular injury it is not possible to accurately predict whether late instability will result in structural malalignment, with or without neurologic deficit. Unfortunately, this goal is not always possible. However, the recent work of White and

Panjabi in establishing guidelines regarding this problem are noteworthy.[12] They have defined stability of the lower cervical spine as "the ability of the spine to limit the patterns of displacement under physiologic stress so as not to damage or irritate the spinal cord or nerve roots."

White and Panjabi performed a series of cadaver studies in which the various supporting structures were systematically cut and resulting instabilities in the spine were noted. The supporting structures of the lower cervical spine can be divided into two groups; anterior and posterior (Fig. 13-14). The anterior group includes both soft tissue supporting structures anterior to and including the posterior longitudinal ligament. These are the anterior and posterior longitudinal ligaments, the intervertebral disc, and the annulus fibrosus. The posterior group consists of the facet capsular ligaments, yellow ligament, and the interspinous and supraspinous ligaments. On the basis of this work, instability occurs when either all the anterior or

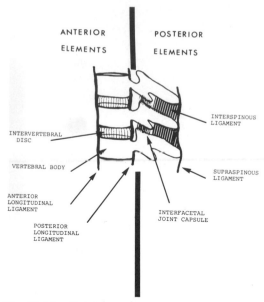

Fig. 13-14. Division of the cervical spine into anterior and posterior supporting elements as described by White and Panjabi.[12]

all the posterior structures are disrupted. Therefore, we may define, on an anatomic basis, an anterior cervical spine instability and a posterior cervical spine instability.

Roentgenographically, cervical spine instability manifests itself by a horizontal translation of one vertebra relative to an adjacent vertebra exceeding 3.5 mm in lateral flexion-extension films. Instability also exists if roentgenograms demonstrate angular displacement of one vertebra relative to another exceeding 11° on the lateral views.

OPERATIVE PRINCIPLES AND TECHNIQUES

In those instances of cervical spine trauma when surgical intervention is indicated for decompression or stabilization, several basic principles must be adhered to.

1. Anterior disc excision and interbody fusion is the procedure of choice for patients with neurologic involvement or persistent disability secondary to traumatic rupture of a cervical disc.

2. In traumatic lesions of the cervical spine in which surgery is indicated, because of either acute or chronic anterior cervical spine instability, an anterior cervical approach and fusion is indicated.

3. Cervical laminectomy for the treatment of fractures and/or dislocations has a limited role and is indicated only in the rare instance when excision of foreign bodies or bony fragments from the spinal canal is necessary.

4. When traumatic lesions of the cervical spine result in acute or chronic posterior instability, posterior stabilization and fusion is indicated.

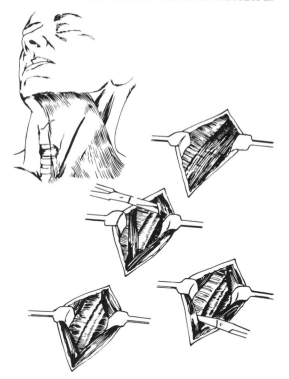

Fig. 13-15. The anterior approach for cervical intervertebral disc excision and interbody fusion begins with the patient supine, the head in slight extension and turned slightly to the right. The cricoid cartilage is opposite C6 and is palpated for orientation. The incision is developed along the anterior border of the sternocleidomastoid muscle, between the carotid sheath and omohyoid muscle, and then through a longitudinal incision in the pretrachial fascia. (Adapted from DePalma, A.F., and Rothman, R.H.: The Intervertebral Disc. Philadelphia, W.B. Saunders, 1970.)

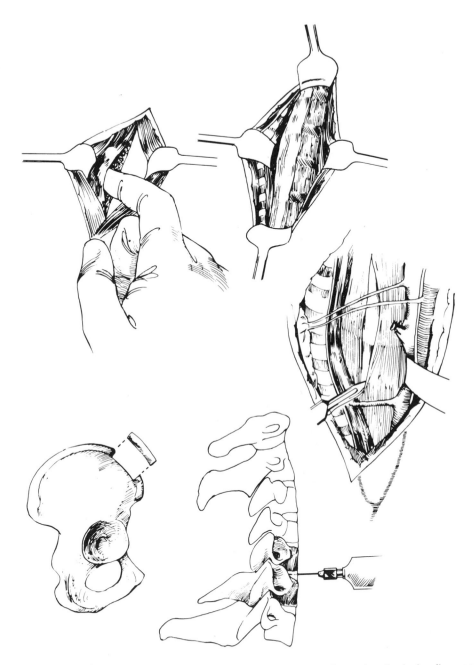

Fig. 13-16.   The retropharyngeal space is developed by blunt dissection using the index finger exposing the prevertebral fascia over the vertebral bodies. At the C2-C3 level, the superior thyroid artery and vein and superior laryngeal nerve were encountered and protected. In lower incisions, it may be necessary to divide the inferior thyroid artery and vein. The desired disc space is identified. A block of bone from the anterior iliac crest is removed. (Adapted from DePalma, A.F., and Rothman, R.H.: The Intervertebral Disc. Philadelphia, W.B. Saunders, 1970.)

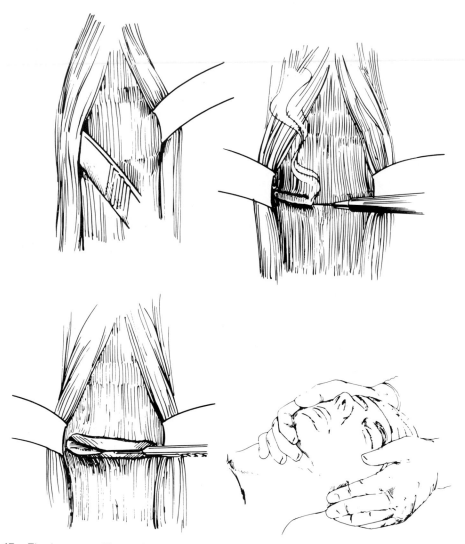

Fig. 13-17. The longus colli muscles are retracted, the disc space is exposed by electrocautery and the annulus fibrosus is incised. Traction is applied to open the disc space. (Adapted from DePalma, A.F., and Rothman, R.H.: The Intervertebral Disc. Philadelphia, W.B. Saunders, 1970.)

Approaching the cervical spine from the posterior aspect and detaching the posterior supporting ligamentous structures when anterior instability exists, compounds the problem and creates an iatrogenic combined anterior and posterior instability. Conversely, an anterior approach, when a posterior instability is the problem, likewise compounds the problem and creates an iatrogenic anterior and posterior instability.

Operative Procedures

Anterior Intervertebral Disc Excision and Interbody Fusion. This procedure, when performed with proper indications by experienced spine surgeons, is the operative treatment of choice for cervical intervertebral disc herniation secondary to trauma. DePalma and Rothman have defined both the advantages and disadvantages.[4] The most advantageous features are:

1. The source of the pathologic process, the disc, can be readily excised in its entirety with immediate relief of pain and reasonable assurance against further occurrence of disc extrusion.
2. The interbody bone graft restores the height of the disc space, thus bringing into normal alignment all the components of the cervical spine. By doing so, subluxation of the apophyseal joints is also corrected.
3. The intervertebral foramina are opened, thus allowing room for their contents.
4. The interbody graft wedged between superior and inferior vertebrae provides immediate stabilization.
5. The operation can be performed from C2 to T1; however, it should be noted that the extremes of the cervical spine exposure may be more difficult to attain than in the midportion.
6. A solid bony fusion is attained in a relatively short period of time, usually 6 to 8 weeks, and the postoperative period of convalescence is relatively short.

The few disadvantages are:

1. The possibility of damage to the anterior surface of the cord and nerve roots.
2. Insertion of large interbody grafts may exert undue pressure on the discs above and below, predisposing them to degeneration.
3. The bone graft may extrude anteriorly.
4. The anterior approach does not permit exploration of the spinal canal and cord at other levels.

The procedure is performed with the patient in a supine position with the head supported in slight hyperextension and turned 15 to 20° to the right. A vertical incision is made along the anterior border of the sternocleidomastoid muscle extending 2 in. above and 2 in. below the desired

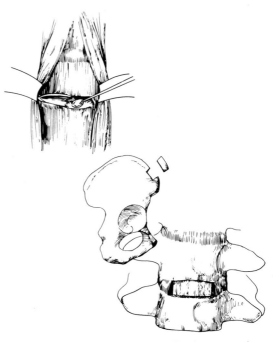

Fig. 13-18. Using a curette, the disc is removed as well as the superior and inferior articular plates, and the prepared bone block is gently tapped into position. (Adapted from DePalma, A.F., and Rothman, R.H.: The Intervertebral Disc. Philadelphia, W.B. Saunders, 1970.)

level. The platysma is cut in the same line as the skin incision. The anterior layer of the cervical fascia is then divided longitudinally along the anterior border of the sternocleidomastoid muscle. Utilizing scissor dissection, the anterior margin of the sternocleidomastoid muscle is then mobilized and gently retracted laterally. The carotid sheath and the omohyoid muscle are then visualized, and by blunt dissection the interval medial to the carotid sheath is developed with the omohyoid muscle retracted medially. The pretracheal fascia is exposed and a small longitudinal incision is made in this structure (Fig. 13-15).

The index finger is placed into the retropharyngeal space, which is developed the full length of the incision. The thyroid gland, trachea, and esophagus are gently retracted medially and the carotid sheath retracted laterally. The prevertebral fascia is then exposed as it covers the vertebral bodies, the anterior longitudinal ligament,

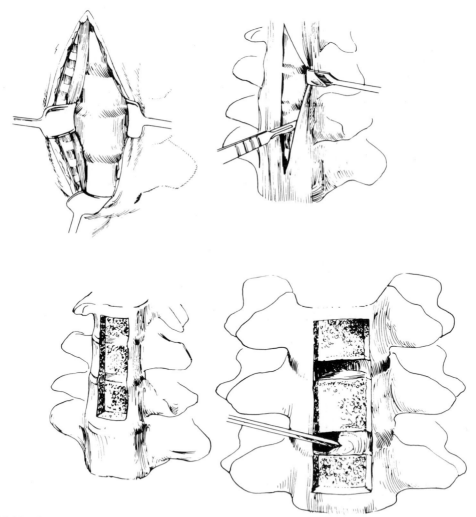

Fig. 13-19. The approach for anterior cervical spine fusion is similar to that for intervertebral disc excision. After the vertebrae to be included in the fusion are identified, a trough is cut in the anterior aspect of the vertebral bodies and intervertebral disc material, and bony fragments are removed. (Adapted from DePalma, A.F., and Rothman, R.H.: The Intervertebral Disc. Philadelphia, W.B. Saunders, 1970.)

and longus colli muscles. The intervertebral disc spaces are clearly visualized through the prevertebral fascia.

When dividing the pretracheal fascia, the middle thyroid vein should be identified, divided, and ligated. In high incisions at the C2-C3 level, the superior thyroid artery and vein and the superior laryngeal nerve are encountered, and should be retracted proximally. It may be necessary to divide these vessels. In low incisions at the C6-T1 level it may be

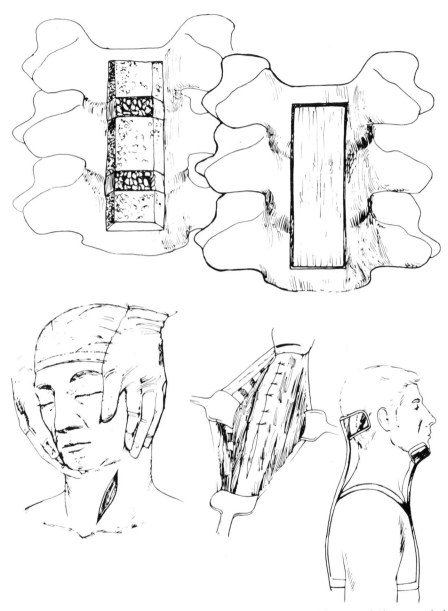

Fig. 13-20. The graft is fitted snugly in the trough, the neck is placed in neutral, the wound closed, and depending on the degree of instability, appropriate immobilization is applied and maintained until healing occurs. (Adapted from DePalma, A.F., and Rothman, R.H.: The Intervertebral Disc. Philadelphia, W.B. Saunders, 1970.)

necessary to divide the inferior thyroid artery and vein. Also, caution should be taken in low incisions to protect the recurrent laryngeal nerve, which descends along the carotid sheath and ascends between the esophagus and trachea.

Localization and identification of the intervertebral disc are accomplished by inserting a straight needle into the disc space and taking a lateral roentgenogram. While the roentgenographic film is being developed, a bone block is removed from the iliac crest. The piece of bone should comprise the full thickness of the crest of the ilium (Fig. 13-16).

By blunt dissection and taking care not to traumatize the sympathetic chain, the longus colli muscles are mobilized and displaced laterally at the level of the disc to be removed. A flat blade retractor is used. The tissues over the intervertebral disc are divided transversely with an electrocau-

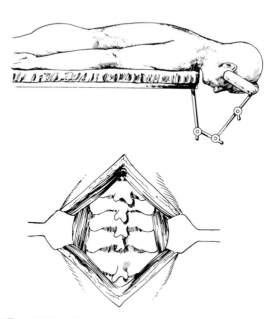

Fig. 13-21. Posterior cervical spine fusion is performed with the patient in the prone position, and the head supported by a headrest. The posterior elements are then exposed to a midline skin incision developed by sharp periosteal dissection exposing the lamina and carried laterally to the margins of the apophyseal joints. (Adapted from DePalma, A.F. and Rothman, R.H.: The Intervertebral Disc. Philadelphia, W.B. Saunders, 1970.)

tery. Note that there is no need to preserve the edges of the divided pretracheal fascia. The bone block fits snugly between the vertebrae and chances for displacement are minimal.

The annulus fibrosus is cut across the entire width of the disc with a scalpel. Manual traction is then applied to the head to open the disc space.

Fifteen pounds of skeletal traction is maintained during operations performed to stabilize fractures and/or dislocations. The weight can be increased if widening of the disc space is desired (Fig. 13-17).

The entire disc is removed with a curette. Also, the articular plate above and below are denuded to subchondral bone. The bone block is then prepared. The width of the graft should be the same as the width of the intervertebral space exposed between the longus colli muscles. The height of the graft should be such that it fits snugly between the two vertebrae. The graft should have cortical bone on both sides. While traction is applied to open the disc space, the graft is gently tapped into position (Fig. 13-18). The anterior surface of the graft should be behind the anterior margins of the superior and inferior vertebrae. The head is then brought into a slightly flexed position and the wounds are closed in layers. At the end of the operation a soft cervical collar is applied. Subsequently the patient is outfitted with a cervical brace that is worn for 6 to 8 weeks, or until the fusion is solid.

Anterior Cervical Spine Fusion. Comminuted cervical vertebral body fractures with anterior instability are effectively managed utilizing the anterior cervical spine fusion technique of Bailey and Badgley. The anterior aspect of the cervical spine is approached through the vertical incision as previously described (Figs. 13-15 and 13-16).

In the usual instance of vertebral body comminuted burst fractures, localization of the level of the lesion is not a problem. However, if there is any question, insert a straight needle into a disc space and take a lateral roentgenogram.

After the vertebra to be included in the fusion has been identified, the prevertebral fascia is incised longitudinally in the midline. The fascia is then reflected off of the vertebral bodies utilizing an elevator.

Decompression of the spinal canal, in instances of Types II and III compression fractures, requires removing all the vertebral body comminuted fragments. All bone violating the spinal canal must be removed. The lateral portions of the vertebral bodies are resected to the pedicles. The disc above and below the level of the lesion, as well as vertebral body end-plates are removed. Using a fine sharp osteotome or an electric drill a trough is cut in the inferior end of the superior vertebra and the superior aspect of the inferior vertebra. After the disc spaces have been evacuated, the articular cartilage is removed from the articular end-plates down to subchondral bone (Fig. 13-19).

The full-thickness iliac crest graft is then cut so that it fits snugly into the trough. Skeletal traction is then adjusted so that the graft is seated firmly in its bed. The prevertebral fascia is closed over the graft. Depending on the degree of preoperative instability, external support in the form of a halo cast or cervical brace must be worn until the fusion is solid (Fig. 13-20). This usually takes from 4 to 6 months. Roentgenograms should be taken frequently to determine the state of the fusion.

Posterior Spine Fusion.   When cervical spine instability involves the posterior element, or in those few instances where laminectomy is indicated, a posterior approach and spine fusion is the surgical procedure of choice.

The patient is placed prone with the head supported by a headrest fixed so that the neck is slightly flexed. A longitudinal midline incision is made over the spinous processes of the involved vertebrae. This should extend one vertebra

above and one vertebra below the proposed laminectomy-fusion area. By sharp periosteal dissection, the lamina are exposed and the dissection is carried laterally to the margins of the apophyseal joint (Fig. 13-21).

If laminectomy is not indicated and a fusion is to be performed for purposes of stabilization, the spinous processes of the vertebrae superior and inferior to the level of subluxation or dislocation are secured with a figure 8 wire, after reduction has been obtained by extension of the neck. The lamina of the two vertebrae superior to and inferior to the level of subluxation or dislocation are denuded of cortical bone out to and including the posterior aspect of the apophyseal joint. With a 7/64 inch drill a hole is made through the inferior facet of the vertebra above, with the drill pointed obliquely downward. This process is performed on the inferior process of all vertebrae to be included in the fusion. No. 20

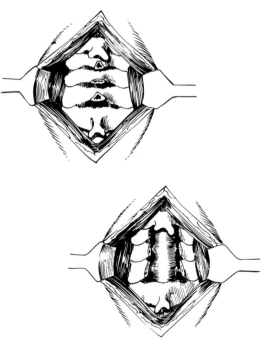

Fig. 13-22.   If indicated, the laminae of the vertebrae to be included in the fusion are removed exposing the spinal canal and its contents. (Adapted from DePalma, A.F., and Rothman, R.H.: The Intervertebral Disc. Philadelphia, W.B. Saunders, 1970.)

stainless steel wire is passed through the drill hole. The wires are then passed around to secure the corticocancellous graft obtained from the posterior iliac crest. The grafts are secured snugly against the facet joint. The grafts should extend from the top of the lamina of the most proximal vertebra to the bottom of the lamina of the most distal vertebra (Fig. 13-22).

In those instances where a laminectomy is indicated, the lamina of the vertebrae to be included in the fusion area are removed as far laterally as the apophyseal joint (Fig. 13-23). The seating of the bone graft is performed as described above.

The wound is closed, and depending on the degree of preoperative instability, external support is maintained in the form of a halo-cast brace or cervical collar until the fusion is solid.

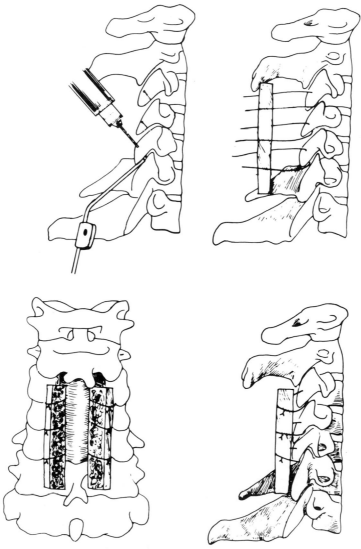

Fig. 13-23. The bone grafts extend from the top of the lamina of the most proximal vertebra to the bottom of the lamina of the most distal vertebra and are stabilized to the inferior facets with a No. 20 stainless steel wire, as illustrated. (Adapted from DePalma, A.F., and Rothman, R.H.: The Intervertebral Disc. Philadelphia, W.B. Saunders, 1970.)

ACTIVITY RESTRICTIONS

Physicians who are involved in the management of athletes who have sustained significant cervical spine injuries are ultimately faced with the question of whether or not the patient can return to his former activity. To be emphasized is the fact that few if any attempts have been made to formally address this question. However, the following guidelines are offered, which are based on clinical experience.

Youngsters who have been diagnosed and successfully treated for cervical sprains, intervertebral disc injuries without neurologic involvement, and stable wedge compression fractures may return to all activities when they are symptom-free, have full range of cervical motion, full muscle strength, and stability of the cervical spine as demonstrated by flexion and extension films.

Those with lesions of the cervical spine resulting in subluxation without fracture should be precluded from further participation in contact sports despite lack of motion on lateral flexion-extension films. Flexion and extension films, a static demonstration of stability, are not an adequate measure of the stability of the spine when exposed to the forces involved in contact sports.

Individuals who have undergone a successful one-level anterior interbody decompression and fusion for herniated nucleus pulposus or anterior instability may return to all activity provided they have full range of motion and strength. However, they should be fully apprised of the possibility of intervertebral disc herniation at an adjacent level.

Individuals who undergo more than one-level anterior fusion or posterior fusion for cervical spine injury should be evaluated on an individual basis with regard to return to noncontact sports. However, these individuals should not be permitted to return to contact activity regardless of how "solid" the fusion appears on roentgenograms. Altered biomechanics of the cervical spine with more than a two level fusion presents several problems. The decrease in motion will, in itself, deprive the spine of its capability of dissipating force through motion. Also, it would appear that there is a higher risk of injury because of the increased torque on the lever arm on the level above and below the fusion mass. The effect of cervical fusion as a precipitating cause of degenerative disease at other levels is also a question that is unanswered, but should be considered.

REFERENCES

1. Albright, J.P., et al.: Nonfatal cervical spine injuries in interscholastic football. J.A.M.A., *236*:1243, 1976.
2. Anderson, L.D., and D'Alonzo, R.T.: Fractures of the odontoid process of the axis. J. Bone Joint Surg., *56A*:1663, 1974.
3. Cloward, R.B.: Acute cervical spine injuries. Ciba Clin. Symp., *32*:2, 1980.
4. DePalma, A.F., and Rothman, R.H.: The Intervertebral Disc. Philadelphia, W.B. Saunders, 1970.
5. Fielding, J.W., et al.: Athletic injuries to the atlanto-axial articulation. Am. J. Sports Med., *6*:226, 1978.
6. Jefferson, G.: Fracture of the atlas vertebra. Br. J. Surg., *7*:407, 1920.
7. Roaf, R.: A st 6. Jefferson, G.: Fracture of the atlas vertebra. Br. J. Surg., *7*:407, 1920.
7. Roaf, R.: A study of the mechanics of spinal injuries. J. Bone Joint Surg., *42B*:810, 1960.
8. Roaf, R.: International classification of spinal injuries. Paraplegia, *10*:78, 1972.
9. Schneider, R.C.: The syndrome of acute anterior cervical spinal cord injury. J. Neurosurg., *12*:95, 1955.
10. Thompson, R.C., et al.: Current concepts in management of cervical spine fractures and dislocations. Am. J. Sports Med., *3*:159, 1975.
11. Torg, J.S., et al.: Spinal injury at the level of the third and fourth cervical vertebrae from football. J. Bone Joint Surg., *59A*:1015, 1977.
12. White, A.A., and Panjabi, M.M.: Clinical Biomechanics of the Spine. Philadelphia, J.B. Lippincott, 1978.

Chapter 14

Anatomy of the Innervation of the Upper Extremity

Carson D. Schneck

THE PLEXUS CONCEPT

The typical spinal nerve, formed by the union of dorsal and ventral roots, divides outside the intervertebral foramen into a dorsal and a ventral ramus.

In general, the *dorsal rami* of spinal nerves supply the skin of the medial two thirds of the back from the top of the head to the coccyx, the deep (intrinsic) muscles of the back, and the zygapophyseal vertebral joints. Each dorsal ramus supplies the strip of skin and muscle and the zygapophyseal joint located at the level of its origin.

The *ventral rami* of spinal nerves supply the rest of the spinally innervated muscles and the skin and joints of the neck, trunk, and extremities. The ventral rami, except those from T2 to T11 form plexi, i.e., they join with higher or lower ventral rami to form networks from which peripheral nerves may arise, which contain nerve fibers derived from more than one spinal cord segment. This is in contrast to the dorsal rami, which generally do not form plexi, and are therefore themselves unisegmental peripheral nerves.

GENERAL MAKEUP OF THE BRACHIAL PLEXUS

The brachial plexus is usually formed from the ventral rami of spinal nerves C5 to T1 (Fig. 14-1). The ventral rami of C5 and C6 fuse to form the superior *trunk,* while the ventral ramus of C7 continues on as the middle trunk, and the ventral rami of C8 and T1 form the inferior trunk. Each trunk divides into an anterior and posterior division. The anterior divisions of the superior and middle trunks join to become the lateral *cord,* while the anterior division of the inferior trunk becomes the medial cord. The posterior divisions of all three trunks unite to form the posterior cord. The cords are named according to their relation to the axillary artery. The cords end by dividing into five *terminal nerves.* The lateral cord gives off the lateral root of the median nerve and then continues as the musculocutaneous nerve. The medial cord gives off the medial root of the median nerve and then continues as the ulnar nerve. The posterior cord terminates by dividing into the axillary and radial nerves. Other nerves arise from the plexus at the levels of the ventral rami, trunks, and cords, and the most important of these nerves are indicated in Figure 14-1.

APPLIED ASPECTS OF THE INNERVATION OF THE UPPER EXTREMITY

In considering the innervation of the upper extremity one should think of three

BRACHIAL PLEXUS

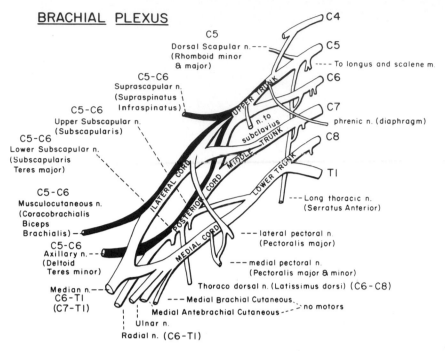

Fig. 14-1. Brachial plexus.

general levels of nerve lesions and the resulting motor and sensory deficits.

Injuries may occur *distal to the plexus* and involve one or more *peripheral nerves* somewhere along their course. Depending on the level of injury, a complete or partial deficit occurs in the distribution of that peripheral nerve. To identify this type of involvement one must appreciate the general distribution of the peripheral nerves derived from the brachial plexus.

Note that the *anterior divisions* of the trunks formed the lateral and medial cords, which in turn gave rise to the musculocutaneous, median, and ulnar nerves. These terminal nerves innervate *all* of the *anterior (flexor) muscles* of the arm, forearm, and hand.

The *musculocutaneous nerve* innervates the muscles of the anterior or flexor compartment of the arm (major elbow flexors and major supinator of the forearm) and the skin of the lateral aspect of the forearm.

The *median nerve* innervates all the muscles of the forearm (major wrist and finger flexors, and forearm pronators) with the exception of the flexor carpi ulnaris and the ulnar half of the flexor digitorum profundus. It also innervates the radial two lumbricals, all the intrinsic muscles of the thumb (thumb opposition) except the adductor pollicis, and the skin on the thumb side of the palm of the hand and the palmar aspect of the radial 3½ digits, as well as the dorsal surface of their terminal phalanges.

The *ulnar nerve* innervates the flexor carpi ulnaris, the ulnar half of the flexor digitorum profundus, all the intrinsics of the little finger, the ulnar two lumbricals, the adductor pollicis, and all the interossei (major abductors and adductors of the fingers). It also innervates the skin on the ulnar side of the palm, dorsum of the hand, and the palmar and dorsal aspects of the ulnar 1½ digits.

The *radial nerve,* which is the major continuation of the posterior cord, supplies all the posterior or extensor muscles of the arm and forearm, and the skin of the posterior aspect of the arm, forearm, and lateral two thirds of the hand distally to about the distal interphalangeal joints.

The *axillary nerve* supplies the deltoid (major shoulder abductor and hyperextender), the teres minor, and the skin over the insertion of the deltoid.

The *pectoral nerves* innervate pectoralis major, and the medial pectoral also supplies the pectoralis minor.

The *medial brachial and antebrachial cutaneous nerves* supply their indicated skin areas.

The *upper subscapular nerve* supplies the upper part of the subscapularis muscle. The *lower subscapular nerve* supplies the lower part of subscapularis muscle and teres major. The *thoracodorsal nerve* innervates the latissimus dorsi; the *suprascapular nerve*, the supraspinatus and infraspinatus muscles; the *dorsal scapular nerve*, the rhomboids (and levator scapulae); and the *long thoracic nerve*, the serratus anterior.

Lesions may occur proximal to the plexus either at the spinal cord, root, or spinal nerve and cause sensory and motor deficits on a segmental basis. The cutaneous area innervated by one spinal cord segment is called a *dermatome*. Since there is considerable overlap between adjacent dermatomes, a given dermatomal loss may be difficult to identify unless adjacent spinal cord segments are also involved. The general dermatomal distribution in the upper extremity is as follows:

C4	Shoulder pad area
C5	Lateral aspect of arm
C6	Lateral aspect of forearm, hand, and the radial two digits
C7	Middle finger
C8	Ulnar two digits and medial aspect of hand and wrist
T1	Medial aspect of forearm
T2	Medial aspect of arm

The segmental motor innervation in the upper extremity is:

C5, C6	Deltoid and other intrinsic muscles of the shoulder (abduction, hyperextension, and external rotation at shoulder)
C5, C6	Biceps, brachialis, and supinator (elbow flexion and supination of forearm)
C6, C7	Pronators of forearm
C7 (C6, C8)	Triceps and extensors of wrist and of fingers at the metacarpophalangeal joints
C8, T1	Intrinsic muscles of hand

The segmental levels of deep reflexes are:

Biceps	C5 (C6)
Triceps	C7 (C6)
Radial jerk (supinator reflex)	C5 (C6, C7)
Ulnar jerk (pronator reflex)	C6 (C7, C8)

Lesions may also involve the plexus itself. For example, the upper plexus may be injured in forcible separation of the head and shoulders during collision; the lower part of the plexus may be injured in forcible abduction of the arm; or mixed types of plexus injuries may follow any type of traction trauma to the extremity. Depending upon whether rami, trunks, or cords are injured, these types of injuries cause various segmental deficits.

The ventral rami and trunks of the plexus, as well as the subclavian artery, emerge from the narrow triangular interval between the anterior and middle scalene muscles and the clavicle below. At this point the plexus and artery may be encroached upon by a number of lesions, such as a cervical rib or an anterior scalene muscle spasm, that narrow this interval. These lesions may cause a neurocirculatory compression (anterior scalene) syndrome with peripheral paresthesia, hypesthesia, weakness, and vascular insufficiency. To test for this syndrome, the head is turned to the side of the symptoms and extended, and a deep inspiration is taken (Adson's test). This narrows the interval, stretches the neurovascular structures, reproduces the symptoms and obliterates the radial pulse.

MAJOR EXTRINSIC MUSCLES OF THE SHOULDER

The major extrinsic muscles of the shoulder are the muscles that arise from the axial skeleton and insert on the shoulder girdle or humerus.

The *latissimus dorsi* is innervated by the thoracodorsal nerve (C6, C7, C8). This muscle extends from the lower-back region to the front of the upper end of the humerus. It participates in extension, adduction, and internal rotation at the shoulder, and its downward pull resists upward displacement of the humerus and scapula as in crutch-walking. It may also act to pull the trunk upward as in climbing. Its function can be checked by performing its movements against resistance and palpating its contraction over the lower back or in the posterior axillary fold.

The *rhomboids* (dorsal scapular nerve, C5) are primarily adductors of the scapula.

The course of the *serratus anterior* (long thoracic nerve, C5, C6, C7) over the apex of the lung exposes it to involvement by apical lung disease. Then its course along the medial axillary wall exposes it to trauma in axillary surgery. This muscle is an abductor and upward rotator of the scapula, and it keeps the vertebral border of the scapula closely applied to the thoracic wall. Paralysis causes winging of the scapula, which can be accentuated by pushing with the arms against a wall.

The *pectoralis major* (medial and lateral pectoral nerves, C5-T1) is the principal adductor of the arm and also flexes and internally rotates the arm. It draws the chest upward as in climbing, and prevents upward displacement of the humerus and scapula as in crutch-walking.

INTRINSIC MUSCLES OF THE SHOULDER

The intrinsic muscles arise from the shoulder girdle and insert on the humerus. They are all innervated by C5, C6 cord segments.

The axillary nerve (C5, C6) winds around the surgical neck of the humerus and thus may be traumatized in shoulder dislocations or fractures of the surgical neck. The deltoid muscle's primary function is abduction of the arm, but its posterior part is also an important hyperextensor, and its various parts may participate in all movements of the arm. In paralysis, the normal shoulder contour may be flattened and normal abduction and hyperextension are considerably weakened.

The teres minor (axillary nerve) is primarily an external rotator and functions as part of the rotator cuff mechanism.

The supraspinatus muscle (suprascapular nerve, C5, C6) abducts and participates in rotator cuff functions. Its function is more commonly impaired by tendinitis and tendon rupture than by denervation.

The infraspinatus muscle (suprascapular nerve) is the primary external rotator and functions as part of the rotator cuff.

The subscapularis muscle (upper- and lower-subscapular nerves, C5, C6) is an internal rotator and a cuff muscle.

Like the latissimus dorsi, with which this muscle helps to form the posterior axillary fold, the teres major (lower-subscapular nerve) is an internal rotator, extensor, and adductor of the arm.

A C5-C6 lesion of the plexus or spinal cord causes loss of abduction and all external rotation so that the arm is held in adduction and internal rotation.

Chapter 15

Brachial Plexus and Upper Extremity Peripheral Nerve Injuries

William G. Clancy, Jr.

Because of their catastrophic sequelae, neck fractures and dislocations sustained in contact sports have gained much attention recently. However, far more common shoulder and neck injuries, those to the brachial plexus, have received far less attention. Often the extent of these seemingly minimal injuries may not be fully appreciated by the player, coach, or physician.

In this discussion, brachial plexus injuries are classified as first, second, and third degree. The clinical manifestations of each correspond to Seddon's classification of nerve injuries.[12] Since the brachial plexus contains many thousands of nerve fibers, any significant injury to the plexus probably produces a spectrum of symptoms including neurapraxia, axonotmesis, and neurotmesis. Our classification is, therefore, based on the most predominant aspect, as determined by both clinical and electromyographic evaluation.

A Grade I injury corresponding to Seddon's definition of a neurapraxia,[12] means that theoretically, a physiologic interruption has occurred without anatomic damage to the brachial plexus. This results in a transitory loss of motor and sensory functions, which may last for minutes or several hours; complete recovery occurs within two weeks. An electromyographic evaluation performed two to three weeks after this type of injury does not demonstrate any signs of axonal injury. A Grade II injury is an injury that produces significant motor weakness, and perhaps some sensory deficit lasting at least two weeks. After two to three weeks, electromyography demonstrates that some significant axonal injury has occurred. This Grade II brachial plexus injury would correspond with Seddon's definition of axonotmesis. A Grade III injury produces motor and sensory deficits of at least one year's duration with no appreciable clinical improvement during this period. This state corresponds with Seddon's definition of neurotmesis.

GRADE I BRACHIAL PLEXUS INJURY (NEURAPRAXIA)

This is the most common injury seen in contact sports. It is often referred to as a "burner" or "stinger" by coaches and players because the player experiences a severe burning pain while making a block or tackle. The pain starts in the shoulder area and radiates down the arm and into the hand. This is then followed by numbness or tingling in the arm and hand. This entity has been frequently referred to in the medical literature as the "cervical nerve pinch syndrome."[1,3,9] Usually there is full recovery of motor and sensory function within several minutes. The athlete frequently develops a significant palpable area of tenderness in the upper or middle portion of the anterior aspect of the trapezius, which persists for several days. The cause of this is unknown.

Since cervical nerve pinch syndrome frequently does not preclude continued participation, the overall incidence of this type of injury in high school and collegiate football is unknown. However, an in-depth study of the 1974 United States Naval Academy and the 1976 University of Wisconsin football teams revealed that over 50% of the players of each team had sustained at least one significant Grade I injury during their playing careers.[4] Approximately 30% sustained their first injury in high school, while the remainder sustained their first injury in college. The number of episodes varied from one/year to at least one/week. Those who sustained at least 10 to 20/year had invariably sustained their first episode in their second or third year of high school football, and the frequency progressed almost geometrically with each year of competition. Quarterbacks, running backs, and receivers developed few or none of these injuries, while defensive backs and defensive linemen had the highest incidence.

Careful questioning of these athletes revealed that the majority held their head laterally flexed away from the side of the injury, and the involved shoulder was driven downward or backward while they were either blocking or tackling. However, a significant number did state that their head and neck were laterally flexed toward the side of the injury. Additionally, a smaller number stated that they had developed "burners" with forced hyperextension of their head and neck.

As soon as he has sustained a "burner," it is our policy to examine the athlete on the field and then to re-examine him when he feels that he has completely recovered. One must always be aware of a possible neck fracture, but neck pain is rarely associated with "burners," and when present, should alert one to a more serious injury. The examination on the field should consist of having the athlete put his head and neck through range of motion against resistance if there is no pain present. Then the internal and external shoulder rotators are tested against resistance while the shoulder is abducted 90°. The deltoid, biceps, and triceps as well as the forearm muscles are then tested against resistance. If there is no subjective pain or weakness, and none demonstrated on examination, the player is then allowed to return to the competition. He is re-examined after the game and the next day.

GRADE II BRACHIAL PLEXUS INJURY (AXONOTMESIS)

In 1973, three football players from the United States Naval Academy presented initially with what appeared to be a cervical nerve pinch syndrome or "burner." However, these athletes failed to regain even reasonable strength of their deltoid, infraspinatus, supraspinatus, and biceps muscles after three weeks. Electromyography revealed changes consistent with significant axonotmesis involving the upper trunk of the brachial plexus without involvement of the rhomboids (dorsal scapular nerve), the serratus anterior (long thoracic nerve), or the posterior paraspinal muscles. This pinpointed the upper trunk as the most likely site of the lesion. All players recovered completely after approximately six months, although there were still some changes present on electromyograms. During the past six years we have seen over 40 athletes who have sustained Grade II brachial plexus injuries, most of which have been documented by electromyography.[10]

All patients complained of a burning pain which "shot down their arm." They were almost completely unable to use the injured upper extremity for several minutes, but strength gradually returned over the next few minutes. However, in most cases there was not full return of strength.

Some players could not actively abduct their shoulders past 45°, and few could abduct past 90°. I personally examined four within one or two hours of their injury and found normal strength. However, within three days, they developed significant weakness and inability to abduct past 45°. None had returned to competition in the interim. Clinical examination revealed that the deltoid, infraspinatus, supraspinatus, and biceps muscles were involved in all cases. Many also displayed involvement of the brachioradialis, pronator teres, and wrist extensors. Electromyography on the majority of these patients confirmed the involvement of the deltoid, supraspinatus, and infraspinatus in all cases.

The mechanism and the pathophysiology of these injuries are still debatable. Although the majority of the athletes held their head flexed laterally to the side opposite the injury while the affected shoulder was being driven downward and backward, a significant number held their head flexed laterally to the side of the injury, and a small number hyperextended their head and neck.

Electromyography has demonstrated that in all cases tested there was no involvement of the muscles innervated by the roots of C5, C6, or C7. This strongly suggests that this is a lesion involving at least the upper trunk (see Fig. 14-1). As noted by Schneider[11] and Maroon,[8] there

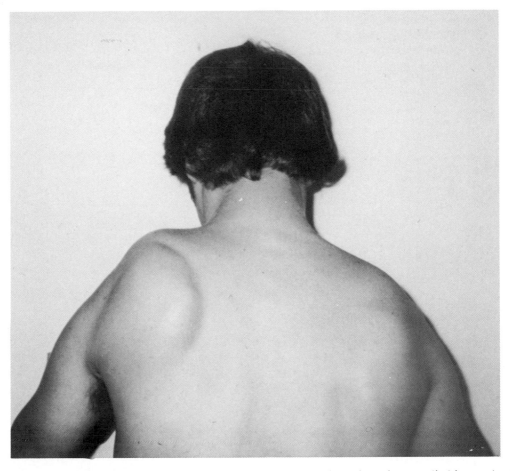

Fig. 15-1. Winging of the left scapula secondary to injury to the long thoracic nerve that innervates the serratus anterior muscle. On examination, the winging is accentuated by having the patient push against the wall. Characteristically, the winging disappears; however, this may take up to 18 months.

was no evidence of disc herniation or central cord injury. It has been postulated that these brachial plexus injuries result from contusion of the roots at the foramen by either vertical compression or by entrapment or contusion due to a subluxating facet. It is certainly possible for injuries to result from the above mechanisms. However, one would expect that if the trauma was sufficient to produce a multiple level root injury, there would be some involvement of the posterior paraspinal muscles, the rhomboids, or the serratus anterior muscle. This did not occur in any of our patients. Further, it is unusual for these athletes to have associated significant cervical spine pain.

The extent of the axonotmesis is probably significantly less than one initially assumes. In the majority of our cases, clinical examination showed there was marked weakness for three to four weeks, but within four to six weeks the athletes usually had recovered full normal strength.

Although, it usually took six months to develop normal strength and endurance, Cybex and barbell testing revealed generally 80 to 90% return of strength and endurance after six weeks. This certainly suggests that the lesion is a combination of neurapraxia and axonotmesis, since axon regeneration requires at least six months, and this regeneration cannot account for the significant return of strength in the four- to five-week interval postinjury. This unusual return of strength over a four- to five-week period strongly suggests that neurapraxia may indeed involve some structural injury to the axon without leading to Wallerian degeneration. As suggested by the work of Denny-Brown, the lesion may be a demyelination of the nerve fibers.[5, 6, 7]

GRADE III BRACHIAL PLEXUS INJURY (NEUROTMESIS)

Only one of the three athletes did not fully recover from his injury. This athlete

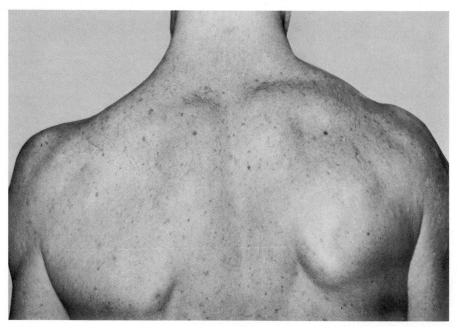

Fig. 15-2. A suprascapulae nerve injury in a 22-year-old intercollegiate basketball player who sustained a direct blow injury across his shoulders followed by ''weakness.'' Examination revealed marked atrophy of both the supraspinatus and infraspinatus, as well as pectoralis major muscles. Differential diagnosis should include a Grade II brachial plexus injury or rotator cuff tear. This particular patient regained full muscle strength and function over several months.

still had severe involvement of the deltoid and supraspinatus and infraspinatus muscles after one and one-half years, but was subsequently lost to follow-up. One cannot categorically state that in the Grade II injuries some neurotmesis has not occurred. It is possible that some neurotmesis may have occurred, but was so minimal that it could not be detected.

A recent paper on brachial plexus injuries expressed concern about the possible increase in Grades I and II injuries due to the change in the high-school rule on blocking.[1] A slight increase in the incidence of Grade I "burners" was noticed, but to date no significant increase in Grade II injuries.

Athletes who have sustained a Grade I injury are allowed to return to competition when their subjective symptoms completely resolve and there is no weakness on clinical examination. We recommend a routine cervical film survey on all those who sustain their first injury, and a repeat clinical evaluation four or five days after their injury.

Athletes who have sustained a Grade II injury should initially have routine cervical spine roentgenograms and an electromyogram after three weeks. They are withheld from contact sports until they have achieved full normal strength and endurance on specific neck and upper extremity muscle testing and after a repeat electromyogram has been obtained when indicated.

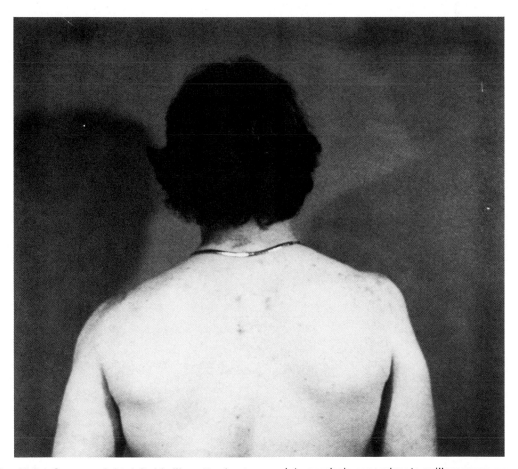

Fig. 15-3. Concave right deltoid silhouette due to complete paralysis secondary to axillary nerve neurotmesis. Injury was associated with a glenohumeral joint dislocation.

Starting from the third week, the athlete is placed on a specific upper body and neck strengthening program. When returning to competition, we strongly recommend the use of a large neck roll.[2] Those athletes with a history of frequent "burners" are placed on a similar program.

PERIPHERAL NERVE INJURIES ABOUT THE SHOULDER

These injuries may involve the spinal accessory nerve (trapezius muscle), the suprascapular nerve (the supraspinatus, the infraspinatus, and the teres major), the axillary nerve (deltoid and teres minor), and the long thoracic nerve (serratus anterior) (see Fig. 14-1).

The spinal accessory nerve is vulnerable anteriorly, just proximal to its entrance into the undersurface of the trapezius, approximately one inch above the clavicle. It can be injured by a direct blow from a hockey or lacrosse stick, or a shoulder pad could be forced against it. With significant trauma, there may be weakness when lifting the arm or shrugging the shoulders, and there may be a rotatory winging of the scapula (Fig. 15-1). This injury should be followed by electromyography. If there is no recovery within six months, the nerve should be explored.

The suprascapular nerve may be injured by a direct blow to the base of the neck (Fig. 15-2). This causes shoulder weakness, which is noticeable at 90° abduction. This injury must be differentiated from a resolving Grade II brachial plexus injury. In followup of Grade II brachial plexus injuries we have noted that the biceps and deltoid functions return to normal significantly faster than the supraspinatus and infraspinatus. Hence, a Grade II plexus injury, if seen late, may readily appear as an isolated suprascapular nerve injury. Careful questioning and electromyographic evaluation often helps differentiate between the two. This differential diagnosis is particularly important, since suprascapular nerve injury without significant return of strength after six months may warrant surgical exploration. Without a concomitant shoulder dislocation, an axillary nerve injury (Fig. 15-3) is an uncommon finding in football players since the shoulder pad usually prevents a direct blow to this nerve.

Several months after the injury it may be difficult to distinguish between a partially recovered brachial plexus injury and a peripheral nerve injury. An awareness of the clinical manifestations and the electromyographic findings at serial intervals may help to differentiate between the two entities.

REFERENCES

1. Alley, R.H.: Head and neck injuries in high school football. J.A.M.A., *188*:418, 1964.
2. Andrish, J., Bergfeld, J.A., and Romo, R.: A method for the management of cervical injuries in football. A preliminary report. Am. J. Sports Med., 5:89, 1977.
3. Chrisman, O.D., and Snook, G.A.: Lateral-flexion neck injuries in athletic competition. J.A.M.A., 192:117, 1965.
4. Clancy, W.G., Jr., Brand, R.L., and Bergfeld, J.A.: Upper trunk brachial plexus injuries in contact sports. Am. J. Sports Med., 5:209, 1977.
5. Denny-Brown, D.E., and Brenner, C.: Paralysis of nerve induced by direct pressure and by tourniquet. Arch. Neurol. Psychiatr., 51:1, 1944.
6. Denny-Brown, D.E., and Brenner, C.: Lesion in peripheral nerve resulting from compression by spring clip. Arch. Neurol. Psychiatr., 52:1, 1944.
7. Denny-Brown, D.E., and Doherty, M.M.: Effects of transient stretching of peripheral nerve. Arch. Neurol. Psychiatr., 54:116, 1945.
8. Maroon, J.C.: "Burning hands" in football spinal cord injuries. J.A.M.A., *238*:2049, 1977.
9. O'Donoghue, D.H.: Treatment of Injuries to Athletes. Philadelphia, W.B. Saunders, 1970.
10. Robertson, W.C., Jr., Eichman, P.L., and Clancy, W.G.: Upper trunk brachial plexopathy in football players. J.A.M.A., 241:1480, 1979.
11. Schneider, R.C.: Head and Neck Injuries in Football. Baltimore, Williams & Wilkins, 1973.
12. Seddon, H.: Surgical Disorders of the Peripheral Nerves. Edinburgh, Churchill-Livingstone, 1972.

Section IV

Facial, Oral and Eye Injuries

Chapter 16

Diagnosis and Management of Maxillofacial Injuries

Steven D. Handler

Sports-related activities account for approximately 12% of maxillofacial injuries seen in large trauma centers.[2,6] Despite the increased use of faceguards and masks, facial and cervical trauma continue to present significant problems in diagnosis and treatment.

GENERAL PRINCIPLES

There are important factors that are common to the management of significant maxillofacial injuries. While these injuries most often occur as isolated trauma, one must be aware of the possibility of associated injuries. Trauma to the chest, abdomen, musculoskeletal, or central nervous systems may be present in the injured athlete. Attention to these problems often takes priority over the management of the maxillofacial injuries.

Infection is an important factor influencing the ultimate healing of maxillofacial injuries. Antibiotics are frequently given on a prophylactic basis because of the contamination of the wound with intraoral flora and the risk of perichondritis in injuries of the cartilaginous nose and ear.

If the skin has been broken in an injury, protection against tetanus should be assessed. Tetanus toxoid is given if the last immunization was more than ten years ago (five years if the wound is deep and con-taminated), or if the status of tetanus immunization is unknown. In the latter case, tetanus antitoxin may also be required.

Dental occlusion is an important concept in evaluating jaw fractures and dislocations. In normal occlusion (neutroclusion) (Fig. 16-1), the anterior upper incisors are slightly anterior to the lower incisors. The midlines (spaces between central incisors) of the maxillary and mandibular dental arches line up with each other. The outer or buccal cusps of the upper molar teeth are slightly lateral to their lower counterparts. While deviations from these relationships may be normal for any one individual, they may indicate a misalignment secondary to a jaw fracture or dislocation.

SOFT-TISSUE INJURY

Contusions, abrasions, and lacerations comprise the majority of soft-tissue injuries of the face and neck. Facial contusions usually resolve spontaneously. However, they must be differentiated from the facial edema associated with a hematoma or underlying facial fracture, which requires further attention and treatment.

Abraded skin surfaces are gently cleansed and antibiotic ointment is

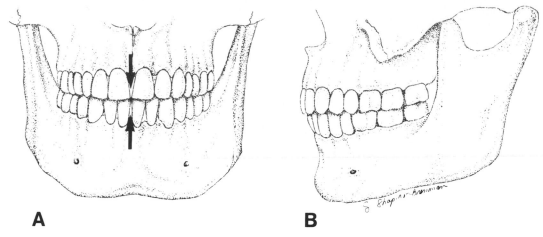

A　　　　　　　　　　　　　　**B**

Fig. 16-1. Normal occlusion. *A*, Frontal view. *B*, Lateral view. The midlines of the upper and lower dental arch (arrows) line up with each other. The outer cusps of the upper molars are more lateral than those of the mandibular arch, and the maxillary incisors are anterior to the mandibular incisors.

applied; the wound is covered with a small protective bandage. Injuries resulting from falls on asphalt or gravel surfaces may cause small foreign bodies to become embedded in the dermal layers. These must be removed to prevent permanent tattooing of the skin. A surgical scrub brush can be helpful in removing these particles. A local, or occasionally a general anesthetic is necessary to permit adequate cleansing of the area.. Grease or oil embedded in the wound may be dissolved and removed with small amounts of ether or acetone.

Linear lacerations, puncture wounds, and avulsion injuries are caused by contact with sharp objects such as ice-skate blades or shoe cleats. Blunt trauma to the cheek or forehead may cause a burst type of laceration, which is frequently stellate in appearance. In evaluating the facial lacerations, one must be certain that there has not been damage to the deeper structures such as the parotid duct, facial nerve, vascular structures of the neck, or facial skeleton.

If the laceration is small, superficial, and uncomplicated, the player may continue playing after application of a sterile dressing. Prepare the skin with tincture of benzoin so that the tape will adhere, taking care to protect the eyes and nasal mucous membrane.

Extensive lacerations may require immediate suturing before the player returns to the playing field. Bleeding can usually be stopped with simple pressure on the wound. Ligation of bleeding vessels is rarely required. Injection of 1% lidocaine (Xylocaine) with 1:100,000 epinephrine solution can be used, if necessary, to control bleeding. After adequate cleansing with saline and bland soap, full-thickness lacerations should be reapproximated by suture. Use of small adhesive strips is contraindicated in the definitive treatment of lacerations because the athlete will be expected to practice and play before wound healing occurs. A definitive "plastic" closure using 5-0 nylon suture is preferred in managing facial lacerations. To a large extent suture removal should be determined by the athlete's activity schedule. Care should be taken to avoid premature removal of all sutures and risking the chance of the wound separating. As a general rule, remove every other suture at four days and the remainder at seven.

Large or complicated injuries require more immediate attention. The presence of damage to underlying neural, vascular, and bony structures must be determined prior to definitive repair of these wounds. Any avulsed or loosely pedicled tissue

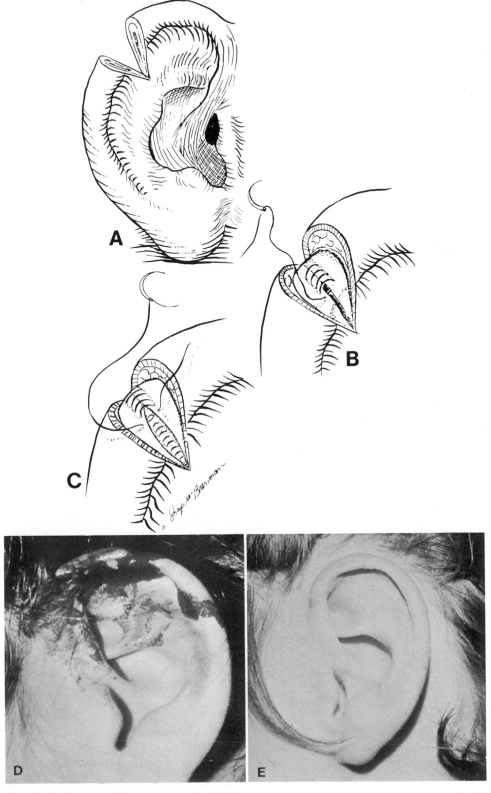

Fig. 16-2. *A*, Auricular cartilage laceration. *B*, Careful reapproximation of the cartilage edges. *C*, The overlying perichondrium is closed over the cartilage repair. *D*, Acute laceration of ear cartilage. *E*, Result of careful reapproximation, 6 weeks later.

should be preserved and protected for possible inclusion in the final repair. The
wound is usually covered with a sterile
gauze dressing until the repair can be undertaken. Wound closure should be accomplished using standard sterile plastic
surgical techniques. Depending on the
depth of the injury, a one- or two-layer
closure is performed. Lacerations through
cartilage require careful approximation of
the cartilage edges (trimmed, if necessary)
and the overlying perichondrium. This is
especially important when reattaching
avulsed portions of the nose or ear (Fig.
16-2). In large, deep wounds, a small rubber drain may be required to prevent blood
accumulation under the skin closure.

If avulsed or pedicled portions of skin
cannot be incorporated into the repair, a
skin defect can be closed by wide under-
mining of the wound edges, local flaps, or
skin grafts. Skin sutures are generally removed in five days to prevent formation of
suture track marks. Plastic revision of an
unsightly scar may be performed at any
time after the injury, but it is usually best to
wait at least one year to allow for maximal
normal healing to occur.

Hematomas of the subcutaneous tissue
of the face occur as a result of blunt trauma.
Swelling, pain, and discoloration are the
common signs of a hematoma. If the
hematoma is small and stable, it usually
resolves spontaneously. Larger hema-

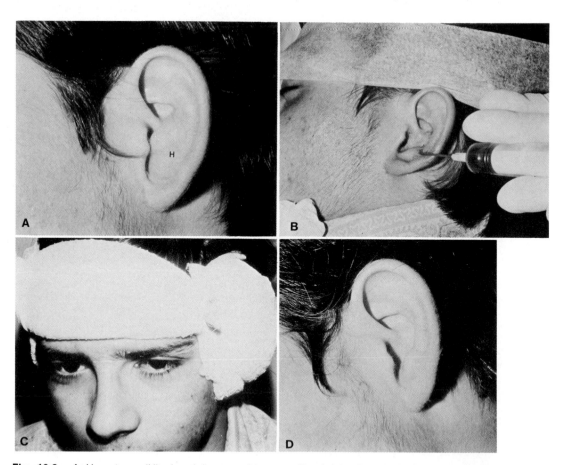

Fig. 16-3. *A,* Hematoma (H) of auricle caused by wrestling injury. *B,* Hematoma being aspirated. *C,* Contoured head dressing to force perichondrium back against auricular cartilage. *D,* Good result 4 weeks
postinjury.

tomas often require a drainage procedure. Soon after the injury, a small incision can be made in the skin overlying the hematoma; the jelly-like hematoma is then manually expressed from the wound. If one waits until the hematoma liquifies (five to seven days), the blood can be aspirated with a syringe and needle. After evacuation of the hematoma, a pressure dressing is usually applied to the wound to prevent reaccumulation of the blood or serum in the hematoma cavity. Progressively enlarging hematomas indicate persistent vascular damage, which may require angiography and surgical exploration.

Hematoma of the Auricle

Hematomas of the auricle pose a special problem that requires prompt attention (Fig. 16-3). This injury occurs as a result of blunt trauma to the exposed auricle from activities such as wrestling or boxing. The hematoma forms between the perichondrium and the cartilage of the ear. This compromises the blood supply to the cartilage, which is derived from the perichondrium. The blood clot should be aspirated as soon as possible to prevent a cosmetic deformity of the auricle. After aspirating the hematoma, a contoured pressure dressing of cotton impregnated with mineral oil is applied to the auricle and held in place with a snug head dressing. This forces the perichondrium back against the underlying cartilage, prevents reaccumulation of the hematoma, and re-establishes the blood supply to the cartilage.

During this time of healing, the hematoma is prone to redevelop if repeated trauma occurs.

If the hematoma is not evacuated, the blood begins to organize, and fibrosis of the overlying skin and pressure necrosis of the auricular cartilage occurs. The end result is the "cauliflower ear" (Fig. 16-4), in which the delicate cartilaginous contours of the auricle are lost. Treatment of this complication of an auricular hematoma is difficult and usually unsatisfactory.

Intraoral Trauma

Intraoral trauma is usually the result of a self-inflicted bite of the tongue or buccal mucosa. If there has been no damage to any intraoral structures, intraoral lacerations may be managed conservatively. Large, gaping lacerations should be reapproximated to restore normal functional anatomy and to aid the healing process. Through-and-through lacerations of the cheek should be carefully reapproximated with at least a two-layer closure. Large lacerations may require a small rubber drain for 24 hours. Antibiotics are given to prevent infection from intraoral flora.

Significant bleeding may occur with intraoral trauma. In the extreme case

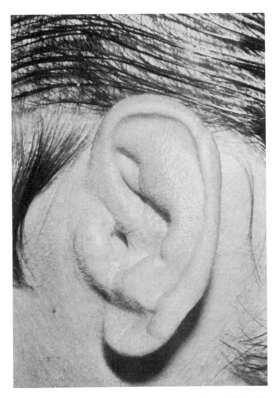

Fig. 16-4. Cauliflower ear. Thickened and fibrotic ear as a result of cartilage necrosis caused by an untreated auricular hematoma.

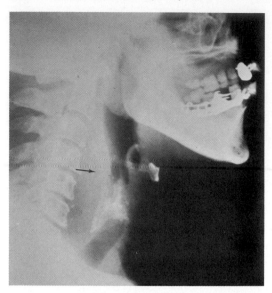

Fig. 16-5. Lateral neck radiograph demonstrating retropharyngeal abscess (arrow) that occurred as a complication of a pharyngeal injury.

where direct pressure or suture ligature is unsuccessful in stopping the bleeding, ligation of the external carotid artery may be necessary. If the mouth is filled with blood or packing, respiratory embarassment can occur.

Patients with lacerations of the pharynx should be examined for signs of perforation. Odynophagia (pain on swallowing) and cervical crepitus are early signs of a perforated viscus. Lateral neck radiographs will show free air in the soft tissues of the neck. The patient with crepitus is placed on antibiotics and observed in the hospital. While cervical free air often resolves spontaneously, endoscopy and repair of larger perforations may be required. Spiking fevers, dysphagia, and increasing respiratory distress may indicate the development of a lateral or posterior pharyngeal abscess. Lateral neck radiographs (Fig. 16-5) or CT scans can help to identify and localize the abscess site. Treatment consists of surgical drainage of the abscess, usually by an external approach.

FACIAL FRACTURES

Nasal Trauma

The most common sequelae of blunt nasal trauma is epistaxis (nosebleed). This usually occurs from a mucosal laceration in the interior of the nose. Bleeding most often originates from Kiesselbach's plexus, a network of prominent superficial blood vessels on the anterior nasal septum. Most instances of epistaxis stop spontaneously. Pressure applied by squeezing the nostrils together often stops persistent bleeding. Topical vasoconstrictors such as ½% phenylephrine hydrochloride (Neo-Synephrine) nose spray may also be useful. Cauterizing the bleeding site or packing the nasal cavity with cotton or vaseline-impregnated gauze is rarely required for the treatment of any but the most profuse nosebleeds. When the bleeding has stopped, and there is no sign of a more serious nasal injury, the player may return to the game.

Nasal fractures account for over 50% of all maxillofacial fractures that occur from sports-related injuries.[6] While facemasks and guards have decreased the incidence of nasal injuries, fractures continue to occur in significant numbers. Direct-blunt trauma may cause a nasal contusion with swelling and ecchymosis, or a fracture of the nasal skeleton. In most instances, the diagnosis of nasal fracture is obvious on clinical examination. The nasal bones are deviated to one side or depressed onto the face. Step-offs (bony irregularities) may be palpated at the fracture site (Fig. 16-6). However, because of the edema common to facial injuries, it may be difficult to determine the presence of a nasal fracture or the degree of nasal deformity at the initial clinical examination. In cases in which a fracture is not clinically apparent, radiographs are extremely useful in determining the existence of a fracture and the amount of displacement of the nasal bones. Lateral and base views of the nasal bones and the

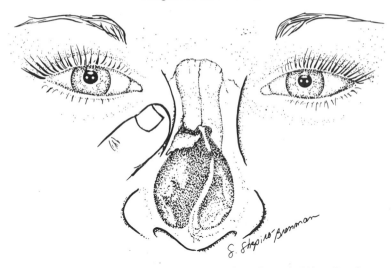

Fig. 16-6. Bony irregularities (step-offs) can often be palpated at the site of a nasal fracture.

upright Waters' view of the facial bones demonstrate the nasal skeleton most effectively (Fig. 16-7).

If a nasal fracture is suspected, a complete examination of the nose and surrounding structures must be performed. If present, associated injuries to the orbit must be identified and treated. The epistaxis that often accompanies these injuries usually stops spontaneously or with compression of the anterior nares; rarely is nasal packing necessary. The interior of the nose should be examined to evaluate the nasal septum. The trauma may have caused a fracture or dislocation of the septum, which must be recognized and treated together with any external deformity. If a septal hematoma has occurred, prompt treatment (described in a later section in this chapter) must be instituted to prevent permanent damage to the nasal structures. External lacerations can be sutured or taped as necessary.

Reduction of a displaced nasal fracture should be performed within seven days of the injury. After this time the fibrosis that has occurred makes it difficult to manipulate the fracture fragments. Severely comminuted or compound fractures are repaired as soon as possible. Open reduction

with interosseous wires, external splints, and intranasal packing may be necessary to restore normal anatomy in severely injured noses. If the nasal bones are obviously deviated on the initial evaluation, and there is minimal edema of the overlying soft tissue, the reduction can be per-

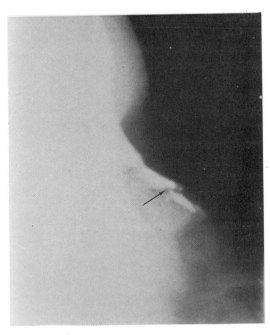

Fig. 16-7. Lateral radiograph of the nasal bones demonstrating a nasal fracture (arrow).

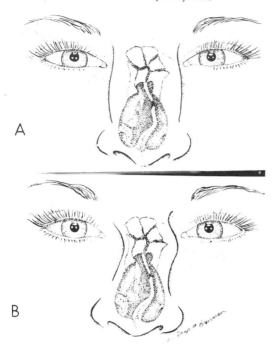

Fig. 16-8. Nasal fracture. *A,* Marked edema associated with the injury may mask the deviation of the nasal bones. *B,* Deviation of the nasal skeleton becomes manifest when edema subsides, approximately 5 to 7 days.

formed at any time. If there is sufficient edema that the presence of a fracture or the degree of deformity is masked, it is best to wait several days before making a decision regarding the necessity of a nasal reduction (Fig. 16-8). If, after the edema subsides, the fracture appears nondisplaced and has not caused any external deformity, no further treatment is required. If there is a visible external deformity, reduction of the fragments should be undertaken. A local anesthetic is required to permit the instrumentation necessary to replace the nasal bones and septum back into their normal anatomic positions (Fig. 16-9). Nasal packing is inserted if there has been significant hemorrhage associated with the reduction, or if internal support is required for the nasal bones. A protective cast of plaster or metal is applied for one week, and the athlete should avoid contact sports for two to three weeks to allow proper healing to occur.

Nasal deformities that persist after the initial reduction, or those that have not

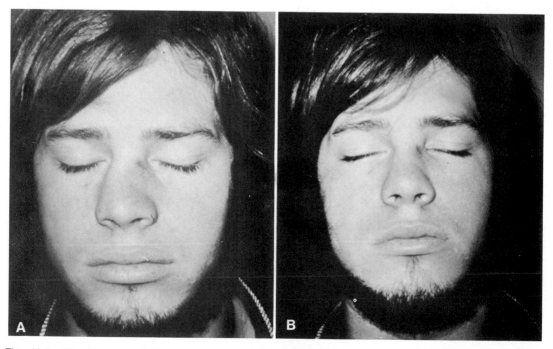

Fig. 16-9. Nasal fracture. *A,* Pre-reduction with obvious deformity of nasal bones. *B,* Post-reduction showing good cosmetic result.

been treated within ten days of the injury, require a formal elective rhinoplastic procedure for their correction. While this can be performed at any time after the injury, most surgeons prefer to wait at least six weeks to allow for complete stabilization of the nasal skeleton.

Septal Hematoma. Septal hematomas are usually associated with nasal fractures, but they may occur as isolated injuries. The patient presents with unilateral or bilateral collections of blood between the septal cartilage and its overlying mucoperichondrium (Fig. 16-10). If a septal hematoma occurs as a result of nasal trauma, it must be recognized early and treated promptly to prevent permanent deformity of the nose (Fig. 16-11). Incisions should be made through the mucosa

overlying the hematoma, and the clot evacuated as soon as possible. A small drain is placed in the wound, and the nasal cavity is packed to force the mucoperichondrium back against the septal cartilage. The packing remains in place three to five days. If the hematoma is not evacuated, necrosis of the septal cartilage with abscess formation can develop. The loss of this portion of the support to the external nose results in a saddlenose deformity (Fig. 16-12). Late correction of this problem is difficult and often unsatisfactory.

Maxillary Trauma

Zygoma Fractures. Fractures of the zygoma (or malar bone) account for approximately 10% of the maxillofacial frac-

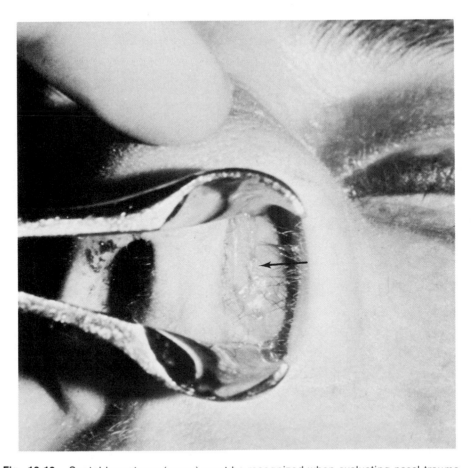

Fig. 16-10. Septal hematoma (arrow) must be recognized when evaluating nasal trauma.

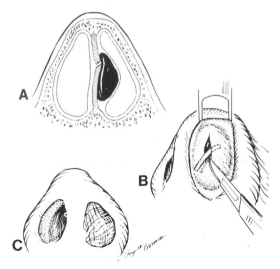

Fig. 16-11. Septal hematoma. *A,* Blood collects between the cartilage and overlying mucoperichondrium. *B,* Incision in nasal mucosa to drain hematoma. Often a drain is inserted to assure complete evacuation of hematoma. *C,* The perichondrium is forced back against the septal cartilage with nasal packing.

tures seen in sports injuries. These occur as a result of direct-blunt trauma to the malar eminence or cheekbone. The zygoma usually fractures at its attachments to the temporal, frontal, and maxillary bones (Fig. 16-13*A*). Because of the three commonly identified fracture sites, this injury is often called a tripod or trimalar fracture. Depending upon the type of mechanism of injury, a varying degree of rotation and inward displacement of the fragment is present. While the resultant facial asymmetry and depression of the malar eminence can often be seen upon viewing the front of the face, the deformity is usually best detected by looking at both cheeks from the top of the patient's head (Fig. 16-13*B*).

Step-offs can often be palpated over the fracture sites at the frontozygomatic suture line and at the inferior orbital rim. Intraorbital hypesthesia is usually present secondary to injury to the infraorbital nerve as it exits on the anterior wall of the maxillary sinus. If the orbital floor has been fractured and orbital soft tissue has become en-

trapped, restriction of ocular mobility may be present.

The edema of the cheek, common in these injuries, may often mask the presence of a facial deformity and prevent recognition of a zygoma fracture. In these cases, radiographs are indispensable in detecting or confirming the presence of a fracture. The sites of fractures and the degree of displacement can be determined best on the Waters' and Caldwell views (Fig. 16-14). The maxillary sinus is often opacified with blood on the side of the injury. This usually indicates that the orbital floor has been fractured, but does not necessarily mean that there is a defect in the floor with herniation of orbital tissue (a blow-out fracture). Tomograms are usually necessary to demonstrate the bony defect and soft-tissue herniation into the sinus, which occur in a blow-out fracture.

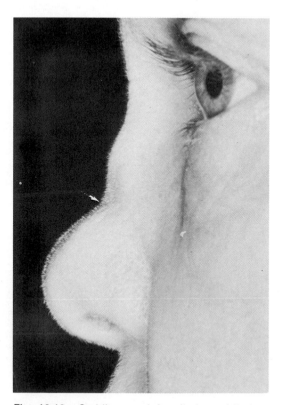

Fig. 16-12. Saddle nose deformity (arrow) that occurred as a result of loss of septal cartilage support secondary to septal hematoma and abscess.

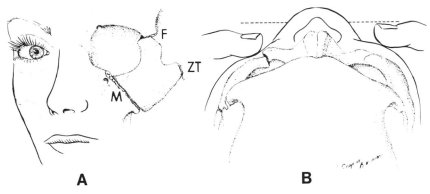

A   **B**

Fig. 16-13. Zygoma (trimalar) fracture. *A*, The zygoma fractures at its attachments to the maxilla (M), frontal bone (F), and the zygomatic process of the temporal bone (ZT). *B*, The best way to evaluate a zygoma fracture is to view both cheeks from the top of the patient's head as one is palpating to determine presence and degree of depression.

Immediate treatment of these injuries includes assessing the condition of the affected eye and an ophthalmologic consultation, if necessary. Antibiotics are given routinely, because the blood in the maxillary sinus is an excellent culture medium. The decision to explore the fracture may have to be delayed for several days to allow

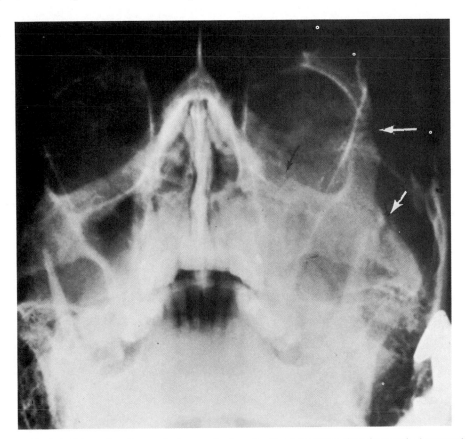

Fig. 16-14. Upright Waters' radiograph demonstrating the three fracture sites (arrows) characteristic of a zygoma fracture.

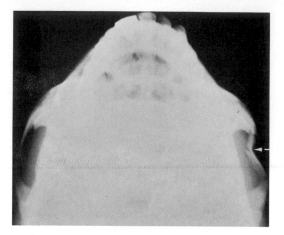

Fig. 16-15. Depressed zygomatic arch fracture (arrow) is best seen on a submental-vertex view.

edema to subside so that an accurate determination of the cosmetic deformity can be made. If there is depression of the malar eminence greater than one cm, enophthalmos, or restriction of ocular mobility, the fracture should be explored. The fracture is reduced and fixed with interosseous wires or antral packing. The orbital floor is examined and any herniation of orbital soft tissue is reduced. Bony defects

should be repaired with bone, alloplastic, or gelatin film implants.[1] The procedure can be performed through external incisions (lower lid and eyebrow), or by means of a sublabial (Caldwell-Luc) approach. The patient should refrain from sports activities for three to four weeks to allow adequate healing.

Some zygoma injuries may involve fracture of only the zygomatic arch. If these fragments are displaced inwardly, they can impinge upon the mandible, resulting in trismus (inability to open the jaw). Depression of the arch may be masked by postinjury edema, and radiographs are often necessary to make the diagnosis. The submental-vertex view is the most suitable for evaluating the zygomatic arch (Fig. 16-15). Reduction of this fracture is performed through an incision in the brow or in the buccal mucosa. The arch may require packing for seven to ten days to maintain its reduction.

Orbital Blow-Out Fractures. Direct trauma to the eye can result in the transmission of the force of the blow through the globe to fracture the bony walls of the

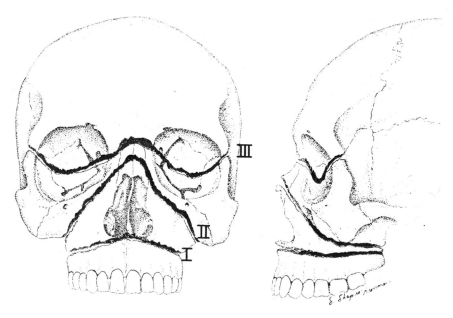

Fig. 16-16. Le Fort maxillary fractures are classified by type and severity: I involves separation of palate from midface; II fracture extends above nasal pyramid; III complete craniofacial disassociation.

orbit. The orbital floor or, less commonly, the medial wall of the orbit fractures leaving the orbital rim intact. Herniation of orbital fat or muscle through the bony defect results in the classic blow-out fracture. Enophthalmos, diplopia, and restriction of ocular mobility are the common findings. The management of these injuries will be discussed in detail in Chapter 18.

Le Fort Fractures. Significant force is required to create the maxillary fractures described by René Le Fort in the early 1900s. Because of this, they are uncommon in sports-related injuries. High-velocity impact to the midface can cause fractures of the maxilla with varying degrees of deformity and mobility of the maxilla with respect to the cranium and upper face (Fig. 16-16). The least severe fracture (Le Fort I) is a fracture above the alveolar ridge, thus mobilizing the palate from the face. The more severe fractures (Le Fort II and III) involve more complete craniofacial disas-

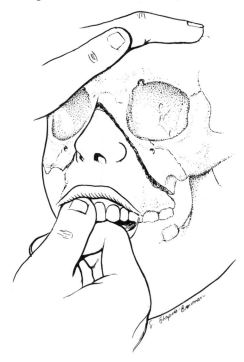

Fig. 16-17. With the head stabilized, mobility of the maxilla is pathognomonic of a Le Fort fracture.

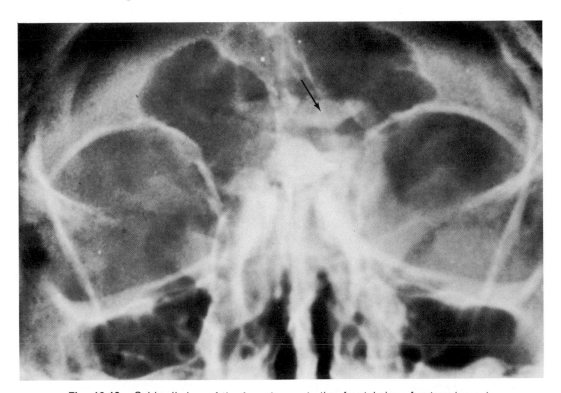

Fig. 16-18. Caldwell view of the face demonstrating frontal sinus fracture (arrow).

sociations. Patients with these injuries usually present with obviously depressed or mobile facial fragments. They may be in respiratory distress from associated intraoral bleeding and tissue edema. Mobility of the maxilla with respect to the upper face is pathognomonic of a Le Fort fracture (Fig. 16-17). Malocclusion is also a common finding on physical examination. In the more severe injuries cerebrospinal fluid (CSF) rhinorrhea may result from disruption of the cribriform plate.

After the initial evaluation and stabilization of the patient, radiographs (plain and tomograms) are taken to determine the fracture sites and the degree of deformity. Reduction and fixation of the fractures are usually undertaken within the first seven days. Intermaxillary fixation is maintained for six weeks, and during this period the player should avoid contact sports. The CSF rhinorrhea associated with Le Fort III fractures usually resolves with conservative treatment. The player is hospitalized and placed at bed rest with his head elevated. Persistent leaks require formal exploration and repair of cribriform plate defects.

Sinus Fractures

Fractures of the facial bones that extend into the paranasal sinuses present special problems in diagnosis and management. Fractures of the walls of the maxillary sinus can occur as isolated entities or as a part of a maxillofacial injury previously discussed, e.g., zygomatic or blow-out fractures. Blunt or penetrating trauma to the cheek can fracture the anterior or lateral walls of the maxillary sinus. The patient presents with pain and swelling of the anterior cheek. Crepitus may be present in soft tissue overlying the sinus. Radiographs are usually needed to confirm the diagnosis and to rule out other injuries. Fractures of the maxillary sinus walls are best seen on the Waters', Caldwell, or lateral views of the face. The maxillary sinus usually appears opacified, because it is

filled with blood. Often, air can be seen in the soft tissues of the cheek or orbit.

If there has been no damage to surrounding structures such as the orbit or zygoma, treatment is conservative. Antibiotics are given to prevent infection in the blood-filled sinus. The patient is observed for signs of increasing swelling or tenderness that could indicate development of a facial abscess. Under normal circumstances the athlete can resume his activities within a week, depending upon the degree of his discomfort. Long-term complications of these fractures, such as chronic sinusitis with obstruction of the maxillary sinus or osteomyelitis of the maxilla, are uncommon.

Fractures of the frontal sinus often present significant immediate and long-term problems. Blunt or sharp trauma to the forehead can fracture the anterior or posterior sinus walls. Pain and swelling of the forehead are the most common findings on physical examination. The deformity of the forehead caused by a depressed frontal sinus fracture may be masked by the immediate postinjury edema. Epistaxis frequently accompanies these injuries. Clear fluid draining from the nose may be CSF, indicating a fracture of the posterior table of the frontal sinus. Initial evaluation should involve inspection for associated cranial or orbital injuries. Radiographs are usually necessary to make the diagnosis of a frontal sinus fracture. Posteroanterior and lateral views in the upright position are the most helpful (Fig. 16-18). In addition to the bony fractures, opacification of the sinus or an air-fluid level is usually seen.

Management of these fractures depends upon the degree of cosmetic deformity and the presence of associated injuries.[5] A fracture through the posterior wall of the frontal sinus allows communication between the sinus and the anterior cranial fossa, and should be treated as a compound skull fracture. The patient should be hospitalized and kept at bed rest with his head elevated to decrease CSF rhinorrhea. He is

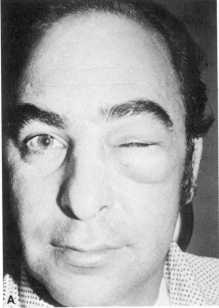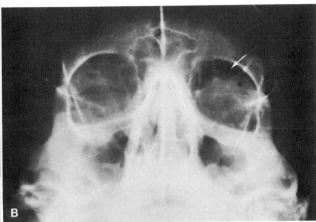

Fig. 16-19. *A,* Patient with swelling and palpable crepitus in orbit secondary to ethmoid sinus fracture. *B,* Waters' radiograph demonstrating air (arrow) in the orbit as a sign of this patient's ethmoid fracture.

then observed for signs of meningitis or other intracranial problems. The sinus should be explored if there is a cosmetic deformity of the forehead, a posterior table fracture, or possible injury to the nasofrontal duct. Exploration can be undertaken through a brow incision or by elevating a large scalp flap downward from above. The bony fragments are reduced and held in place with interosseous wires, if necessary, and dural lacerations are repaired. If the fracture has damaged the nasofrontal duct, thus impairing drainage of the sinus, the sinus should be stripped of all mucosa and the cavity obliterated with abdominal wall fat. This is done to prevent late complications of nasofrontal duct obstruction such as chronic sinusitis, osteomyelitis of the frontal bone, or mucocele formation.

The ethmoid sinuses are spared from direct trauma by their relatively protected position on the face. However, they can be injured by forces transmitted through more exposed structures, such as the orbit and the nasal bones. The presenting signs of ethmoid fractures are swelling and palpable crepitus in the medial portion of the orbit (Fig. 16-19). This results from escape of air from the ethmoid sinuses into

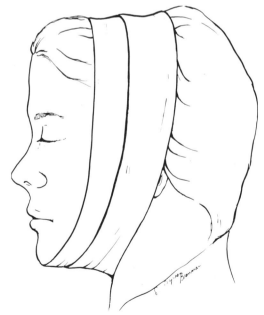

Fig. 16-20. Circumferential head dressing (Barton bandage) is helpful in restricting jaw movement and minimizing pain associated with mandible fractures.

the adjacent soft tissues of the orbit and face. If there has not been any associated injury to the nose or eye, fractures of the ethmoid sinus are managed conservatively. The patient is placed on antibiotics and observed for signs of orbital infection. He should be cautioned not to blow his nose until the crepitus resolves (about five to seven days). By blowing his nose, he could force more air and bacteria-laden

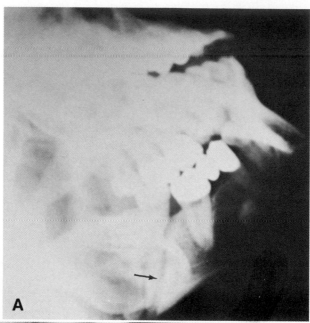

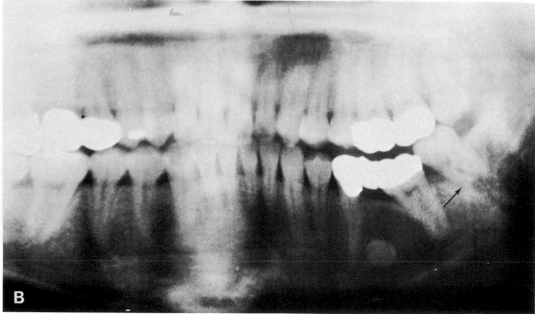

Fig. 16-21.   *A,* Angle fracture of mandible (arrow) is well seen in standard mandible view. *B,* Panoramic dental film is necessary to detect fractured tooth root (arrow) necessitating extraction prior to reduction of fracture.

sinus secretions into the facial soft tissues and increase the risk of an orbital infection. Contact sports should be avoided for about the same length of time.

Mandible Trauma

Fractures. Mandible fractures account for approximately 10% of maxillofacial fractures seen in sports-related accidents.[6] Most commonly the athlete falls and strikes the mandible against a hard playing surface. Occasionally, the fracture results from contact with another player or equipment. Pain and swelling of the lower face are the usual presenting symptoms. If the fracture extends through the intraoral mucosa, as almost all of them do, bleeding may occur from the mouth. The patient complains that his bite feels uncomfortable and that he has pain upon attempting to move his jaw. Malocclusion and abnormal mobility of the mandible are the most common findings on physical examination.

If a mandible fracture has occurred, airway management is the most important aspect of the immediate treatment. Blood, avulsed teeth or fragments of teeth, and saliva should be carefully cleared from the mouth. Prolapse of the tongue with airway obstruction often occurs as a result of mandibular arch instability. The mobile jaw fragments may require support either manually or with a snug head dressing (Barton bandage) (Fig. 16-20). This dressing also helps to reduce the pain associated with these fractures by restricting jaw movement. Radiographs are extremely useful in evaluating these fractures. Plain mandibular views show most fractures well, but panoramic dental films (Fig. 16-21) may be necessary to evaluate the position of the fragments and the status of the involved teeth.

The parts of the mandible most frequently fractured are the subcondylar area (40%), body (20%), angle (20%), and symphysis (15%).[3] Because of the structure of the mandibular arch, fractures often occur at two sites. Therefore, when a mandible

fracture has been identified, it is important to search for a second fracture site (Fig. 16-22).

If there is no compromise of the airway, the patient can be managed initially with a liquid diet. Since these fractures almost always extend through the oral mucosa or the periodontal ligament surrounding a tooth root, and are therefore compound fractures, antibiotics are given routinely. Simple, uncomplicated fractures of the subcondylar area may be managed with soft diet alone if the patient has good occlusion (Fig. 16-23). This continues for about six weeks until the patient can move his jaw normally without pain. If fragments are displaced by their attached muscles or there is evidence of malocclusion, stabilization of the fracture by open or closed reduction and placement of intermaxillary fixation becomes necessary (Fig. 16-24). Fractured or devitalized teeth in the fracture line are removed. Dental splints can be utilized to provide better fixation in occlusion, especially in patients with poor dentition. Fixation is maintained for six weeks. The athlete can resume sports activities once he is out of

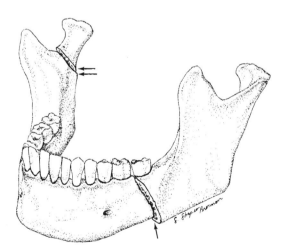

Fig. 16-22. The arch-shaped structures of the mandible are responsible for the common occurrence of two fracture sites in traumatic injuries. This figure illustrates one such injury with a body fracture (arrow) and contralateral subcondylar fracture (double arrows).

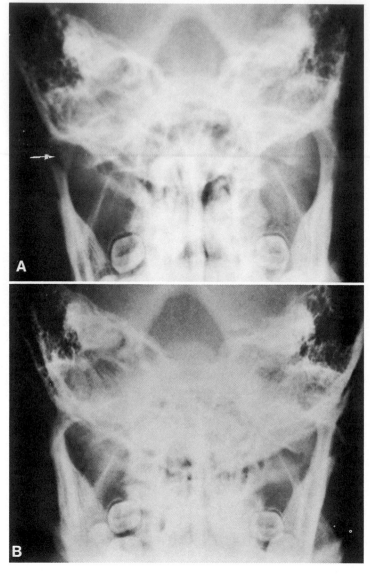

Fig. 16-23. *A*, Subcondylar fracture (arrow) in a patient with good occlusion. *B*, Fracture site healed after six weeks on a soft diet.

fixation and there is good evidence that the fracture has healed.

Mandibular trauma may transmit significant forces through the condylar joint and into the external auditory canal. Patients with mandible fractures should have a thorough examination of the external ears to determine if the bony ear canal has fractured. Packing of the ear canal may be required to stabilize the bony fragments and to keep the canal patent.

Dislocation of the Mandible. If the lower jaw is suddenly depressed in a sports activity, dislocation of the mandible can occur. The mandibular condyle comes to rest anterior to the articular eminence of the glenoid fossa and is held there by spasm of the masticatory muscles. The chin tends to deviate to the side opposite the dislocation, and the patient is unable to close his mouth (open-bite deformity) (Fig. 16-25*A*). Radiographs are necessary to dif-

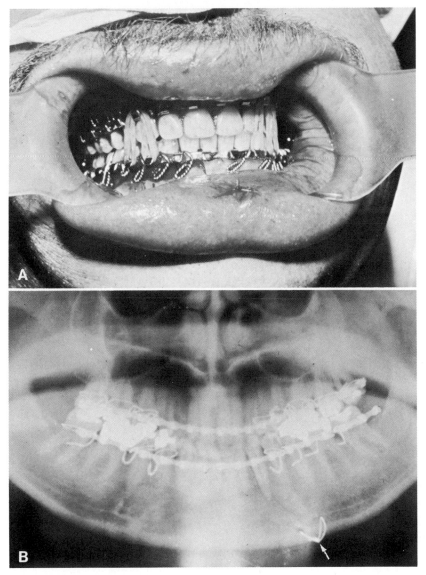

Fig. 16-24. *A,* Arch bars and rubberbands are used to provide intermaxillary fixation. *B,* Radiograph showing intermaxillary fixation and interosseous wire (arrow).

ferentiate this condition from a fractured mandible or to determine if a fracture has accompanied a traumatic dislocation.

The mandible should be repositioned as soon as possible (Fig. 16-25*B*). Postinjury edema and muscle spasm may make this difficult to perform without some form of muscle relaxant, sedative, or occasionally a general anesthetic. The patient is usually in the sitting position with his head sup-

ported. The physician's thumbs are placed on the mandibular body lateral to the lower molars, and his fingers grasp the mandibular body. Wrapping the physician's thumbs with cloth helps to prevent injury to his hand. The posterior portion of the mandible is depressed downward and posteriorly so that the condyle can slip under the articular eminence and return to the glenoid fossa. Once the reduction is ac-

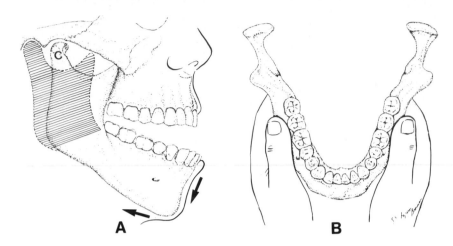

Fig. 16-25. Dislocation of mandible. *A,* Mandibular condyle (C) is displaced anteriorly from its normal position (striped lines). *B,* To replace mandible, physician's hands are placed on mandible as shown, and downward and backward forces are exerted (indicated in *A*) to allow the condyle to slip back into its normal position.

complished, the patient is placed on a soft diet and should refrain from contact sports for two to three weeks to allow healing of the muscles and ligaments that were stretched during the dislocation. Chronic or recurrent dislocations may require formal surgical procedures, such as placement of intermaxillary fixation or exploration of the temporomandibular joint.

NECK TRAUMA

Blunt Trauma

Blunt trauma can cause a hematoma in the soft tissues of the neck. The patient presents with a painful, ecchymotic swelling that appears soon after the injury. Initially, one should evaluate the size, location, and progression of the hematoma and the patency of the airway. Small, stable hematomas are usually caused by venous tears and are self-limited. They resolve spontaneously as the blood is resorbed. Larger hematomas may require evacuation to aid in their resolution. The clot can be expressed out through a small incision made over the hematoma, or it can be aspirated after the clot has liquified. Progressively enlarging hematomas may endanger the airway, and usually require surgical

intervention. Following arteriography to determine the source of the hemorrhage, neck exploration and ligation of the bleeding vessel is indicated in these cases. An anteriovenous fistula may occur as a late complication of large vascular injuries if they are not recognized and repaired early.

Lacerations

Lacerations of the neck may range from small superficial cuts to large gaping wounds. They are often caused by contact with sharp playing equipment such as ice skates. The diagnosis is usually obvious on initial examination. The initial evaluation should include a search for associated injuries of the cervical spine, upper airway, and underlying vascular and neural structures. Hemorrhage is usually mild in nature and stops spontaneously, or with mild pressure. Rarely is the bleeding so brisk that surgical exploration and ligation of a small vessel is required. If the laceration is small and uncomplicated, the wound edges may be reapproximated with Steri-Strips, and the player can resume his activities. Larger lacerations may require formal repair as described in the section on soft-tissue injury.

Any laceration or puncture wound that

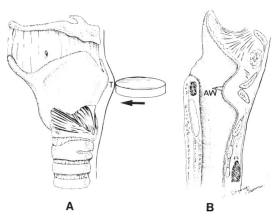

A   **B**

Fig. 16-26. Blunt trauma to the larynx. *A,* Normal anterior prominence of the thyroid cartilage (T) prior to trauma. *B,* Acute trauma with laryngeal fracture. Note depression of cartilage and absence of thyroid prominence. Airway (AW) is markedly decreased.

penetrates the platysma muscle can potentially produce an associated neural, vascular, or aerodigestive tract injury. While some authors recommend routine surgical exploration of these wounds, I feel that each case should be individually evaluated and treated.[4] If the injury is not associated with neural deficits, absent or diminished pulses, expanding hematoma, or signs of injury to the aerodigestive tract, it may be repaired without formal surgical exploration. If any of the conditions mentioned are present, further evaluation by angiography, endoscopy, and neck exploration may be indicated. The wounds are generally closed in layers, and a small rubber drain is utilized. Unless the wound is in continuity with the aerodigestive tract, antibiotics are not given.

INJURIES OF THE UPPER AERODIGESTIVE TRACT

Blunt Trauma

Blunt trauma to the aerodigestive tract occurs most frequently in high-velocity sports such as hockey. Direct trauma to the exposed neck can crush the larynx and upper trachea and cause airway embarrassment. The esophagus is rarely involved in these injuries. The athlete with

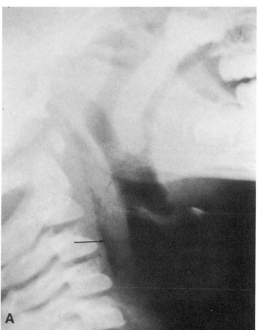

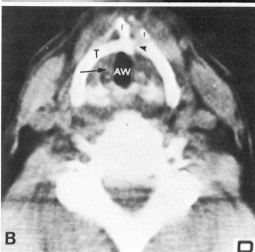

Fig. 16-27. Laryngeal injury. *A,* Lateral neck radiograph demonstrating free air in the neck (arrow) as a result of laryngeal disruption. *B,* Horizontal CT scan of same patient showing fracture of the thyroid cartilage (T) with multiple fragments (f). Airway (AW) is markedly compromised by the edema and hemorrhage caused by this injury. (CT scan courtesy of Drs. Anthony Mancuso and William Hanafee, UCLA Department of Radiology.)

significant injury to the larynx presents with neck pain, odynophagia (pain on swallowing), and dyspnea. Hemoptysis usually accompanies laryngeal trauma.

The voice can be normal, hoarse, or absent (aphonia). The severity of respiratory obstruction is dependent upon the type and extent of the injury. Ecchymosis and crepitus are usually noted over the anterior neck. The absence of the normal prominence of the thyroid cartilage ("Adam's apple") indicates a significant crush injury of the larynx (Fig. 16-26). In severe injuries in which airway obstruction is complete, endotracheal intubation and even emergency tracheostomy may become life-saving maneuvers in the first few minutes after the injury.

Once the diagnosis of blunt trauma to the larynx or trachea has been made, the patient should be transferred to a medical facility for further evaluation and treatment. Radiographs (plain films and CT) are useful in detecting the presence and degree of injuries to the larynx or esophagus (Fig. 16-27). Otolaryngic consultation should be obtained to evaluate the status of the airway and vocal cord function. Nondisplaced laryngeal fractures or small hematomas of the vocal cords may not require any further intervention. The patient should be hospitalized and observed for development of respiratory distress. Intubation or tracheostomy may become necessary as postinjury edema can obstruct the upper airway. More severe injuries require endoscopy to evaluate the integrity of the larynx and upper trachea. Formal neck exploration and fixation of laryngeal fragments may be necessary in the more comminuted or depressed fractures. The patient is placed on antibiotics, and the neck wounds are routinely drained. While many with mild injuries may return to activities within six to eight weeks, those with a history of severe laryngeal injuries should probably refrain from contact sports in the future.

Penetrating Trauma

Penetrating injuries of the aerodigestive tract in the neck are uncommon. They are freak accidents, such as when a player is "speared" in the neck by a sharp piece of sports equipment. The player with this injury complains of neck pain, dysphagia, and occasionally dyspnea. Physical examination reveals crepitus in the soft tissues of the neck, and the player often has hemoptysis. Changes in the voice, such as hoarseness or aphonia, are indicators of laryngeal trauma. Patency of the upper airway is the prime concern, and intubation or tracheostomy may be required. Secretions should be gently cleared from the mouth and pharynx, and the player transferred to a medical facility for observation and treatment. Lateral neck radiographs often demonstrate free air in the soft tissues of the neck indicating perforation of the aerodigestive tract. The severity of the injury determines the treatment, which may consist of close observation, endoscopy, or surgical exploration and repair of the perforation.

REFERENCES

1. Canalis, R.F., et al.: Complications of orbital floor implants. Trans. Pac. Coast Otoophthalmol. Soc. Annu. Meet., 61:81, 1978.
2. Converse, J.M.: Surgical Treatment of Facial Injuries. 3rd Ed. Baltimore, Williams & Wilkins, 1974.
3. Dingman, R.O., and Natvig, R.: Surgery of Facial Fractures. Philadelphia, W.B. Saunders, 1964.
4. May, M.: Penetrating neck wounds. Laryngoscope, 85:57, 1975.
5. Newman, M.H., and Travis, L.W.: Frontal sinus fractures. Laryngoscope, 85:1, 1975.
6. Schultz, R.C.: Facial Injuries. 2nd Ed. Chicago, Yearbook Medical Publishers, 1977.

Chapter 17

Diagnosis and Management of Oral Injuries

Martin S. Greenberg
Philip S. Springer

DENTAL INJURIES

Injuries to the teeth are common in sports. The picture of a smiling face devoid of maxillary anterior teeth has become synonymous with hockey, although elbows in basketball, high-bouncing ground balls in baseball, fists, knees, hardwood floors, and pavements are all common causes of lifelong dental injury and malformation. Approximately 15% of school children have significant dental injuries before the age of 18.[3] The major cause of these injuries is sports and games. Studies performed to date show that these injuries occur twice as often in males.[4] However, with the recent increase in female participation in sports, including contact sports, one can expect an increase in the number of women receiving dental injuries.

In Hawke's study of rugby players, 62% of the players interviewed had a history of oral injury.[9] The most common, which occurred in 50% of all rugby players, was injury to the lip. The second most common, which occurred in 26% of the players, was dental injury requiring the services of a dentist. About one half of these dental injuries were accompanied by lip injuries. Tongue injuries occurred in about 21% of the players.

Depending on the direction of the trauma, injuries to the teeth can be divided into two categories. Direct trauma to the teeth by a stick, ball, or bat frequently fractures the maxillary anterior teeth. Direct trauma to the lip reduces the frequency of tooth fracture by cushioning the blow, but increases the incidence of luxation of the tooth.

Indirect trauma is caused by upward force on the mandible. This occurs in boxing or sports where falling is frequent, such as football, lacrosse, or hockey. In these instances, the mandibular teeth are suddenly forced into the maxillary teeth causing injury to the posterior teeth, which support the bite. Teeth with large fillings or previous root canal treatment are particularly susceptible to fractures from indirect trauma.

Dental injuries can occur alone or in conjunction with other injuries to the maxillofacial region. Multiple injuries are particularly common in high-speed sports, such as hockey, skiing, or auto racing.

The physician or dentist attending the injured athlete with an obvious dental injury must consider other maxillofacial injuries. Limitation in opening the mandible or malocclusion may indicate a fracture of the mandible, maxilla, zygomatic arch, or injury to the temporomandibular joint. The patient should be examined for anesthesia or paresthesia of the lip or cheek and mobility of jaw fragments. Examination for a maxillary fracture should include placing a finger in the middle of the hard palate and pressing it in all directions while looking for both intra- and extra-oral mobility. The presence of diplopia often indicates a fracture involving the orbit. Mobility of a single tooth may indicate a root fracture or avulsion of the tooth. Adjacent teeth moving together suggest a fracture of the alveolar bone. If a tooth fracture is accompanied by an adjacent laceration of the lip, the fragments of the tooth should be accounted for. If this cannot be done, a roentgenogram of the lip should be taken to look for fragments.

Avulsed Teeth

Avulsed teeth that have been completely extruded from the socket due to trauma can often be found lying in the patient's mouth or on the ground (Fig. 17-1A-D). These teeth can be saved, but speed is an important factor. Studies of reimplantation of

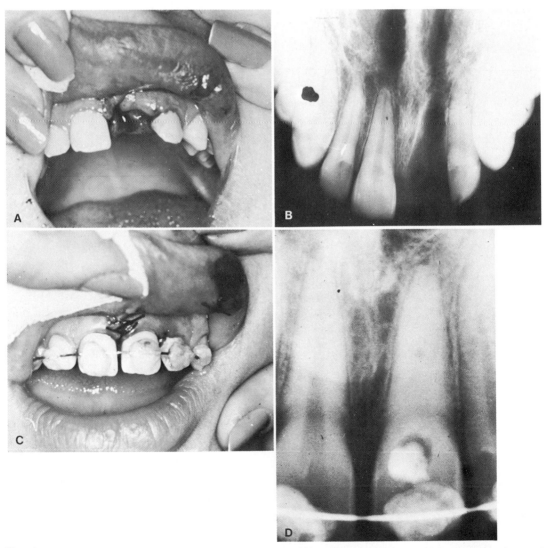

Fig. 17-1. *A,* A nine-year-old girl tripped while playing softball. She avulsed a maxillary central incisor and sustained lacerations of her lip and gingiva. *B,* Radiograph of avulsion site. *C,* Incisor reimplanted and stabilized with wire and acid etch resin. *D,* Radiograph of reimplanted incisor.

avulsed teeth conclude that the sooner the tooth is reimplanted, the higher the success rate.[4] The team physician or trainer should institute treatment immediately by replacing the tooth in the socket instead of waiting for a dentist.

If a tooth has been out of the socket for less than one hour, wash the tooth with cool water and attempt to replace it in its normal position in the socket. If the tooth has been positioned properly, the patient should be able to close his teeth normally. If the patient's teeth close on the reimplanted tooth first, it has not been completely seated in the socket. Avoid touching the roots. If the tooth cannot be replaced by gentle pressure, place it under the patient's tongue and take him to a dentist skilled in emergency dental procedures as soon as possible. While waiting, do not allow the tooth to dry since this decreases the chance of a successful result. When a tooth has been out of the socket for over one hour, it should not be reimplanted; but the patient, with the tooth under his tongue or wrapped in moist gauze, should be taken to the dentist as soon as possible. The dentist then performs immediate root canal treatment on the avulsed tooth to remove necrosing pulp tissue and then reimplants the tooth. All reimplanted avulsed teeth must be splinted with arch bars, orthodontic appliances, wires, acrylic, or resin. The dentist should reexamine the patient every two to four weeks to rule out complications

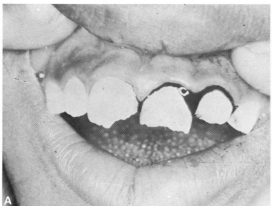

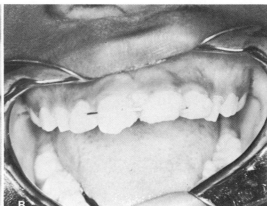

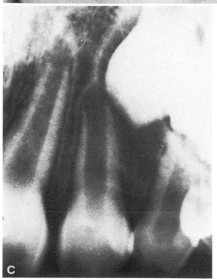

Fig. 17-2. A nine-year-old boy was hit in the mouth with a ball while playing baseball. The right maxillary central and lateral incisors were avulsed and chipped. The left maxillary central incisor was chipped. *A,* Avulsed teeth reimplanted with finger pressure. *B,* Wire and resin splint placed. *C,* Radiograph of root canal with wide-opened apex. Reimplanted quickly, these teeth may not require root canal treatment.

such as periapical abscesses and root resorption. Treatment for these complications consists of root canal therapy. In
young patients whose teeth have opened,
developing apices, normal circulation may
be restored after implantation, and root
canal treatment may not be necessary (Fig.
17-2*A-C*). In older patients, root canal
treatment is done, in most cases, to prevent
root resorption and periapical abscesses.

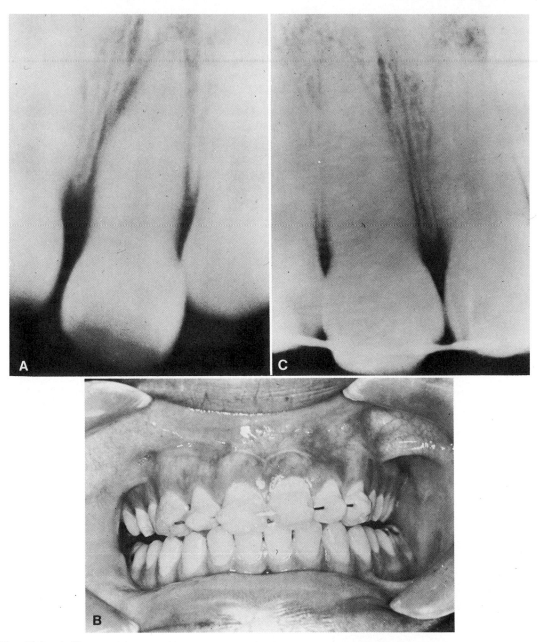

Fig. 17-3. A 19-year-old man with an extruded, subluxated maxillary central incisor. *A,* Radiograph of
extruded incisor. *B,* Clinical photograph of tooth stabilized with wire and resin. *C,* Radiograph of proper
placement of tooth.

Luxated Teeth

A luxated tooth is one that has been displaced from its normal position within the socket. The tooth may be intruded, extruded, or laterally displaced (Fig. 17-3A-C). Extruded teeth are those that have been partially displaced outward from the socket. If this occurs during a sporting event in which a team dentist is not present, the team trainer or physician should not wait for a dentist to perform initial treatment. An immediate attempt should be made to place the tooth into its normal position in the socket with firm finger pressure. The patient should then be taken to the dentist for final treatment. The dentist should take a dental radiograph to insure that the tooth has been completely replaced, and then firmly splint the tooth to the surrounding teeth with wires, arch bars, resin, or acrylic. If personnel administering dental first aid are unable to replace the tooth in the socket completely, firmer pressure requiring local anesthesia

may be necessary. Occasionally, a blood clot forms between the apex of the tooth and the alveolar bone. In these cases, the tip of the root may be removed or a surgical vent may be cut in the gingiva and the alveolar bone to the apex of the tooth. This releases the blood clot, enabling the tooth to be pushed back to its normal position. The tooth should then be splinted in place for approximately four weeks. During this time, the tooth should be completely out of occlusion, even if it is necessary to relieve the bite on the opposing tooth with a dental stone or bur.

The same principles apply to laterally luxated teeth. The teeth should be replaced into their normal position in the dental arch, splinted in place, and ground away from direct biting forces.

Teeth that are intruded, or driven further into the socket by injury, should be treated in a different manner. No immediate treatment is necessary at the time of injury. No attempt should be made to suddenly pull intruded teeth into their correct position. This maneuver often results in the permanent loss of the tooth. Some intruded teeth will re-erupt on their own with no treatment. If several weeks pass and no movement of the tooth is noted,

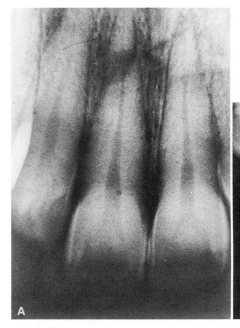
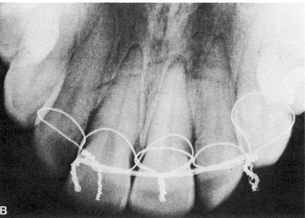

Fig. 17-4. A 35-year-old woman was hit in the mouth by a ball while a spectator at a baseball game. *A,* Radiograph demonstrating alveolar fracture of maxillary anterior region and fracture of apical one third of maxillary central incisor root. *B,* Teeth and fragment stabilized with ligation wire and quick-cure acrylic.

slow movement with orthodontic appliances should be considered.

Patients with a history of luxated teeth should be examined clinically and radiographically at three month intervals for at least two years after the injury to insure that there is no evidence of pulpal necrosis or root resorption. Teeth with pulp necrosis or root resorption require endodontic therapy.

Alveolar Fractures

Alveolar fractures can be diagnosed clinically. The diagnosis is obvious when two or more adjacent teeth move as a unit. Proper treatment for alveolar fracture is immediate rigid splinting of the teeth (Fig. 17-4A, B). Unsuccessful treatment is directly related to delay in stabilizing the fragments. Continued mobility of the fragments compromises the blood supply to the teeth, and causes necrosis. Andreasen studied a large series of alveolar fractures;[3] pulpal necrosis requiring root canal treatment was necessary in 75% of the cases. Pulp necrosis did not occur in those cases in which the fragment was immediately reduced and rigidly splinted. Root resorption occurred in a little over 10% of the cases of alveolar fracture. Unlike root resorption secondary to avulsion, root resorption in patients with alveolar fractures appears to be self-limiting and superficial.

Tooth Trauma Without Fracture or Displacement

When a tooth is traumatized without fracture, check for mobility to rule out subluxation or alveolar fracture. If this examination is negative, no immediate treatment is necessary, but the patient should be referred to a dentist skilled in managing these injuries for adequate follow-up. Trauma to the tooth may lead to bleeding into the pulp chamber, and result in necrosis. This problem may not become apparent for several weeks or even months.

Signs and symptoms of pulpal necrosis secondary to trauma are: increased sensitivity of the tooth to heat or cold, sensitivity to percussion, discoloration, and swelling above the apex of the tooth.

There are several radiographic signs of pulp necrosis. Radiolucency at the apex of the tooth indicates granuloma or cyst formation. In younger patients there occurs interruption of normal root development. An increase in odontoblastic activity in response to inflammation results in obliteration of the pulp. External root resorption is caused by traumatic stimulation of osteoclastic activity in the periodontal membrane. Internal root resorption on the other hand is caused by osteoclastic activity within the pulp chamber.

Proper treatment for all these conditions with the exception of pulp obliteration is root canal therapy. Asymptomatic teeth without pulps, and no radiographic evidence of granuloma or cyst may be left untreated.

Crown Fractured, Pulp Not Exposed

Fractures of the enamel cause few or no symptoms; however, sharp edges of the tooth should be smoothed to prevent further injury to the lips and oral mucosa. Fractures that involve the dentin cause pain and should be referred to a dentist. Proper treatment consists of placing a sedative dressing over the exposed dentin. This dressing consists of a zinc oxide and eugenol paste.

Aesthetic restoration of fractured anterior teeth is now possible. Tolerating untreated fractured anterior teeth until one becomes "old enough" for a full crown is no longer necessary. Materials are now available that can aesthetically repair the teeth prior to, or instead of, a permanent full crown. Among the most important of these materials is a composite resin, which physically bonds to the tooth after the surrounding enamel is etched with a dilute acid.

Crown Fractured With Pulp Exposure

Teeth with pulp exposures should not be extracted, and the patient should be referred to a dentist immediately. Reducing the contamination of the exposed pulp by the oral flora improves the prognosis.

Pulp exposures can be treated by one of three techniques. If the pulp exposure is small, a pulp capping procedure may be attempted. This procedure should be attempted within two to three hours of the injury. This technique involves the placement of calcium hydroxide on the area of the exposure. This medication stimulates the formation of a new odontoblastic layer, which bridges the exposed portion of the pulp chamber. If this treatment is successful it eliminates the necessity for root canal treatment.

The second treatment that can be used for teeth with exposed pulp is pulpotomy. This involves removing the vital pulp tissue in the coronal portion of the root canal leaving the vital uninjured pulp present in the root. This is a particularly good form of treatment in young patients whose roots have not fully formed. If successful, it maintains the vitality of the pulp tissue until root formation is complete.

The third treatment for an exposed pulp is complete pulpectomy, the removal of the entire pulpal contents of both the crown and the root. In uncomplicated cases with vital pulps, the entire root canal treatment can be completed in one visit. If the root canal has been contaminated, two or more visits may be necessary.

One treatment which has recently been studied in the management of vital pulp-exposed teeth is the technique of partial pulpotomy. This consists of removing only part of the vital pulp tissue near the injury and placing calcium hydroxide over the exposed area. In a recent study by Cuek, 80 traumatized teeth were treated with partial pulpotomy.[6] He reported successful healing requiring no further treatment in 96% of the cases.

Subgingival Coronal Fractures

In the past, teeth fractured below the gingiva were usually extracted. This is no longer necessary. These teeth can now be restored in one of two ways. In the first technique, sufficient gingiva and bone are removed to expose the root. Standard root canal treatment is performed on the tooth and the tooth is restored with a full crown using a post into the root canal to increase retention. A newer technique involves the use of an orthodontic appliance, which can extrude the tooth prior to root canal treatment and restoration.[7, 14] This technique is preferable in a cooperative patient since surgery is not necessary, aesthetics are improved, and the prognosis for the long-term retention of the tooth is increased.

Root Fractures

Root fractures are commonly seen in adolescent males who are active in sports (see Fig. 11-5*A*, *B*). The chief clinical sign of root fracture is mobility. The clinician should also examine the teeth adjacent to the obviously mobile tooth because root fractures are often associated with alveolar bone fractures.

Remember that routine jaw films may not show root fractures. If a root fracture is suspected, periapical dental films should be taken of the area. Dental films taken too soon after the injury may not show the fracture clearly, and these films may have to be repeated in one or two days when inflammation separates the fragments. Teeth with vertical fractures involving the entire length of the crown and root require extraction. More frequently, the root fracture is horizontal. Some clinicians automatically extract these teeth, although many can be saved by proper management. If the horizontal fracture is in the apical one half of the tooth, the prognosis is good. The tooth may remain vital with healing of the root fragments. Roots, like bone, may heal with deposition of new dentin or connective tissue. The proper treatment for a

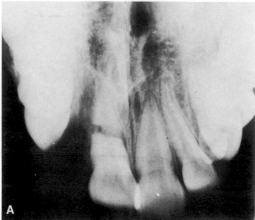

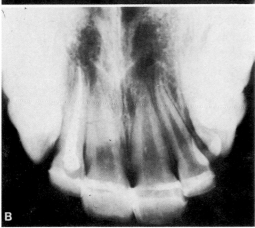

Fig. 17-5. A 10-year-old boy sustained a horizontal root fracture during a neighborhood football game. *A,* Pretreatment radiograph showing midroot fracture. *B,* Proper reduction of root fracture using arch bar and resin.

horizontal fracture consists of splinting the tooth in its proper position. Splinting can be successfully accomplished using arch bars, orthodontic bands, wires, acrylic, or composite resin (Fig. 17-6A-D). A ,splint should remain in place for approximately six weeks. If infection or sensitivity of the tooth occurs during this period, the tooth should not be removed but treated with endodontic therapy. If root healing does not take place, the apical fragment of the root may have to be removed surgically. These procedures are preferable to removing the tooth and replacing it with a fixed or removable bridge.

TEMPOROMANDIBULAR JOINT INJURIES

Post-traumatic facial pain is frequently misdiagnosed and mistreated. In particular, mistakes are made in the management of patients with facial pain related to injuries of the temporomandibular joint (TMJ) and its associated structures. These injuries are common sequelae of trauma to the mouth, chin, or side of the face.

There is a tendency to lump together all injuries occurring in the area of the TMJ, without making a specific diagnosis. To treat these patients correctly, it is important to differentiate between disorders affecting the joint.[2] The severity of such sports-related injuries can be reduced by the shock-absorbing qualities of a custom-fitted mouth protector.

Traumatic Arthritis

A patient with mild, acute traumatic arthritis of the TMJ has pre-auricular pain (usually unilateral), limitation of mandibular opening, difficulty chewing, and a deviation of the mandible to the affected side. The involved joint is also tender to palpation and may appear swollen.[5] Radiographically, limited movement of the condyle on a TMJ series (opened and closed views) is apparent. A widening of the space between the condyle and the temporal bone may reflect edema.

The use of aspirin for its anti-inflammatory and mild analgesic actions is beneficial in the treatment of mild, acute traumatic arthritis. Cold compresses to the TMJ during the first 24 hours after injury and a relative decrease in joint function for two or three days are also helpful. Most symptoms resolve in one to two weeks.[5]

Symptoms may be more severe when extensive damage to the joint occurs. This may involve tearing, crushing, or dislocation of the articular disc. The use of interarticular steroids may be indicated in the treatment of moderate to severe, acute traumatic arthritis.

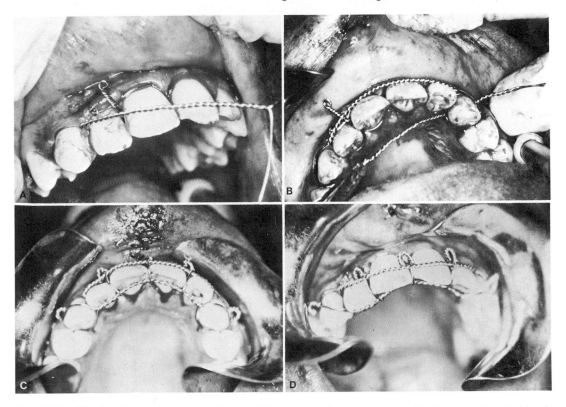

Fig. 17-6. Wire ligation technique used to stabilize alveolar fractures, avulsed teeth, or subluxated teeth. *A,* Double twisted wire placed across labial surface of involved to uninvolved teeth. *B,* Same wire placed through the interproximal space and across the lingual surfaces of the teeth. *C,* Interproximal wires placed between each tooth and twisted around labial and lingual wire. *D,* Completed splint in place.

A chronic decrease in function often results because the disc does not heal spontaneously. Surgery, involving meniscectomy or high condylectomy, should be considered when conservative measures fail to alleviate the pain or when function is dramatically affected.[13]

Bony or fibrous ankylosis of the condyle is a possible complication of trauma to the TMJ. Limited movement of the condyle and deviation of the mandible to the affected side on opening are characteristic. Because of increased osseous and fibrotic activity, ankylosis is more likely to be seen in injuries to children. If the growth center of the condyle is disturbed, asymmetry may result. Surgery is indicated when bony ankylosis occurs.[2, 5, 13]

Spasm of the Muscles of Mastication

Myofascial pain caused by spasm of the muscles of mastication is a finding often observed following injuries to the mandible. Classically, the patient complains of unilateral facial pain, limitation of motion, deviation of the mandible, muscle tenderness, and frequently clicking of the TMJ.[11] The muscles most often noted to be in spasm are the lateral pterygoid and masseter muscles. The temporalis and medial pterygoid muscles may also be involved.[1, 2, 11] The key to making the diagnosis is detecting tenderness and spasm on palpation of these muscles. No radiographic evidence of changes in the TMJ is apparent in myofascial pain.

Conservative therapy is usually successful in relieving the symptoms. First, the patient should be reassured that the problem appears to be only muscle spasm and not something more serious. Applying warm, moist compresses, eating a relatively soft diet, limiting wide opening, and taking acetaminophen (Tylenol) or aspirin for pain relief are helpful recommendations. The ability of ethyl chloride refrigerant spray to break up muscle spasm makes it useful in both the diagnosis and treatment of myofascial pain. Similarly, injection of the involved muscles with a local anesthetic, such as 2% lidocaine (Xylocaine) without epinephrine, is usually beneficial. Diazepam (Valium) and other muscle relaxants may also be effective.[1, 2]

It should be noted that clenching and grinding of the teeth, secondary to stress, are the principal causes of myofascial pain in the general population.[11]

Condylar Fractures

Condylar fractures often result from a blow to the chin. These injuries include fractures of the condylar head and neck, in addition to fractures of the subcondylar region.[13] The patient with a condylar fracture usually shows limitation and deviation of the mandible to the injured side on opening. A traumatic arthritis, with edema and pain, is also evident. Bilateral condylar fractures can result in an anterior open bite.[5, 13] Radiographs provide the definite diagnosis.

Intracapsular, nondisplaced fractures of the condylar head are usually left untreated. Early mobilization of the mandible is emphasized so as to prevent a bony or fibrotic ankylosis.[13]

The indication for surgical intervention increases as the site of the fracture occurs further below the condylar head and as the extent of displacement of the fractured segment increases.[13]

Dislocation

Acute dislocation of the mandible usually results from excessive opening of the mandible during eating or yawning, and less commonly from trauma.[2, 5] In dislocation, the condyle is positioned anterior to the articular eminence and cannot return to its normal position without assistance. Dislocations of the mandible may be unilateral or bilateral in presentation.

Alderman notes certain signs and symptoms classically associated with dislocations.[2] These include inability to close the mouth, acute pain due to muscle fatigue and ligament stretch, deep facial depression in pretragus area, deviation of mandible with unilateral dislocation, and sharp clicking. These patients often show evidence of panic.

The condyle can usually be repositioned without the use of muscle relaxants or general anesthetics. If muscle spasms are severe and reduction is difficult, the use of intravenous diazepam (Valium) can be beneficial.

The practitioner who is repositioning the mandible should stand in front of the seated patient. He then should place his thumbs lateral to the mandibular molars on the buccal shelf of bone; the remaining fingers of each hand should be placed under the chin. The condyle is repositioned by a downward and backward movement. This is achieved by simultaneously pressing down on the posterior part of the mandible while raising the chin. As the condyle reaches the height of the eminence, it can usually be guided posterior to its normal position.

Postreduction management consists of decreasing mandibular motion and use of aspirin to lessen inflammation. The patient should be cautioned not to open wide in eating or yawning, because recurrence is common. Long periods of immobilization, however, are not advised because of the possibility of ankylosis.

PREVENTION OF ORAL INJURIES

Mouth injuries were once considered to be an inevitable by-product of participation in many sports. Missing teeth and oral lacerations were accepted risks of athletic competition. Today, however, there exists the technology to produce mouth protectors that can prevent or lessen such injuries.

Mouth protectors were used initially in boxing in the early part of this century. Besides their acceptance by amateur and professional boxers, mouth protectors have gained popularity in football, rugby, and to a lesser extent, in ice hockey. Since 1974, it has been mandatory for all college and high school football players in the United States to wear mouth protectors.[8, 17, 19] Dental and oral injuries comprised 50% of all football injuries before faceguards and mouth protectors were employed. The use of faceguards reduced these injuries by half, and mouth protectors have almost eliminated them.[8]

The results of studies conducted during the 1960s implied that mouth protectors provide more than just protection against injuries to the oral tissues. Stenger provided mouth protectors to the Notre Dame football team for five years. In addition to the expected decrease in dental injuries, he observed a significant reduction in the number of concussions and neck injuries experienced by the players.[15] A British study conducted in 1969 found that mouth protectors reduced the incidence of fractured jaws in rugby players.[16]

Hickey studied the effect of a blow to the chin on intracranial pressure and bone deformation. He found that such an injury can cause deformation of the bones of the skull, an increase in intracranial pressure, and an acceleration of the head itself. He noted that each of these changes was capable of producing brain damage.[10] Hickey then demonstrated that the amplitude of the intracranial pressure wave was significantly reduced and bone deformation was also moderately decreased by using custom-made mouth protectors. He concluded that some mouth protectors can prevent concussions by decreasing the shock transmitted through the TMJ to the skull.[10]

A properly constructed mouth protector should provide maximum protection of the lips, teeth, and gums by absorbing energy, spreading impact, and cushioning contacts between the upper and lower teeth.[18, 19] The appliance should also be durable, retentive, resilient, inexpensive, easy to fabricate, tasteless, odorless, and not bulky. It must not encroach on the airway, affect speech, or be uncomfortable.[8, 12, 19]

An external type of mouth protector is widely used in amateur ice hockey, especially in the junior levels.[18] The apparatus attaches to the helmet in place of the chinstrap. The advantages of this piece of equipment are its strength, malleability, and lack of odor and taste. Also, no impressions need to be taken. The external type of mouth protector has been recommended for children under 13 years of age. Rapid changes in dentition and bone growth in children make a custom intraoral appliance impractical. An external mouth protector, when used by itself, does not provide protection against concussions resulting from a blow to the chin.

The most commonly used devices for preventing oral injuries are intraoral mouth protectors. There are three basic types of intraoral mouth protectors: stock, mouth-formed, and custom.

Stock mouth protectors are usually made of latex rubber. They are available at most sporting goods stores in small, medium, and large sizes. These protectors are ready to be used, as bought, without any further preparation. Stock mouth protectors must be held in place by constant occlusal pressure and tend to interfere with speech and breathing. They are also bulky and lack retention. These disadvantages have made the stock protectors the least acceptable among players.

Mouth-formed protectors are also commercially available. They usually consist of a firm outer shell, which is filled with a softer inner material.[12, 19] The softer material is thermally or chemically set after being molded over the individual player's teeth. Ideally, the liner remains resilient at mouth temperature to provide the shock-absorbing quality of the protector. Thermoplastic material, soft acrylic resins, and silicone have been used as the inner material. The thermoplastic materials have the drawback of losing their elasticity at mouth temperature causing the protector to loosen. Mouth-formed protectors lack extension into the labial and buccal vestibules. Therefore, they do not provide adequate protection for the oral soft tissues. These devices must be centered properly over the dental arch during initial fabrication in order to be effective; they usually cannot be resoftened to make corrections. Mouth-formed protectors also tend to be excessively bulky.

Custom-fitted mouth protectors require a dentist for their fabrication. The dentist takes an impression, usually of the maxillary teeth, of each player. A model is then made. Over the model a material such as thermoplastic vinyl (i.e., polyvinyl acetate-polyethylene) is then vacuum-adapted.[8] Custom mouth protectors are retentive, tasteless, odorless, tear resistant, resilient, inexpensive, translucent, and of uniform thickness. Custom protectors are generally considered comfortable and have little effect on speaking, drinking, or breathing. These appliances are fabricated with adequate extension to provide protection to the gingival tissues.[17] Most custom mouth protectors last one or two years. As previously mentioned, they have been shown to be effective in reducing oral injuries, concussions, and neck injuries.

Although boxing, football, hockey, and rugby have been the predominant sports in which mouth protectors have been employed, participants in any activity in which there is occasional trauma to the mouth or jaws would benefit. Mouth protectors could also be used in lacrosse, wrestling, soccer, karate, judo, gymnastics, and basketball.[8]

REFERENCES

1. Alderman, M.M.: Disorders of the temporomandibular joint and related structures. Rationale for diagnosis, etiology, management. Alpha Omegan, 69:12, 1976.
2. Alderman, M.M.: Disorders of the temporomandibular joint and related structures. *In* Burkett's Oral Medicine. Edited by M. Lynch. Philadelphia, J.B. Lippincott, 1977.
3. Andreasen, J.O.: Fractures of the alveolar process of the jaw. Scand. J. Dent. Res. 78:263, 1970.
4. Andreasen, J.O.: Traumatic Injuries of the Teeth. St. Louis, C.V. Mosby, 1972.
5. Carlsson, G.E., et al.: Arthritis and allied diseases of the temporomandibular joint. *In* Temporomandibular Joint—Function and Dysfunction. Edited by G.A. Zarb, and G.E. Carlsson. St. Louis, C.V. Mosby, 1979.
6. Cuek, M.: A clinical report on partial pulpotomy and capping with calcium hydroxide in permanent incisors with complicated crown fracture. J. Endo. 4:232, 1978.
7. Delevanes, P., Delevanes, H., and Kuftinec, M.M.: Endodontic-orthodontic management of fractured anterior teeth. J. Am. Dent. Assoc., 97:483, 1978.
8. Going, R.E., et al.: Mouthguard materials: their physical and mechanical properties. J. Am. Dent. Assoc., 89:132, 1974.
9. Hawke, J.L., and Nicholes, N.K.: Dental injuries in rugby football. N.J. Dent. J., 65:173, 1969.
10. Hickey, J.C., et al.: The relation of mouth protectors to cranial pressure and deformation. J. Am. Dent. Assoc., 74:735, 1967.
11. Laskin, D.M.: Etiology of the pain-dysfunction syndrome. J. Am. Dent. Assoc., 79:147, 1969.
12. Picozzi, A.: Mouth protectors. Dent. Clin. North Am., 19:385, 1975.
13. Shira, R.B., and Alling, C.C.: Traumatic injuries involving the temporomandibular joint articulation. *In* Facial Pain and Mandibular Dysfunction. Edited by L. Schwartz, and C. Choyes. Philadelphia, W.B. Saunders, 1968.
14. Simon, J.H.S., et al.: Extrusion of endodontically treated teeth. J. Am. Dent. Assoc., 97:17, 1978.
15. Stenger, J.M., et al.: Mouthguards: protection against shock to head, neck, and teeth. J. Am. Dent. Assoc., 69:273, 1964.
16. Turner, C.T.: Mouth protectors. Br. Dent. J., 143:82, 1977.
17. Wehner, P.J.: Maximum prevention and preservation: an achievement of intraoral mouth protectors. Dent. Clin. North Am., 9:493, 1965.
18. Wood, A.W.S.: Head protection: cranial, facial, and dental in contact sports. Oral Health, 62:23, 1972.
19. Wood, A.W.S.: Mouth protectors: 11 years later. J. Am. Dent. Assoc., 86:1365, 1973.

Chapter 18

Diagnosis and Management of Injuries to the Eye and Orbit

Alexander J. Brucker

David M. Kozart

Charles W. Nichols

Irving M. Raber

ANATOMY OF THE EYE AND ADNEXA

An awareness of the anatomy of the eye and its surrounding structures is essential to the evaluation of an ocular injury (Fig. 18-1).

The front part of the eye includes the cornea, a crystal clear structure through which light passes on its path to the retina. It is continuous with the sclera, which forms the opaque, tough fibrous outer coat of the eye. The sclera is covered by a layer of loose connective tissue, Tenon's capsule, which is continuous with the dural covering of the optic nerve and the mucosal lining of the sinuses surrounding the orbit. The anterior portion of the sclera and overlying Tenon's capsule also is covered by conjunctiva, which runs as a continuous sheet of tissue from the posterior margin of the lid to the limbus, which is the junction of the cornea and sclera.

The middle coat of the eye is the uveal tract and consists of three parts: the iris, the ciliary body, and the choroid. The iris, or colored part of the eye, functions as a diaphragm regulating the amount of light that passes through the pupil. It is innervated by the third cranial nerve and sympathetic fibers. The ciliary body produces aqueous humor and also regulates the focusing of light by the lens. The choroid furnishes the blood supply to the outer portion of the retina and to the entire macular area. The inner coat of the eye is the retina, which receives the light input and transmits it as an electric impulse through the optic nerve to the brain.

The inside of the eye is divided into three chambers: the anterior chamber, the posterior chamber, and the vitreous cavity. The anterior chamber is bound anteriorly by the cornea and posteriorly by the iris and pupillary space. It contains aqueous humor that drains out of the eye through the canal of Schlemm located in the angle formed by the iris and the corneoscleral junction. The posterior chamber is limited anteriorly by the iris, posteriorly by the vitreous, and centrally by the lens. The ciliary processes (part of the ciliary body), which form the outer limit of the posterior chamber, produce the aqueous humor and give rise to the zonular fibers, which suspend the lens in the pupillary space. The

257

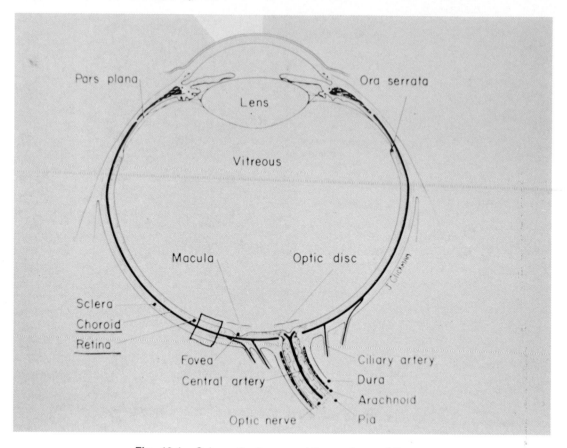

Fig. 18-1. Schematic diagram of the anatomy of the eye.

largest cavity within the eye is the vitreous space which is filled by the vitreous, a clear, jelly-like substance that is in close contact with the retina.

The movement of the eye is produced by six extraocular muscles that attach to the sclera. The inferior oblique, medial, inferior, and superior rectus muscles are innervated by the third cranial nerve; the lateral rectus is innervated by the sixth cranial nerve; and the superior oblique is innervated by the fourth cranial nerve.

The front part of the eye is protected by the lid. The lid is formed by skin and muscle (orbicularis) in its outer half and by a thick, fibrous plate (tarsus) and conjunctiva in its inner half. The tarsus provides the support for the lid, and along with the conjunctiva, produces the tears that normally wet the cornea. The nasal portion of the lids contain the lacrimal punctum and canaliculus, which provide the drainage channel for the tears.

The eyeball is protected by the bony orbit and the cushion of orbital fat. The orbital walls separate the orbit from the sinuses and the cranium.

EXAMINING THE TRAUMATIZED EYE

Although sophisticated instrumentation and expertise are necessary for a thorough eye examination, much useful information can be gleaned from the history and careful inspection of the injured eye.

Often the cause of injury is obvious. However, it is important to determine whether the injury resulted from a blunt force, a sharp implement, or a projectile.

The patient's symptoms may provide an important clue regarding the nature and extent of the injury, and may determine whether referral to an ophthalmologist is indicated. Loss of all or part of the visual field in one or both eyes, persisting blurred or distorted vision, double vision (diplopia), light sensitivity (photophobia), boring or throbbing eye pain or headache around the eye, are all symptoms suggestive of severe ocular injury and dictate immediate referral to an ophthalmologist. Foreign body sensation or blurred vision that clears intermittently with blinking may indicate superficial corneal trauma, and may be diagnosed and managed locally.

The examination of the injured eye ideally begins with an assessment of the visual function of the eye. However, if the lids are swollen shut and the patient cannot voluntarily open them, it is mandatory that no effort be made to mechanically open the lids. This maneuver may lead to further injury and even loss of the eye. Visual function should be evaluated by first asking the patient to compare the vision of the injured eye to the uninvolved eye. If the vision of the injured eye is blurred, then the acuity of that eye may be assessed by noting whether the patient can see light or hand movements in all quadrants of gaze, can count fingers held at a specified distance in front of the eye, or can read print.

The nature and extent of injury should be determined by careful inspection with the aid of a pen light. The following signs suggest significant injury to the eye or adnexal structures and require referral to an ophthalmologist for evaluation and management. Tense, swollen, and ecchymotic lids, which prevent visualization of the eye, may indicate serious ocular injury such as a ruptured globe. Deep lacerations of the lid, with or without involvement of the tarsal plate, and lacerations of the lid margin require meticulous surgical repair. Protrusion (exophthalmos) or posterior displacement (enophthalmos) of the globe may indicate orbital trauma such as fractures or hemorrhage. Injection of the conjunctiva, especially in the limbal area, and a small pupil suggest the presence of an iritis. Loss of corneal clarity, shallowing of the anterior chamber, blood between the cornea and the iris (hyphema), pupillary distortion, irregularity, dilation or constriction (in comparison to the other eye), or the presence of brown tissue (uvea) protruding through the cornea or sclera, are all ominous signs. Restriction of eye movement may be due to an orbital fracture, or may indicate damage to the nerves supplying the extraocular muscles anywhere along their course, from the brain stem to the eye.

Certain ocular findings seen in association with head trauma may indicate serious brain injury. These include loss of vision in one or both eyes in a portion of the visual field, pupillary dilatation, paralysis of eye movement in one or more directions of gaze, and papilledema. The following sections present a brief discussion of commonly seen ocular injuries and their management.

TRAUMA TO THE ANTERIOR SEGMENT OF THE EYE
Subconjunctival Hemorrhage
(Fig. 18-2)

The most common consequence of ocular trauma is a subconjunctival hemorrhage resulting from a blow to the eye.

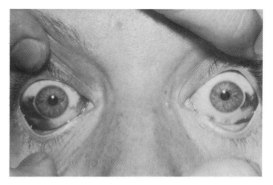

Fig. 18-2. Bilateral subconjunctival hemorrhages sustained while scuba diving.

These types of hemorrhages can also be seen in scuba divers. Spontaneous subconjunctival hemorrhages can also occur spontaneously for no apparent reason. Subconjunctival hemorrhage requires no treatment and resolves spontaneously in one to three weeks. However, if there are associated symptoms such as blurred vision or pain, or signs such as limitation of movement of the eye, marked hemorrhagic chemosis of the conjunctiva, lid swelling, the presence of blood in the anterior chamber, or ocular hypotony, then serious injury to the eye has occurred and the patient should be referred to the ophthalmologist for evaluation.

Conjunctival Foreign Body
(Figs. 18-3 and 18-4)

Foreign matter, such as cinders, dirt, and glass, commonly finds its way into the conjunctival sac of active athletes. There is an immediate sensation of something in the eye, followed by irritation and tearing. Frequently, the profuse tearing itself will wash the foreign body out of the conjunctival sac; however, if symptoms persist, the eye should be examined carefully in an effort to locate and remove the foreign matter. When trying to find foreign material in the conjunctival sac, the simplest procedure is to have the patient move his eye in all directions and attempt to visualize anything on the eye. If a foreign body is found, it sometimes can be gently irrigated out with water or normal saline solution. If this does not work, it should be removed with a sterile cotton swab. If no foreign body is found on initial examination, a more thorough search is required. First, have the patient look in extreme upgaze and pull down his lower lid, thereby exposing the lower fornix of the conjunctiva. Then, have the subject look down and evert the upper lid by grasping the lashes while applying counter-pressure with a cotton swab at the upper edge of the tarsus. The patient should maintain downgaze throughout.

Upon completion of the examination, the lid can be returned to its normal position merely by asking the patient to look up. Double eversion of the upper lid to expose the upper fornix of the conjunctiva may be needed to find the foreign body. If the foreign body is located, it can be wiped away with a sterile cotton applicator. Care must be taken to avoid damaging the cornea while removing the foreign body. Following the removal of the foreign mat-

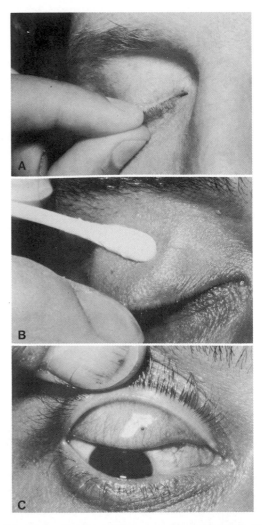

Fig. 18-3. Eversion of the upper lid. *A,* Have patient look down and grasp his lashes. *B,* Apply counter-pressure with a cotton swab at the upper edge of the tarsus. *C,* Evert upper lid by pulling lashes upward. Foreign body embedded in upper tarsal conjunctiva. Patient must maintain downgaze throughout.

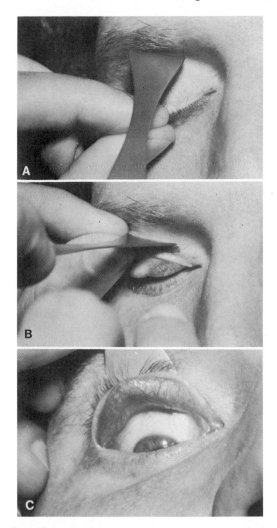

Fig. 18-4. Double eversion of the upper lid. *A,* Have patient look down and grasp his lashes. Use a lid retractor to apply counterpressure. *B,* Evert the upper lid over the retractor. *C,* Lift up on the retractor thereby exposing the upper fornix. Patient must maintain downgaze throughout.

ter, topical antibiotics should be used prophylactically for 24 to 48 hours.

Contact Lens Problems
(Figs. 18-5 and 18-6)

Athletes often wear contact lenses while participating in sports. These lenses normally sit on the cornea, but may become dislodged onto the conjunctiva with a resultant diminution of vision and foreign-body sensation in the eye. This occurs much more commonly with hard than with soft contact lenses. The patient is usually able to tell what has happened and repositions the lens by himself. However, he may need help in finding the lens, which can become lodged under the upper or lower lid. The lens usually can be maneuvered back in place by manipulating the eyelid. Another method for removing displaced hard contact lenses utilizes a small, inexpensive suction cup that can be applied directly to the contact lens. Failure to locate a dislodged contact lens may be due to the lens having fallen out of the eye. Almost everyone has witnessed a sporting event in which play has been interrupted by players crawling on their hands and knees in search of a lost contact lens.

Contact lenses frequently are implicated in corneal abrasions. Foreign material may get underneath the lens and damage the cornea, or the cornea may be scratched

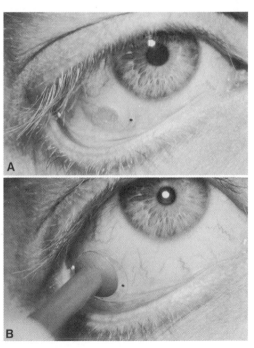

Fig. 18-5. Displaced hard contact lens. *A,* Note the lens in lower fornix, and the air bubble under it. *B,* Remove lens with the aid of a suction cup. Dot on lens marked the lens for the right eye.

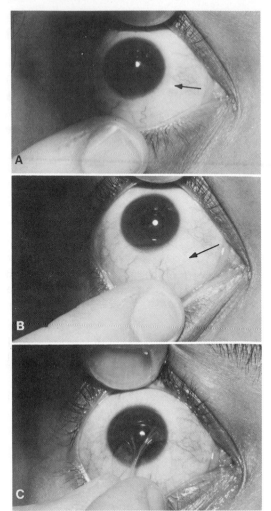

Fig. 18-6. Removing a soft contact lens. *A,* Lens in place. *B,* Patient looks up and lens is maneuvered into the lower fornix. Arrow indicates contact lens edge. *C,* Lens is pinched between two fingers and removed.

while inserting or removing the lens. If a contact lens wearer experiences eye pain or discomfort, the lens should be removed immediately. The patient is usually able to remove the lens himself, but if there is pain or photophobia, he may require assistance. If the patient is wearing a soft contact lens, it may be removed by asking him to look up; the weight of the lens will carry it partly off the cornea onto the lower conjunctival surface. A finger is then applied against the portion of the lens off of the cornea, and the lens is maneuvered into

the lower fornix where it can be pinched between two fingers and removed. One should never try to grasp the lens while it is centered on the cornea, because this may cause a large corneal abrasion. A hard contact lens can be removed by asking the person to open his eyes widely, grasping the outer canthus, and pulling the lids temporally. This tightens the upper and lower lid against the globe. A forcible blink will then pop the lens out of the eye. A hand should be kept under the eye to catch the lens when it comes out. The entire procedure should be carried out over a table or a bench to insure that the lens does not fall on the ground where it can be damaged or lost.

Corneal Abrasion (Fig. 18-7)

A corneal abrasion results in sudden onset of pain, tearing, and photophobia. The discomfort is aggravated by blinking and moving the eye. The patient inevitably complains of an intense foreign-body sensation. Even though a foreign body usually

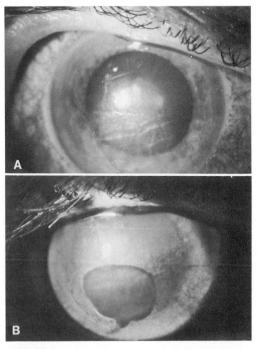

Fig. 18-7. Corneal abrasion. *A,* Without fluorescein. *B,* With fluorescein.

is not found, careful inspection of the eye is indicated to rule out its presence.

The diagnosis of a corneal abrasion is confirmed by instilling fluorescein dye into the conjunctival sac. The fluorescein stains any area devoid of epithelial cells. The green color of the dye is augmented by using a blue light while examining the cornea. The pattern of the fluorescein stain is noteworthy. For example, multiple linear stains in the upper half of the cornea should alert one to the possibility of a foreign body lodged under the upper lid.

Treatment of a corneal abrasion consists of a shortacting topical cycloplegic, such as 1% cyclopentolate, a broad-spectrum topical antibiotic ointment, and a semipressure patch for 24 to 48 hours. The cycloplegic relaxes ciliary muscle spasm resulting from secondary iritis. The antibiotic is used as a prophylaxis against secondary bacterial infection. The patching makes the patient more comfortable and promotes healing of the epithelial defect by splinting the lids. When applying the patch, care must be taken to ensure that the lids are closed beneath the patch, and that the patch is sufficiently firm to prevent the lids from opening and closing beneath it.

Corneal Foreign Body (Fig. 18-8)

Superficial corneal foreign bodies frequently can be removed by irrigation or by gently wiping them away with a sterile cotton swab. However, at times foreign bodies become deeply embedded in the cornea. These are best removed under topical anesthesia with appropriate instrumentation, and with the illumination and magnification of the slit lamp. After removing the foreign body, a rust ring often remains. A small amount of rust left behind is usually of no consequence. However, should it need removal, care must be taken not to be too vigorous, since the more manipulation used, the greater the residual scar. Following removal of the foreign body and rust ring, the eye is treated as for a simple corneal abrasion.

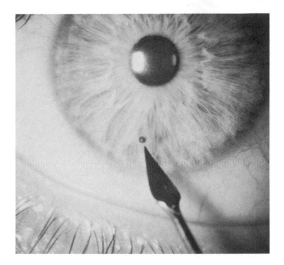

Fig. 18-8. Corneal foreign body about to be removed with a spud.

Chemical Burns

Chemical burns of the athlete's eye may be caused by swimming pool chemicals such as chlorine, or from accidents with some types of lime used to line sports fields. Chemical burns constitute a vision-threatening emergency and require prompt, on-the-spot treatment. Copious irrigation of the eyes should be carried out immediately, using the most readily available source of water. The lids must be held open to allow access to the cornea and conjunctiva. Irrigation should be continued for 20 to 30 minutes before arranging for transfer to a medical facility where more definitive treatment is available. Any particulate chemical matter lodged in the fornices and conjunctival folds should be removed with cotton swabs. It must be emphasized that the initial prompt irrigation of the eyes is the single most important part of the management of these cases.

Hyphema (Fig. 18-9)

A hyphema (hemorrhage in the anterior chamber) may result from blunt trauma to the eye. Squash injuries are a frequent cause of hyphemas. Because of the relatively small size of the court and the speed of the action, there is a moderate risk of

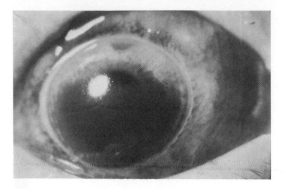

Fig. 18-9. Hyphema. Note that the blood in the anterior chamber obscures the lower half of the iris.

being struck in the eye by a racquet. The ball also represents a direct threat to the globe. Because of its small size, it can fit within the protective bony margins of the orbit, thereby inflicting damage directly upon the eye. This is in contrast to a tennis ball, which rarely causes ocular injury because it is too large to fit within the orbital margins. Hockey is another sport in which ocular trauma is prominent. Injuries inflicted by either the stick or puck are common and frequently result in hyphemas. Any direct blow to the eye can cause a hyphema.

The amount of blood in the anterior chamber varies from case to case and ranges from microscopic amounts to total hyphemas filling the entire chamber. Initially there is a red tinge in the anterior chamber, but within a few hours the blood settles inferiorly. This produces a red fluid layer in the anterior chamber, usually visible with a hand light. Traumatic hyphemas may be associated with other ocular injuries, such as blow-out fractures of the orbital floor, iridodialysis (disinsertion of the iris from the ciliary body), vitreous hemorrhage, concussive injuries to the posterior pole, retinal detachments, or scleral rupture. A thorough ocular examination is required to rule out any associated ocular damage.

Patients with traumatic hyphemas tend to be drowsy. This is especially true in children, although the mechanism is not clear. It is essential to rule out any neurologic deficit before attributing the drowsiness to the hyphema alone.

The conventional treatment of traumatic hyphemas consists of hospitalization, bed rest with elevation of the head of the bed to 30 or 45°, bilateral patching, and sedation. Analgesics are frequently required, but the use of aspirin-containing compounds is to be avoided. Aspirin prolongs the bleeding time and increases the risk of rebleeding.

Elevation of the intraocular pressure is a common problem in hyphemas. Ocular hypertension results from a contusion injury to the trabecular meshwork and blood clogging the outflow pathways. The pressure usually can be controlled with carbonic anhydrase inhibitors such as acetazolamide (Diamox) or with hyperosmotic agents such as mannitol.

The initial hemorrhage usually resorbs in a few days. If the hemorrhage clears uneventfully and there is no associated ocular damage, the prognosis is good. Bleeding recurs in approximately 20% of all hyphemas. This usually occurs between three to five days after the initial trauma, and is an ominous sign with a poor visual prognosis. The intraocular pressure becomes more difficult to control after a secondary hemorrhage.

Surgical intervention is indicated in the presence of medically uncontrolled intraocular pressure and blood in the anterior chamber. Failure to control the pressure may result in blood staining the cornea and irreversible damage to the optic nerve.

Hyphemas frequently are associated with traumatic recession of the anterior chamber angle and subsequent impairment of aqueous outflow. This predisposes the involved eye to the development of chronic glaucoma months or years after the injury; thus, any eye which has sustained a hyphema must be evaluated regularly.

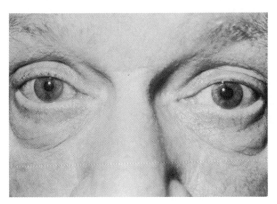

Fig. 18-10. Traumatic iritis. Note the small pupil and injection of the right eye.

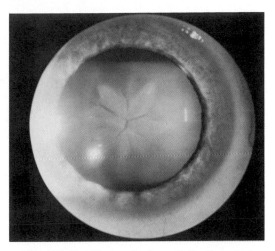

Fig. 18-11. Traumatic "rosette" cataract.

Traumatic Iritis (Fig. 18-10)

Mild trauma to the eye can set up an inflammatory iridocyclitis. The eye becomes injected, and the pupil becomes small. The injection is most intense in the perilimbal area (ciliary flush) in contrast to an infected conjunctivitis in which the reaction is most intense in the palpebral conjunctiva. Depending upon the severity of the inflammatory reaction, the anterior chamber becomes cloudy and the patient complains of blurred vision and photophobia. In certain cases, the pupil becomes dilated instead of miotic. This is a result of contusion injury to the iris sphincter. The pupil reacts minimally and is often slightly irregular. The mydriasis may persist for days to weeks. More severe trauma can produce a tear in the iris sphincter and a permanent pupillary deformity.

The treatment of traumatic iritis includes topical cycloplegic mydriatics to relax ciliary spasm and prevent posterior synechiae formation (inflammatory adhesions between the posterior surface of the iris and lens). Topical corticosteroids are used for their anti-inflammatory effect.

Traumatic Cataract and Dislocated Lens (Figs. 18-11 and 18-12)

Traumatic cataracts may be caused by blunt or perforating injuries. Those result-

ing from perforating injuries are dealt with in the section on corneal lacerations. In blunt trauma, the characteristic lens change is the formation of a rosette-shaped opacity in the anterior or posterior subcapsular area. Other lens changes varying from minimal to total cataract may also be produced by blunt ocular trauma.

Traumatic cataracts secondary to contusion injuries frequently are associated with damage to related ocular structures. The trauma can break the zonular attachments

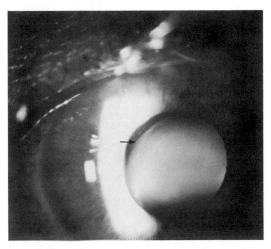

Fig. 18-12. Subluxated cataractous lens. Arrow indicates edge of the lens displaced into the pupillary space.

to the lens with resultant subluxation or dislocation of the lens. Subluxation of the lens is suspected if there is irregularity in the depth of the anterior chamber, or visible trembling of the iris with quick movements of the eye (iridodonesis). The presence of vitreous in the anterior chamber confirms the diagnosis of a subluxated lens.

Surgical intervention for a dislocated lens is hazardous. An emergency operation is indicated when the lens blocks the pupil or is situated in the anterior chamber with secondary acute glaucoma. Surgical intervention may be indicated at a later date if the subluxated lens becomes opacified and interferes with vision or causes phacolytic glaucoma. Even in the absence of a significant opacity, a subluxated lens may cause distressing symptoms such as unstable vision, distortion, or diplopia. Surgical intervention should be approached with great caution because of the attendant hazards and guarded prognosis.

Blunt Corneal Trauma

Severe direct trauma to the cornea can produce marked stromal edema with underlying folds in Descemet's membrane. The patient usually presents with a thickened, central, disc-shaped, corneal haziness with a clear peripheral margin (disciform edema). The edema usually clears within a few weeks leaving little or no permanent opacification. Topical corticosteroids may hasten recovery.

Corneal Lacerations (Fig. 18-13)

Lacerations of the anterior segment of the eye are caused by trauma from sharp objects such as nails, darts, skate blades, or broken glass. Superficial corneal lacerations rarely need suturing unless there is loss of substance or a gaping wound. A pressure patch or "bandage" soft contact lens with concomitant topical antibiotics and cycloplegics is usually all that is required.

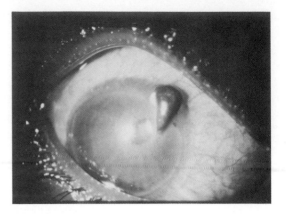

Fig. 18-13. Corneal laceration with flat anterior chamber and iris.

Any time the eye has been lacerated, pressure on the globe must be avoided to prevent extrusion of the intraocular contents. If during an athletic event a penetrating eye injury is suspected, the eye should be covered immediately with a protective shield. Pressure from the shield should be on the bony orbit rather than the eyelid and globe (Fig. 18-14). The athlete should be transferred to the nearest ophthalmic facility for treatment.

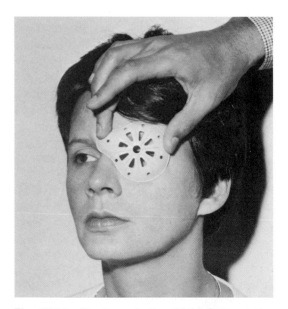

Fig. 18-14. Plastic protective shield. Care must be taken to ensure that no pressure is placed on the globe. Shield may be held in place by tape.

Lid lacerations can be associated with underlying corneal or scleral lacerations. When treating a lid laceration, the physician always should check to make sure that the underlying globe is intact.

Roentgenograms should be taken of all corneal lacerations to rule out any opaque intraocular foreign bodies. Conjunctival smears and cultures should be obtained and systemic antibiotics started.

A corneal laceration associated with loss of the anterior chamber and iris prolapse requires prompt surgical repair.

TRAUMA TO THE OCULAR ADNEXA

Periorbital Ecchymosis (Black Eye)

The black eye is a frequent and obvious consequence of a blunt injury to the periorbital region. Blood from injured vessels dissects in the subcutaneous tissue and produces the violaceous appearance of the skin. Associated edema often restricts lid movement.

Periorbital ecchymosis may be an accompanying manifestation of severe injury to the globe or surrounding facial bones. Roentgenograms of the orbit and facial bones should be obtained to rule out fractures. If the eye itself is not readily visible, no attempt should be made to force the lids apart, since this maneuver may result in expulsion of intraocular contents if there is a serious, coincident ocular injury such as a ruptured globe. If injury to the globe is suspected or if the eye cannot be seen easily, the patient should be referred to an ophthalmologist for evaluation.

In the absence of associated injury to the globe or surrounding structures, the black eye, although temporarily debilitating, is of no lasting consequence. Therapy consists of ice packs to reduce swelling.

Lid Lacerations (Fig. 18-15)

Lid lacerations may result from blunt trauma, sharp trauma, or the impact of a projectile. Frequently the globe also may

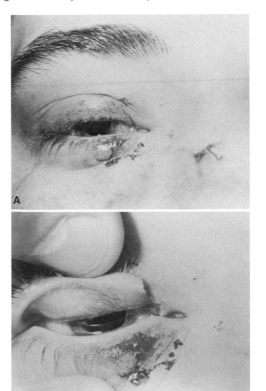

Fig. 18-15. *A,* Laceration of right upper lid. *B,* Only after lid is everted is the extent of injury evident. Laceration involves the full thickness of the lid.

be injured; therefore, a thorough eye examination must be performed as part of the evaluation.

Superficial lacerations of the skin of the lids may be treated with a butterfly bandage to approximate the wound edges. Deeper lacerations and lacerations involving the tarsal plate or the lid margin require meticulous surgical repair in order to minimize functional and cosmetic deformities.

Occasionally, blunt trauma may result in minimal injury to the external surface of the lid, but at times produces an extensive rupture of the tarsal plate, including avulsion of the levator muscle. This type of injury can be detected only if the examination includes careful eversion of the lids.

Special attention should be given to puncture wounds of the lids produced by a projectile or a pointed object. Depending

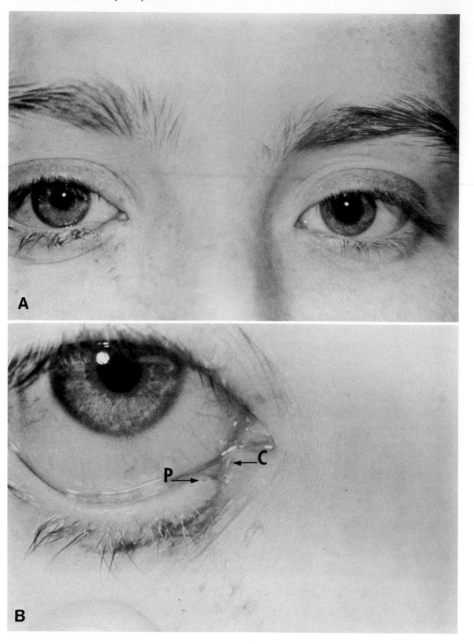

Fig. 18-16.   Laceration of lower lid and canaliculus. *A,* Laceration involving medial aspect of right lower lid. *B,* Lid everted revealing laceration of canaliculus. Lumen of canaliculus (C) visible. Punctum (P).

upon the trajectory of the wound, an occult penetrating injury of the globe can occur, or especially if the path of the wound is directed upward, the orbital roof may be fractured with injury to the frontal cortex. Careful clinical evaluation and roentgenograms to detect a fracture or foreign body are essential.

Injury to the Lacrimal Drainage System (Fig. 18-16)

Traumatic injury to the nasal aspect of the upper or lower lid may produce damage to the lacrimal drainage system. Normally, the tears enter the drainage system at the punctum, a small aperture on the lid margin approximately 6 mm temporal to the medial canthus, and are carried through the canaliculi into the lacrimal sac, the bony nasolacrimal duct, and ultimately into the nose. The most common type of injury to the lacrimal drainage system involves interruption of the continuity of the canaliculus anywhere along its course. Often, in the presence of soft-tissue swelling, it is difficult to diagnose canalicular injury by inspection alone. The diagnosis may require irrigation of the system through the punctum in order to establish the presence of a lacerated canaliculus. Failure to identify injury to the lacrimal system results in obstruction of tear drainage and consequent epiphora. Treatment requires surgical reapproximation of the torn canaliculus and maintenance of a patent lumen.

Trauma to the canalicular portion of the lids often results in associated injury to the medial canthal ligament, a structure important in maintaining the proper position of the puncta in the tear lake. Failure to repair the medial canthal ligament may result in ectropion of the punctum and persisting epiphora despite adequate surgical repair of the canaliculi.

Fracture of the Orbital Floor (Blow-Out Fracture)
(Figs. 18-17 through 18-19)

A blow-out fracture is produced by the impact of a blunt force to the front of the orbit, resulting in a sudden rise in intraorbital pressure. This leads to posterior displacement of the orbital contents and transmission of the force of impact to the orbital walls. Typically, the orbital margin remains intact and the fracture occurs in the area of least resistance, namely the orbital floor. Herniation of the inferior orbital contents through the defect in the floor may occur with incarceration of tissue by bony fragments.

The diagnosis of an orbital floor fracture is based on clinical and roentgenographic findings. Clinical findings suggestive of an orbital floor fracture include diplopia, restricted movement of the globe, enophthalmos and downward displacement of the globe, and anesthesia or hypesthesia in the distribution of the infraorbital branch of the maxillary nerve. The presence of diplopia and restricted movement of the globe does not establish the diagnosis of a fracture, since soft-tissue swelling and hemorrhage, with or without associated fracture, may produce these findings. In the presence of a fracture, the diplopia and restricted movement may be a consequence of herniation and incarceration of the inferior rectus muscle (and less commonly the inferior oblique muscle), damage to the inferior branch of the third cranial nerve to the inferior rectus or oblique muscle, or adhesions and scarring of the orbital tissue to the fracture site. Forced ductions may be useful in determining the presence of mechanical restriction.

Enophthalmos and downward displacement of the globe may be an early or late clinical finding. Commonly, as a result of edema, the injury may initially produce proptosis. With time, the edema resolves and because of herniation or scarring the diminution of orbital fat leads to backward and downward displacement of the globe. This may produce a cosmetic deformity with or without functional derangement.

Hypesthesia or anesthesia of the skin of the malar region, upper lid, or upper gum and teeth on the involved side is often as-

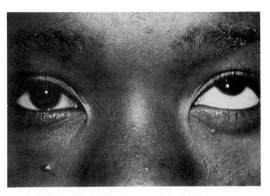

Fig. 18-17. Right orbital floor fracture with entrapment of inferior rectus muscle and inability to elevate the eye.

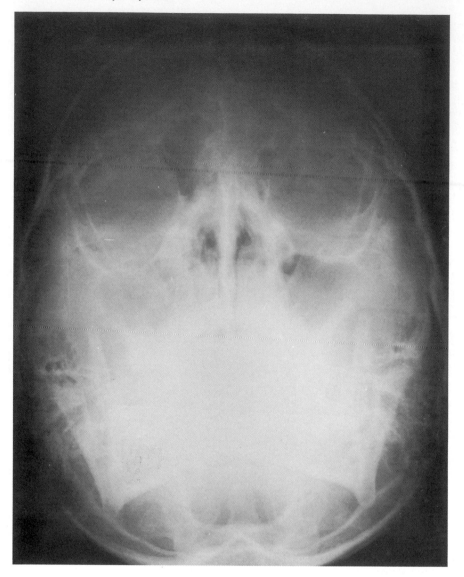

Fig. 18-18. Waters' view of patient in Figure 18-17 showing clouding of right maxillary sinus.

sociated with an orbital floor fracture. This occurs as a conseqence of trauma to the infraorbital nerve in its course through the orbital floor.

Roentgenograms of the orbit (stereoscopic Waters' and Caldwell views) are useful in the diagnosis of an orbital floor fracture. The presence of clouding of the maxillary sinus is suggestive of an orbital floor fracture. However, the radiographic diagnosis can be made with certainty only with the finding of tissue herniated into the maxillary sinus. Often tomograms are necessary to visualize this.

Trauma sufficiently severe to cause a fracture, frequently also produces injury to the eye itself. Thus, a thorough eye examination must be a part of the evaluation of the patient with a suspected fracture. The absence of diplopia in a patient with a blow-out fracture may in fact be due to loss of vision in the involved eye, rather than to absence of muscle involvement.

The initial treatment of an orbital floor

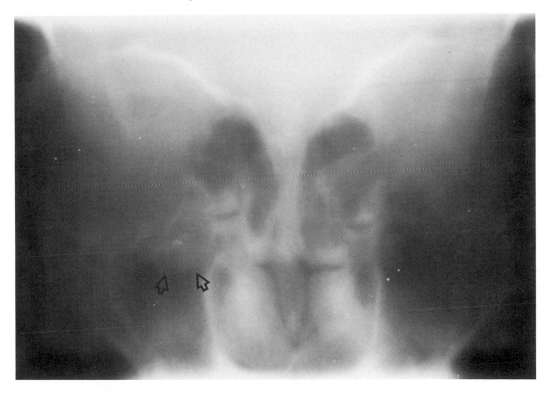

Fig. 18-19. Tomogram of patient in Figure 18-17 showing prolapse of orbital tissue (arrows) into right maxillary sinus.

fracture consists of systemic antibiotics administered prophylactically to decrease the likelihood of an orbital cellulitis. A fracture of the orbital floor provides communication between the potentially contaminated maxillary sinus and the orbit. Some difference of opinion exists regarding the surgical repair of orbital floor fractures. Some surgeons advocate surgical intervention for all fractures associated with herniation of soft tissue into the maxillary sinus, while other surgeons prefer to defer an operation for five to ten days in order to determine the extent of spontaneous resolution of diplopia. An operation is then indicated for persisting, incapacitating diplopia.

Medial Wall Fracture

Blunt trauma to the orbit may result in a fracture of the medial wall, thus producing a communication between the orbit and the ethmoid sinus. In the absence of incarceration of the medial rectus muscle, diplopia usually is absent. Subcutaneous emphysema, detected by palpating the lids and noting crepitation, is a frequent finding and may be accentuated by blowing the nose. The diagnosis is supported by the roentgenographic findings of air in the orbit and by tomographic evidence of a fracture of the ethmoid bone. Treatment consists of systemic antibiotics. Surgery is not indicated unless there is entrapment of the medial rectus muscle.

Retrobulbar (Orbital) Hemorrhage

Hemorrhage into the orbit can occur as a consequence of fractured orbital bones or direct or indirect trauma to the orbital vessels. Bleeding may occur at the time of trauma or be delayed for several days. If the hemorrhage is extensive, it may lead to proptosis of the globe with corneal exposure, restriction of eye movement, increase of intraocular pressure, and compromise of the blood supply to the optic nerve and internal structures of the eye. The patient may complain of pain, decreased vision, and diplopia. If the integrity of the eye is threatened, surgical decompression of the orbit is indicated.

TRAUMA TO THE POSTERIOR SEGMENT OF THE EYE

Damage to the posterior segment of the eye (sclera, choroid, retina, optic nerve, and vitreous) may occur with or without injury to the anterior segment. Although trauma to this part of the eye requires referral to an ophthalmologist, an understanding of the nature of these types of injuries is useful in facilitating proper management.

Retinal Edema

Blunt trauma to the eye may produce retinal edema. When the edema involves the peripheral retina, the patient may be asymptomatic. The edema usually subsides spontaneously and without any permanent retinal damage. However, occasionally the edema may lead to serious retinal complications, such as retinal holes and detachment.

Edema involving the macular area produces immediate symptoms of blurred or distorted vision. Although normal function usually returns, occasionally severe damage to the macula can occur, leading to permanent visual loss. Clinically, retinal edema produces a white appearance to the involved areas, in contrast to the reddish-orange appearance of the healthy retina. Although systemic steroids and other anti-inflammatory agents such as indomethacin have been employed, there is no proof that they are therapeutically useful.

Retinal Breaks

Peripheral retinal tears following blunt trauma may be associated with symptoms of floaters (black dots, dust, or smoke). Retinal breaks can exist with or without symptoms, and their occurrence may be a late consequence of blunt injury; therefore,

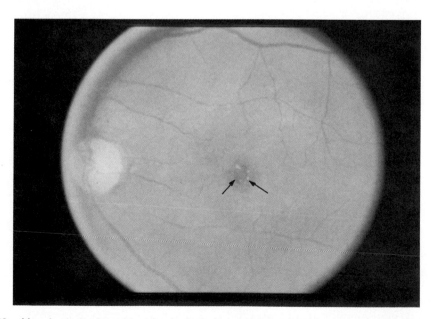

Fig. 18-20. Macular hole. Atrophic macular hole (arrows) following blunt trauma and macular edema.

the sudden onset of such symptoms requires prompt referral to an ophthalmologist. Peripheral retinal breaks following injury should be treated surgically to prevent the development of retinal detachment. A variety of therapeutic modalities is available and includes cryotherapy, laser, or diathermy.

Macular hole formation usually occurs as consequence of severe macular edema and produces profound, irreversible loss of central vision. Macular holes rarely lead to retinal detachment, and no treatment is indicated (Figs. 18-20 and 18-21).

Retinal Detachment

Retinal detachment is a consequence of fluid seeping through a retinal break and separating the neurosensory retina from the retinal pigment epithelium. If the retinal separation extends into the macula, there is severe loss of vision. However, if the macula is spared, central vision may be normal, but a field defect or blurred vision will be noted in the quadrant opposite from the location of the detachment. In some cases, a peripheral retinal detachment may be asymptomatic. The presence of light flashes or floaters may precede or accompany the development of the detachment.

A retinal detachment requires surgical correction.

Vitreous Hemorrhage

Blunt trauma to the eye can produce hemorrhage from vessels in the choroid or the retina. If blood spreads into the vitreous, the patient will note floaters. Occasionally, vitreous hemorrhage may be sufficiently severe as to significantly decrease vision. The presence of a vitreous hemorrhage frequently indicates significant retinal damage, and a careful search for retinal breaks and detachment must be made. If the vitreous hemorrhage is dense enough to preclude direct visualization of the retina with an ophthalmoscope, then ultrasonography may be used to detect the presence of retinal detachment. Vitreous hemorrhage frequently clears spontaneously over a period of weeks to months.

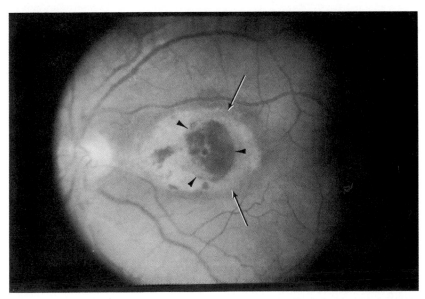

Fig. 18-21. Macular hole and pigment epithelial abnormalities. Typical macular hole (arrowheads) and secondary retinal pigment epithelial changes (arrows) secondary to blunt trauma with macular edema and subretinal hemorrhage.

lenses. If corrective lenses are not needed, protective goggles or rims should be worn in certain sports such as squash. Properly designed facemasks should be employed in all appropriate sports.

REFERENCES

1. Bronchoff, S.A. (ed.): Practical Management of Ocular Injuries. Int. Ophthalmol. Clin., 14:4, 1974.

2. Ophthalmology Study Guide for Students and Practitioners of Medicine. 3rd Ed. American Academy of Ophthalmology and Otolaryngology, 1976.

3. Paton, D., and Goldberg, M.D.: Management of Ocular Injuries. 2nd Ed. Philadelphia, W.B. Saunders, 1976.

4. Zayora, E.: Eye Injuries. Springfield, Charles C Thomas, 1970.

Appendix I

The Heimlich Maneuver

Airway obstruction occurs when a foreign object is sucked against or into the larynx during inspiration. Thus, at the time of obstruction, the lungs are expanded. The Heimlich maneuver produces pressure on the upper abdomen, which is transmitted upward to the lungs. Heimlich states, "Sudden elevation of the diaphragm compresses the lungs within the confines of the rib cage, increasing the air pressure within the tracheobronchial tree. This pressure is forced out through the trachea and will eject food or other objects that are occluding the airway. The action can be simulated by inserting a cork in the mouth of an inflated balloon or compressi-

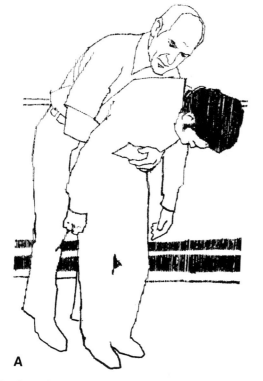

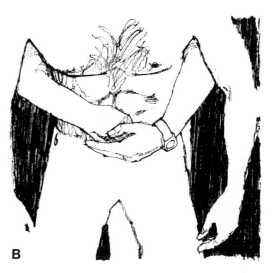

Fig. I-1. *A,* Application of Heimlich maneuver when the victim is standing. *B,* Position of rescuer's hands. (From Heimlich, H.J.: The Heimlich maneuver to prevent food choking. J.A.M.A., *234*:399, 1975. Copyright 1975, American Medical Association.)

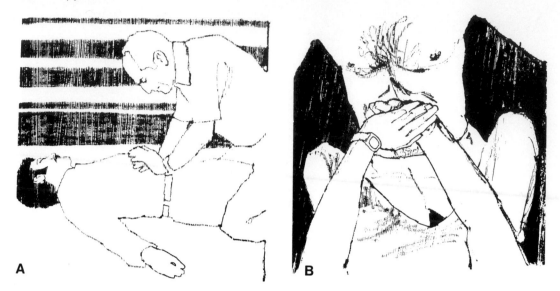

A

B

Fig. I-2. *A,* Application of Heimlich maneuver when the victim is lying on back. *B,* Position of rescuer's hands. (From Heimlich, H.J.: The Heimlich maneuver to prevent food choking. J.A.M.A., *234*:400, 1975. Copyright 1975, American Medical Association.)

ble plastic bottle, then squeezing the balloon or bottle suddenly. The cork flies out due to the increased pressure, similar to the forceful 'pop' of a champagne cork."[1] In the emergency situation, the maneuver can be performed with the victim standing, sitting, or supine.

Rescuer Standing. The rescuer should stand behind the victim and wrap his arms around the victim's waist (Fig. I-1*A*). The rescuer then grasps his fist with his other hand and places the thumb side of his fist against the victim's abdomen, slightly above the navel and below the rib cage (Fig. I-1*B*). The rescuer presses his fist into the victim's abdomen with a quick upward thrust. This should be repeated several times if necessary. When the victim is sitting, the rescuer stands behind the victim's chair and performs the maneuver in the same manner.

Rescuer Kneeling. A variation of the maneuver can be performed when the victim has collapsed or the rescuer is unable to lift him. The victim is lying on his back (Fig. I-2*A*). Facing the victim, the rescuer should kneel astride his hips. With one of

his hands on top of the other, the rescuer places the heel of his bottom hand on the abdomen slightly above the navel and below the rib cage (Fig. I-2*B*). The rescuer then presses into the victim's abdomen with a quick upward thrust. This thrust should be repeated several times if necessary. Should the victim vomit, the rescuer should quickly place him on his side and wipe out his mouth to prevent aspiration (inhalation of foreign material).

On very rare occasions, obstruction can result from a blow to the larynx that fractures or deforms it. This type of obstruction is not cleared by the Heimlich maneuver. A physician may choose to create an air passage into the larynx by putting a tube or large needle through the cricothyroid membrane of the larynx. An emergency tracheostomy (incision into the trachea) is not generally done because it usually creates more problems than it solves.

REFERENCE

1. Heimlich, H.J.: The Heimlich maneuver to prevent food choking. J.A.M.A., *234*:398-401, 1975.

Appendix II

Cardiopulmonary Resuscitation *

In cases of collapsed or unconscious persons, the adequacy or absence of breathing and circulation must be determined immediately. If breathing alone is inadequate or absent, rescue breathing may be all that is necessary. If circulation is also absent, artificial circulation must be started in combination with rescue breathing. The methods of recognizing adequacy or absence of breathing or circulation and the recommended techniques for performing artificial ventilation and artificial circulation are presented below.

ARTIFICIAL VENTILATION

Opening the airway and restoring breathing are the basic steps of artificial ventilation. The steps can be performed quickly under almost any circumstances and without adjunctive equipment or help from another person. They constitute emergency first aid for airway obstruction and respiratory inadequacy or arrest. Respiratory inadequacy may result from an obstruction of the airway or from respiratory failure. An obstructed airway is sometimes difficult to recognize until the air-

way is opened. At other times, a partially obstructed airway is recognized by labored breathing or excessive respiratory efforts, often involving accessory muscles of respiration, and by soft-tissue retractions of the intercostal, supraclavicular, and suprasternal spaces. Respiratory failure is characterized by minimal or absent respiratory effort, failure of the chest or upper abdomen to move, and inability to detect air movement through the nose or mouth.

AIRWAY

Opening the Airway

The most important action for successful resuscitation is immediate opening of the airway. The tongue is the most common cause of airway obstruction in the unconscious victim. Since the tongue is attached to the lower jaw, moving the lower jaw forward will lift the tongue away from the back of the throat and open the airway. As long as there is enough tone in the muscles of the jaw, tilting the head back will cause the lower jaw to move forward and open the airway. In the absence of sufficient muscle tone, head tilt alone may be insufficient to open the airway, and a technique that will move the jaw forward will be necessary. In addition to passive obstruc-

* Reprinted from The Journal of the American Medical Association, August 1, 1980. Copyright 1980, the American Medical Association. Reprinted with permission from the American Heart Association.

tion by the tongue, another important mechanism of airway obstruction by the tongue is the negative pressure created in the airway during inspiration. For an unconscious person making inspiratory effort and creating negative pressure in the airway, the tongue, which is close to the posterior wall of the airway, may act as a valve and occlude the airway during inspiratory effort. Even though the head is tilted back and the neck extended, the lower jaw may need support to lift adequately the tongue and provide an open airway. Head tilt combined with neck lift has been the principal method taught to open the airway. Head tilt with chin lift has been used successfully in place of neck lift and has some advantages especially in the unconscious spontaneously breathing victim.

Head Tilt. Head tilt is the initial and most important step in opening the airway, and this procedure is augmented by either chin lift or neck lift. Head tilt is accomplished by placing the hand on the victim's forehead and applying firm, backward pressure with the palm, resulting in tipping the victim's head maximally backward. Since optimal and effective head tilt may be difficult to obtain using one hand on the forehead, additional assistance is gained in opening the airway by using either chin lift or neck lift with head tilt as described below (Fig. II-1).

Head Tilt–Neck Lift. The rescuer places one hand on the forehead to apply backward pressure and the other hand beneath the neck to lift and support it upward. Excess force in performing this maneuver may cause cervical spine injury. Since the specific movement used is extension of the head at the junction of the neck rather than hyperextension of the cervical vertebrae, the hand lifting the neck should be placed close to the back of the head to minimize the cervical spine extension. Emphasis should be placed on the need for gentleness when lifting the neck. If loose dentures are a problem, they may be managed with head tilt–chin lift or

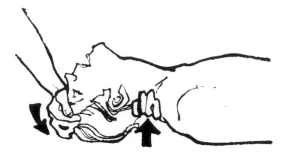

Fig. II-1. Head-tilt method of opening airway. (From Standards for Cardiopulmonary Resuscitation (CPR) and Emergency Cardiac Care (ECC). Reprinted from the Supplement to Journal of the American Medical Association, August 1, 1980. Copyright 1980, the American Medical Association. Reprinted with permission from the American Heart Association.)

may be removed. The fact that layperson-initiated CPR employing neck lift may have a survival rate as high as 61% in selected subgroups attests to the efficacy of head tilt–neck lift (Fig. II-1).

Head Tilt–Chin Lift. Evidence was offered as early as 1960 that head tilt–chin lift offered a greater opening of the airway than head tilt–neck lift. It has been demonstrated that in the unconscious nonbreathing victim additional airways may be opened by chin lift when compared with head tilt–neck lift. In the unconscious victim making spontaneous respiratory effort, chin lift combined with head tilt is highly effective in opening the airway when used initially. In addition, evidence has been offered suggesting that head tilt–chin lift may open the airway in some persons in whom head tilt–neck lift was not successful. Support of the lower jaw may be accomplished by lifting the chin. The tips of the fingers of one hand are placed under the lower jaw on the bony part near the chin bringing the chin forward, supporting the jaw, and helping to tilt the head back. The fingers must not compress the soft tissues under the chin, which might obstruct the airway. The other hand continues to press on the victim's forehead to tilt the head back. The chin should be lifted so the teeth are nearly brought together, but the rescuer should avoid closing the mouth completely. The thumb is used rarely when lifting the chin and then only to depress slightly the lower lip so that the mouth will remain open. If the victim has loose dentures, they can be held in position making obstruction by the lips less likely. If rescue breathing is needed, the mouth-to-mouth seal is easier when dentures are in place. If dentures cannot be managed in place, they should be removed (Fig. 4-12).

Jaw Thrust With Head Tilt. Additional forward displacement of the jaw—jaw thrust—may be required if head tilt–neck lift or head tilt–chin lift is unsuccessful in opening the airway. This can be accomplished by the rescuer's hands at the side of the victim's head grasping the angles of the victim's lower jaw and lifting with both hands, one on each side, displacing the mandible forward while tilting the head backwards. The rescuer's elbows should rest on the surface on which the victim is lying. If the lips close, the lower lip can be retracted with the thumb. If mouth-to-mouth breathing is necessary, close the nostrils by placing the rescuer's cheek tightly against them (Fig. 4-11).

Jaw Thrust Without Head Tilt. This technique is the safest first approach to opening the airway of a victim who has a suspected neck injury, because in most cases it can be accomplished without extending the neck. The head can be carefully supported without tilting it backwards or turning it from side to side. If this is unsuccessful, the head should be tilted back very slightly and another attempt made to ventilate (Fig. 4-11).

Establishing Breathlessness

When maintaining the open airway position, the rescuer places his ear over the victim's mouth and nose, looking toward the victim's chest and stomach. He looks for the chest to rise and fall, listens for air escaping during exhalation, and feels for the flow of air on his cheek.

It should be stressed that although the rescuer may notice that the victim is making respiratory efforts, the airway still may be obstructed. Many times, opening the airway is all that is needed. If the victim resumes breathing, the airway is simply maintained. If the victim is not breathing, apply rescue breathing.

BREATHING

With the thumb and index finger of the hand that is on the forehead, the rescuer gently pinches the nostrils closed so that air will not escape. Then he takes a deep breath, opening his mouth very wide and placing it around the outside of the victim's mouth, making a seal. He blows air into the victim's mouth. Out of the corner of his eye, the rescuer watches to see if the victim's chest is rising. If it is, the lungs are being ventilated. Adequate ventilation is ensured on every breath by the rescuer making the following observations: (1) seeing the chest rise and fall; (2) feeling in his own airway the resistance and compliance of the victim's lungs as they expand; (3) hearing and feeling the air escape during exhalation. The initial ventilatory maneuver should be four quick, full breaths without allowing for full lung deflation between breaths (Fig. II-2).

After delivering each breath, the rescuer quickly turns his head toward the victim's chest to take a breath of fresh air. Throughout the time of giving the four breaths, positive pressure is maintained in the airway. If breathing has stopped, even for a short time, some of the small air sacs of the lung collapse. These are more effectively filled and ventilated by maintaining positive pressure in the lungs during the four initial full breaths.

Two quick full breaths, without allowing time for full lung deflation between breaths, are delivered after each cycle of 15 compressions in single-rescuer CPR. One breath every five seconds is performed either for nonbreathing victims with a pulse (rescue breathing alone), or during

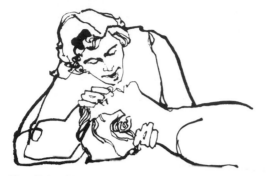

Fig. II-2. Mouth-to-mouth resuscitation. (From Standards for Cardiopulmonary Resuscitation (CPR) and Emergency Cardiac Care (ECC). Reprinted from the Supplement to Journal of the American Medical Association, August 1, 1980. Copyright 1980, the American Medical Association. Reprinted with permission from the American Heart Association.)

two-rescuer CPR. During two-rescuer CPR, the breath is interposed during the upstroke of the fifth chest compression.

In some cases, mouth-to-nose ventilation is more effective than mouth-to-mouth ventilation. The former is recommended when it is impossible to open the victim's mouth, when it is impossible to ventilate through his mouth, when the victim's mouth is seriously injured, and when it is difficult to achieve a tight seal around his mouth. For the mouth-to-nose technique, the rescuer keeps the victim's head tilted back with one hand on the forehead and uses the other hand to lift the victim's lower jaw and close the mouth. The rescuer then takes a deep breath, seals his lips around the victim's nose, and blows in until he feels the lungs expand. The rescuer removes his mouth, and the victim is allowed to exhale passively. The rescuer can see the chest fall when the victim exhales. When mouth-to-nose ventilation is used, it may be necessary to open the victim's mouth or separate his lips to allow the air to escape during exhalation because the soft palate may cause nasopharyngeal obstruction.

No adjuncts are required for effective rescue breathing, so artificial ventilation should never be delayed to obtain or apply adjunctive devices.

Gastric Distention

Artificial ventilation frequently causes distention of the stomach. This occurs most often in children, but it is not uncommon in adults. It is most likely to occur when excessive pressures are used for inflation or if the airway is partially or completely obstructed. The incidence of gastric distention can be minimized by limiting ventilation volumes to that point at which the chest rises, thereby avoiding exceeding esophageal opening pressures.

Marked distention of the stomach may be dangerous because it promotes regurgitation and reduces lung volume by elevation of the diaphragm. If the stomach becomes distended during rescue breathing, recheck and reposition the airway, observe the rise and fall of the chest, and avoid excessive airway pressure. Continue rescue breathing without attempting to expel the stomach contents. Experience in the field has shown that attempting to relieve stomach distention by manual pressure over the victim's upper abdomen may cause him to regurgitate, and when suctioning equipment is not available, aspiration of stomach contents into the lungs may occur. If severe gastric distention results in inadequate ventilation and it cannot be corrected by repositioning the airway, pressure over the epigastrium (after placing the victim on his side) to expel the air from the stomach may be necessary despite the risk of inducing regurgitation and aspiration. If regurgitation does occur whenever performing CPR, turn the victim's entire body on the side, wipe out the mouth, and continue CPR.

ARTIFICIAL CIRCULATION (EXTERNAL CHEST COMPRESSION)

When sudden, unexpected cardiac arrest occurs, all of the ABCs of Basic Life Support (BLS) are required in rapid succession. This includes both artificial ventilation and artificial circulation (external chest compression). Cardiac arrest is recognized by pulselessness in large arteries in an unconscious victim having a death-like appearance and absent breathing. In a cardiac arrest, the rescuer first opens the airway and quickly ventilates the lungs four times. He then maintains the head tilt with one hand on the forehead, and with the tips of the fingers of the other hand gently locates the victim's larynx and slides his fingers into the groove between the trachea and the muscles at the side of the neck where the carotid pulse can be felt. The pulse area must be felt gently, not compressed. There are a number of reasons for recommending palpation of the carotid pulse in the adult rather than other pulses. First, the rescuer already is at the victim's head to perform artificial ventilation, and the carotid pulse is in the same area. Second, the neck area generally is accessible immediately without removal of any clothing. Third, the carotid arteries are central, and sometimes these pulses will persist when more peripheral pulses are no longer palpable. Trainees should practice palpation of the carotid pulse during classes. In hospital situations, palpation of the femoral artery is an acceptable option to use instead of the carotid artery.

Activate EMS (Emergency Medical Services) System

The EMS system should be activated after the pulse check by phoning 911 or another appropriate telephone number. This should be done at this time, after breathing and pulse check, to give useful information to the dispatcher so he can send the appropriate personnel and equipment. The most important information is a complete and correct address together with special instructions pertaining to exact location, i.e., the floor of the building, office number, or other information to identify the specific location of the victim.

If the rescuer is not alone, one person should be sent to call the emergency telephone number to activate the EMS system. The shorter the time interval between collapse and initiation of basic CPR and ACLS [Advanced Cardiac Life Support], the more likely will be the survival of the cardiac arrest victim. If the rescuer is alone, he may perform CPR for one minute and then quickly telephone for help. The decision as to when to telephone for help is affected by a number of variables, including the possibility of someone else arriving on the scene. If no telephone is available, the only option for the rescuer usually is to continue CPR.

Absence or questionable presence of the pulse is the indication for starting artificial circulation by means of external chest compression. External cardiac compression consists of the rhythmic application of pressure over the lower half of the sternum but not over the xiphoid process. The heart lies slightly to the left of the middle of the chest between the lower sternum and the spine. Intermittent pressure applied to the sternum raises intrathoracic pressure and produces cardiac output. Coughing also raises intrathoracic pressure and may produce circulation during early cardiac arrest. During cardiac arrest, properly performed external chest compression can produce systolic blood pressure (BP) peaks of more than 100 mmHg, but the diastolic BP is low and the mean BP seldom exceeds 40 mmHg in the carotid arteries. The carotid artery blood flow resulting from external chest compression on a cardiac arrest victim usually is only one fourth to one third of normal.

External chest compression always must be accompanied by artificial ventilation. Compression of the sternum produces some ventilation, but the volumes are insufficient for adequate oxygenation of the blood. Therefore, artificial ventilation is always required when external chest compression is used.

Technique for External Chest Compression

The patient always must be in the horizontal position when external chest compression is performed. Even during properly performed external chest compression, blood flow to the brain is reduced by gravity or completely prevented with any elevation of the head above the level of the heart. It is imperative, therefore, to get the cardiac arrest victim to a horizontal position as quickly as possible when the head is above the level of the heart, e.g., when the victim is in a dental chair or cardiac arrest occurs in a vehicle, on a telephone pole, or in a stadium seat. Elevation of the lower extremities, while keeping the rest of the body horizontal, may promote venous return and augment artificial circulation during external chest compression.

Effective external chest compression requires sufficient pressure to depress an adult's lower sternum a minimum of 4 to 5 cm (1-½ to 2 in.). For external chest compression to be fully effective, the victim must be on a firm surface. This may be the ground, a floor, or a spineboard on a wheeled litter. If the victim is in bed, a board, preferably the full width of the bed, should be placed under his back. However, chest compression must not be delayed while this support is awaited.

Technique of External Chest Compression. The following 11 points describe the technique of external chest compression in detail:

1. The rescuer positions himself close to the side of the victim's chest. With the middle and index fingers of the hand closest to the feet, the rescuer locates the lower margin of the victim's rib cage on the side next to the rescuer.
2. The fingers are then run up along the rib cage to the notch where the ribs meet the sternum in the center of the lower part of the chest.
3. With one finger on the notch, the other finger is placed next to the first finger on the lower end of the sternum. (Note that the location of the xiphoid is irrelevant if this technique is used.)
4. The heel of the hand closest to the head (which had been used on the victim's forehead to maintain head tilt) is placed on the lower half of the sternum just next to the index finger of the first hand that located the notch. The heel of the rescuer's hand should be placed on the long axis of the breastbone. This maneuver will keep the main line of force of compression on the breastbone and decrease the chance of rib fracture.
5. The first hand is then removed from the notch and placed on the top of the hand on the sternum so that the heels of both hands are parallel and the fingers are directed straight away from the rescuer. (Alternate methods of locating the correct pressure point are acceptable if they accomplish the same hand position on the chest.)
6. The fingers may be either extended or interlaced but must be kept off the chest.
7. An acceptable alternative hand position is grasping the wrist of the hand on the chest with the hand that has been locating the lower end of the breastbone. This technique is helpful for those rescuers with arthritic problems of the hand and wrist.
8. The elbows are straightened by locking them, and the rescuer positions his shoulders directly over his hands so that the thrust for external chest compression is straight down. If the thrust is other than straight down, the torso has a tendency to roll, part of the effort is

lost, and the chest compression is less effective.

9. For a normal-sized adult, the rescuer must apply sufficient force to depress the sternum about 4 to 5 cm (1-½ to 2 in.). Then he must release the pressure completely to allow the heart to refill without losing position on the sternum.

10. Release the pressure completely and allow the chest to return to its normal position. This will allow blood to flow into the heart. The time allowed for release should be equal to the time required for compression. Thus, during two-man CPR with a compression rate of 60 per minute, compression should be sustained for 0.5 second, with relaxation given for an equal period. The compressions must be regular, smooth, and uninterrupted.

11. Do not lift the hands off the chest or change their position in any way because correct hand position may be lost. Bouncing compressions must be avoided, since they are less effective and are more likely to cause injury.

When there is only one rescuer, he should perform both artificial ventilation and artificial circulation using a 15:2 ratio. This consists of two very quick lung inflations after each 15 chest compressions. Because of interruptions for lung inflation, the single rescuer should perform each series of 15 chest compressions at a rate of approximately 80 per minute to deliver close to 60 compressions per minute. The two full lung inflations must be delivered in rapid succession, within a period of four to five seconds, without allowing full exhalation between the breaths. If time for full exhalation were allowed, the additional time required would reduce the number of compressions and ventilations that could be achieved in a one-minute period (Fig. II-3).

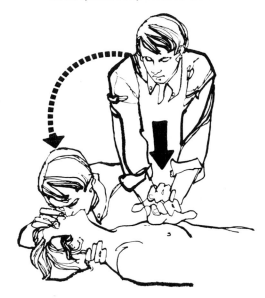

Fig. II-3. One-rescuer cardiopulmonary resuscitation.
15 chest compressions (rate of 80/min)
2 quick lung inflations
(From Standards for Cardiopulmonary Resuscitation (CPR) and Emergency Cardiac Care (ECC). Reprinted from the Supplement to Journal of the American Medical Association, August 1, 1980. Copyright 1980, the American Medical Association. Reprinted with permission from the American Heart Association.)

The carotid pulse should be palpated periodically during CPR to check the effectiveness of external chest compression or the return of a spontaneous effective heartbeat. This should be done after the first minute of CPR and every few minutes thereafter. It should be checked particularly when a second rescuer arrives to determine the effectiveness of external chest compressions and to confirm pulselessness.

Since artificial circulation always must be combined with artificial ventilation, it is preferable to have two rescuers. One rescuer positions himself at the victim's side and performs external chest compression while the other one remains at the victim's head, keeping it tilted back, and continues rescue breathing. The compression rate for two rescuers is 60 per minute. When performed without interruptions, this rate can maintain adequate blood flow and pressure and will allow cardiac refilling. This rate is practical because it avoids fatigue, facilitates timing at a rate of one compression per second, and allows optimal ventilation and circulation by permitting the swift interposition of an inflation at the upstroke of each fifth compression without any pause in compressions (5:1 ratio). The rate of 60 compressions per minute allows breaths to be interposed without any pauses (Fig. II-4).

When a second rescuer becomes available, he should identify himself as a qualified rescuer and let the first rescuer know that he is willing to help. Without stopping CPR, the single rescuer lets the second rescuer know that he wants him to assist and is ready to switch over to two-rescuer CPR. The second rescuer will need to check the victim's pulse himself to assure himself that the first rescuer has correctly interpreted the victim's condition. He should kneel down on the side of the victim opposite the first rescuer, in position for rescue breathing, his fingers in position to feel the victim's carotid pulse. If compressions are adequate, a pulse should be felt; if no pulse is felt, the compressor's technique should be reevaluated. When the second rescuer can feel a pulse with each compression, he calls out "Stop compression." The first rescuer stops compressing for five seconds so that the second rescuer can check if the victim has a spontaneous pulse. If no pulse is found, the rescuers should begin two-rescuer CPR. The second rescuer should deliver a breath to the victim immediately after confirming pulselessness.

This entire process, from the moment the second rescuer arrives to the point where he delivers a full, deep breath, should be done in as little time as possible to ensure that CPR continues effectively. As soon as this breath is delivered to the victim, the first rescuer changes to the two-person rate (60 compressions per minute). Rescue breathing is then interposed during the upstroke of each fifth chest compression.

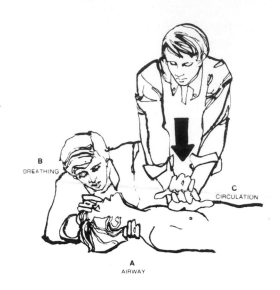

Fig. II-4. Two-rescuer cardiopulmonary resuscitation.
  5 chest compressions
    Rate of 60/minute
    No pause for ventilation
  1 lung inflation
    After each 5 compressions
    Interposed between compressions
(From Standards for Cardiopulmonary Resuscitation (CPR) and Emergency Cardiac Care (ECC). Reprinted from the Supplement to Journal of the American Medical Association, August 1, 1980. Copyright 1980, the American Medical Association. Reprinted with permission from the American Heart Association.)

The CPR can be performed more smoothly and effectively when the two rescuers are on opposite sides of the victim. They can then switch positions when necessary without serious interruption in the 5:1 sequence. The switch is initiated when the rescuer who is performing compressions directs that a switch takes place at the end of a 5:1 sequence. The rescuer who is performing the ventilations, after giving a breath, moves into position to give compressions. The rescuer giving compressions, after giving the fifth compression, moves to the victim's head and checks the pulse for five seconds, but no longer. If no pulse is felt, the rescuer at the head gives a breath and tells the rescuer at the chest to "continue CPR." If there is a pulse but no breathing, he should say there is a pulse and give artificial respiration.

PITFALLS IN PERFORMANCE OF CPR

When CPR is performed improperly or inadequately, artificial ventilation and artificial circulation may be ineffective in supporting life. Enumerated below are important points to remember in performing external chest compression and artificial ventilation.

1. Do not interrupt CPR for more than five seconds except in the following circumstances:

    a. *Endotracheal Intubation.* Under emergency conditions, endotracheal intubation usually cannot be accomplished in five seconds. It should be performed only by those well trained and proficient in the technique. It should be attempted only after the victim has been ventilated and properly positioned and all preparations made. It may take up to 30 seconds, but should never cause suspension of CPR for more than 30 seconds.

    b. *Problems with Transportation.* When there are problems with moving a victim, e.g., up or down a stairway, it is difficult to continue effective CPR. Under these circumstances, it is best to perform effective CPR at the head or foot of the stairs, then interrupt CPR at a given signal, and move quickly to the next level where effective CPR can be resumed. Such interruptions should be as brief as possible and usually should not exceed 30 seconds.

2. Do not move the patient to a more convenient site until he has been stabilized and is ready for transportation or until arrangements have been made for uninterrupted CPR during movement.

3. Never compress the xiphoid process at the tip of the sternum. The xiphoid extends downward over the abdomen. Pressure on it may cause laceration of the liver that can lead to severe internal bleeding.

4. Between compressions, the heel of the hand must completely release its pressure but should remain in constant contact with the chest wall over the lower half of the sternum.

5. The rescuer's fingers should not rest on the victim's ribs during compression. Interlocking the fingers of the two hands may help avoid this. Pressure with fingers on the ribs or lateral pressure increases the possibility of rib fractures and costochondral separation.

6. Sudden or jerking movements should be avoided when compressing the chest. The compression should be smooth, regular, and uninterrupted (50% of the cycle should be compression, and 50% should be relaxation). Quick jabs increase the possibility of injury and produce small jets of flow with the result that the output from the heart per compression may be sharply reduced. The result may be that blood flow may be inadequate to maintain brain viability.

7. It has been recommended in the past that continuous pressure be maintained on the abdomen during CPR to minimize gastric distention. The present recommendation is that continuous pressure on the abdomen not be maintained because of the danger of trapping the liver, which could cause liver rupture. An additional reason to avoid such pressure is that it may lead to regurgitation and aspiration of gastric contents.

8. The shoulders of the rescuer should be directly over the victim's

sternum. The elbows should be straight. Pressure is applied vertically downward on the lower sternum. This technique provides a maximally effective thrust, minimizes rescuer fatigue, and reduces the risk of complications for the victim. When the victim is on the ground or floor, the rescuer can kneel at his side. When the victim is elevated above the ground or floor, as on a bed or high-wheeled litter, the rescuer must stand on a step or chair or kneel on the bed or litter to achieve proper position. With a low-wheeled litter, the rescuer usually can stand at the victim's side. When low-wheeled litters are used in ambulances, special arrangements must be made for proper positioning of the rescuer relative to the design of the ambulance.

9. The lower half of the sternum of an adult must be depressed about 4 to 5 cm (1-½ to 2 in.) by external chest compression. Lesser amounts of compression may be ineffectual.

10. While complications may result from improperly performed external chest compression, even properly performed external chest compression may cause rib fractures in some patients. Other complications that may occur despite proper CPR technique include fracture of the sternum, costochondral separation, pneumothorax, hemothorax, lung contusions, lacerations of the liver, and fat emboli. These complications may be minimized by careful attention to details of performance but cannot be entirely prevented. Accordingly, concern for injuries that may result even from properly performed CPR should not impede prompt and energetic application to the technique in behalf of the cardiac arrest victim. The only alternative to the timely initiation of effective CPR in behalf of the cardiac arrest victim is death.

SPECIAL RESUSCITATION SITUATIONS

Drowning

Extensive research has delineated the pathophysiology of drowning and the differences between fresh water and sea water submersion. However, Basic Life Support resuscitation procedures after drowning are the same as Basic Life Support procedures presented earlier. CPR should be initiated as quickly as possible. The usual circumstances in which the drowning victim is found, i.e., in a body of water, have several important implications regarding CPR performance as follows:

1. When attempting to rescue a drowning victim, the rescuer should get to him as quickly as possible, preferably with some conveyance, i.e., boat, raft, or surfboard. If a conveyance is not available, a flotation device should be carried by the rescuer. *The rescuer should be aware that he may endanger himself and should exercise caution to minimize this risk.*

2. External chest compression should not be attempted in the water unless one has had special training because it is generally impossible to perfuse the brain effectively unless the victim can be maintained in the horizontal position; it is usually not possible to keep the drowning victim's chest at a level with his head and still keep the victim's head above water, in position for rescue breathing.

3. Mouth-to-mouth or mouth-to-nose ventilation may be performed in the water; it is difficult and often impossible in deep water unless the rescuer has some type of flotation device.

4. Artificial ventilation (rescue breathing) should be started as soon as possible, even before the victim is moved out of the water, into a boat, or onto a surfboard. It can almost always be initiated once the rescuer can stand in water, and it should be initiated at this time in preference to efforts aimed exclusively at getting the victim out of the water.

5. In cases of suspected neck injury, the victim's neck should be supported in a neutral position, and the victim should be floated onto a back support before being removed from the water. Careful consideration and effort should be made to maintain the victim in a supine horizontal position with the head, neck, and chest aligned. If artificial respiration is required, the maximal head tilt should not be used. Artificial ventilation should be accomplished with the head maneuver without head tilt, or chin lift without head tilt should be used.

6. When removed from the water, the victim should have, if needed, standard artificial ventilation or CPR performed as described previously. Since successful resuscitation of drowning victims has been reported after prolonged periods of submersion in cold water, efforts at resuscitation should usually be initiated despite documented submersions of 20 to 30 minutes or more.

7. There should be no delay in moving the victim to a life support unit where ACLS capabilities are available. Every submersion victim, even one who requires only minimal resuscitation and regains consciousness at the scene, should be transferred to a medical facility for follow-up care.

Accident Cases

In accident cases, it is imperative that caution be used to avoid inflicting further injury by backward tilt of the head when there is a possibility of neck fracture. The diagnosis of a fractured neck should be suspected in diving accidents and automobile accidents when the victim has evidence of injury to the face or head. If diagnosis of a fracture is suspected, all forward, backward, lateral, or turning movement should be avoided. To open the airway, a modification of the jaw thrust maneuver without backward head tilt should be used. In this variation, the rescuer places his hands on either side of the victim's head so the head is maintained in a fixed, neutral position without the head tilted backward. The index fingers should then be used to displace the mandible forward without tilting the head backward or turning it to either side (jaw thrust without head tilt). If required, artificial ventilation usually can be provided in this position. If this is unsuccessful, the head should be tilted back very slightly and another attempt made to ventilate using the jaw thrust maneuver. To minimize the risk of avoidable, additional injury, keep the head, neck, and chest aligned.

Index

Page numbers in *italics* indicate figures; page numbers followed by "t" indicate tables.